Test Success

Test-Taking Techniques
for Beginning Nursing Students

. . .

FIFTH EDITION

Test Success

Test-Taking Techniques for Beginning Nursing Students

• • •

FIFTH EDITION

Patricia M. Nugent, RN, MA, MS, EdD

Professor Emeritus, Adjunct Professor

Nassau Community College

Garden City, New York

President of Nugent Books, Inc.

Barbara A. Vitale, RN, MA

Professor Emeritus, Adjunct Professor

Nassau Community College

Garden City, New York

President of Professional Resources for Nursing (PRN)

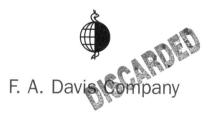

F. A. Davis Company

F. A. Davis Company
1915 Arch Street
Philadelphia, PA 19103
www.fadavis.com

Printed in the United States of America

Last digit indicates print number: 10 9 8 7 6 5 4 3 2 1

Publisher, Nursing: Robert G. Martone
Director of Content Development: Darlene D. Pedersen
Project Editor: Padraic J. Maroney
Art and Illustration Manager: Carolyn O'Brien

As new scientific information becomes available through basic and clinical research, recommended treatments and drug therapies undergo changes. The author(s) and publisher have done everything possible to make this book accurate, up to date, and in accord with accepted standards at the time of publication. The author(s), editors, and publisher are not responsible for errors or omissions or for consequences from application of the book, and make no warranty, expressed or implied, in regard to the contents of the book. Any practice described in this book should be applied by the reader in accordance with professional standards of care used in regard to the unique circumstances that may apply in each situation. The reader is advised always to check product information (package inserts) for changes and new information regarding dose and contraindications before administering any drug. Caution is especially urged when using new or infrequently ordered drugs.

Dedicated to
Joseph Vitale and Neil Nugent
For their love and support,
particularly during the production of this book

Preface

The increase in nursing knowledge and medical technology is accelerating at a breathtaking rate. This places greater stress on nursing students to learn what they need to know to provide safe patient-centered nursing care. Faculty and curricula are stretched to the limit to include all the information students must absorb to successfully complete the requirements to graduate as accountable practitioners. Attrition rates support the fact that academic demands are strenuous. This is compounded by the fact that nursing students arrive with more needs than ever before. An increasing percentage of nursing students are mature individuals who have been out of secondary education for years and need to relearn how to study and take tests, single parents who have the responsibility of supporting children and need to maximize their effectiveness when they study, or persons who speak English as their second language and demonstrate needs in reading and/or writing English. Beginning nursing students may be faced for the first time with multiple-choice questions that require not just regurgitation of information but comprehension, application, or analysis of information. Therefore the level of thinking on nursing examinations requires a high cognitive ability. Needless to say, testing situations induce anxiety for these test takers. Nursing students need supportive textbooks to increase their chances of success.

This book is designed for beginning nursing students who are preparing to take tests at the end of a unit of instruction or at the completion of a fundamentals of nursing course. It also can be used by students in licensed practical nurse programs to prepare for class examinations, NCLEX-PN, or advanced-standing examinations for entry into Registered Nurse programs. Students preparing for the NCLEX-RN may review the book to maximize their success on this national examination. Finally, nursing faculty members may find this book helpful when designing a test-taking workshop for student nurses.

Because it takes nursing students at least 2 years of study to build a body of knowledge from which safe nursing judgments can be made, this book presents only content that is common to meeting patients' basic physical and psychosociocultural needs. The information presented in Chapters 1 through 10 is designed to maximize success by helping students to develop a positive mental attitude; understand critical thinking; manage their time; study and learn more effectively; become test wise by identifying the step in the nursing process being tested to better establish what the question is asking; explore all testing formats, specifically multiple-choice and alternate format questions; appreciate computer applications in nursing education and evaluation; and analyze test performance. In addition, such topics as ethics, rights, common theories, legal issues, the nursing process, pharmacology, community health nursing, and principles related to the management of nursing care are included on a fundamental level.

A variety of tools have been included to allow the student to perform self-assessments and ultimately improve studying and testing performance. Chapter 3 presents three tools (Assessment of Inconsistencies Between Values and Behavior, Personal Time/Activity Journal, and Self-Assessment of Barriers to Productivity) and a guide called Corrective Action Plan to Maximize Your Productivity. These permit the reader to perform a self-assessment of the use of time in relation to personal values and individualize a plan to maximize productivity. Chapter 10 presents two tools (Identify Information Processing Errors and Identify Knowledge Deficits) and a guide called Corrective Action Guide for Information Processing Errors. These allow the reader to perform a self-assessment to determine why questions are answered incorrectly and to personalize a plan to correct test-performance errors that have a negative effect on test success.

In the spring of 2003, the National Council of State Boards of Nursing introduced alternate-format questions on the NCLEX-RN and NCLEX-PN. To address this change, Chapter 8, Testing Formats Other Than Multiple-Choice Questions, includes content called Alternate Question Formats Reflective of NCLEX. Alternate-format questions are discussed and numerous examples are presented using graphic images, charts, flow sheets, pictures, and tables.

Seventy-five questions have been added since the last edition for a total exceeding 825 questions. Chapter 11 contains 400 questions divided into 14 content areas common to nursing practice. Chapter 12 contains a 100-question Comprehensive Final Book Exam. In addition, two 75-item Comprehensive Course Exit Exams are include in the enclosed disk. Rationales for the correct and incorrect answers are included for every question. These rationales should help the learner review some of the basic content in nursing theory and practice and contribute to the mastery of answering questions. In addition, the majority of questions in Chapter 11 include a Test-Taking Tip to emphasize one or more of the test-taking techniques that can be applied when answering a question.

Throughout the textbook, the word "patient" is used to indicate the consumer of health care, although consumers of health care are often referred to elsewhere as "clients" or "residents." The word "nurse" is used consistently to indicate a licensed nurse. It is recognized that this individual may be referred to by other titles such as Patient Care Coordinator or Nurse Manager. The words "Nurse's Aide" or "Nursing Assistant" are used consistently to reflect credentialed or uncredentialed supportive nursing staff members. These individuals are sometimes referred to by other titles such as Patient Care Assistant, Nurse Technician, or Comfort Care Associate. The word "physician" is used consistently when indicating a health-care provider with prescriptive privileges. It is recognized that nurse practitioners, physician's assistants, podiatrists, and dentists also have prescriptive privileges.

Some current study guides provide students with practical skills to help them become more successful learners. However, few books exist that are designed specifically to aid beginning nursing students who are grappling with examination questions created to test fundamental nursing theory and practice. This book was written to fill that void.

We want to thank Bob Martone, Publisher for Nursing, who guided and supported us through the publication process. Our association has spanned over 15 years and we value him not only as a colleague but as a friend. In addition, the collaborative efforts of the F. A. Davis team of Padraic Maroney, Project Editor; Sam Rondinelli, Production Manager; Barbara Tchabovsky, Developmental Editor; and Lisa Thompson, Production Editor, ensured that this project progressed from a manuscript to a book. We appreciated their thoughtful comments, attention to detail, and grace under pressure. Most importantly, we give special thanks to our husbands and our children and their spouses —Joseph Vitale, Neil Nugent, Joseph and Nicole Vitale, John and JoAnne Vitale, Christopher and Whitney Vitale, Kelly and John Dall, and Heather and James McCormack for their love and support. Lastly, special thanks to our grandchildren John and Ava Dall, Aiden, Cade, and Ronan McCormack and Joseph, Andie Grace, and Andrew Vitale who are the best stress reducers. They make our day.

Patricia M. Nugent
Barbara A. Vitale

Reviewers

Teresa Graham, RN, MSN
Director
Holmes Community College
Goodman, Mississippi

Mark Fisher, RN, MSN
Instructor
University of Oklahoma Health Sciences Center
Oklahoma City, Oklahoma

Contents

The Nursing Process 63

Test-Taking Techniques 91

8 *Testing Formats Other Than Multiple-Choice Questions* 117

9 *Computer Applications in Education and Evaluation* 145

How to Use This Book to Maximize Success

It is amazing what **you** can achieve when **you** are tenacious, organized, and determined to attain a goal. By purchasing this book, **you** have demonstrated a beginning commitment to do what **you** have to do to improve your success in nursing examinations. This book is designed to introduce **you** to various techniques that can contribute to a positive mental attitude, promote the development of critical thinking skills, and help **you** become test wise. If you are beginning to get the feeling that "you" is an important word, "you" are right! Learning requires you to be an active participant in your own learning. Your ultimate success can be maximized if you progress through this book in a planned and organized fashion and are willing to practice the techniques suggested. Effort is directly correlated with the benefits you will derive from this book. After you have determined that you are eager and motivated to learn, you are ready to begin.

Chapter content is organized in a specific order to provide you with techniques that will contribute to developing a positive mental attitude, understanding critical thinking, managing your time, studying and learning more effectively, exploring all testing formats with an emphasis on multiple-choice and alternate-format questions, identifying the nursing process as a form of problem solving, becoming test wise, and appreciating computer applications in nursing education and evaluation. More than 825 questions afford you the opportunity to practice test-taking techniques. The correct answers and the rationales for all the options are presented to reinforce the theories and principles of fundamentals of nursing that you have learned in your nursing program. In addition, tools are provided for you to assess your test performance and a guide is presented for studying and improving your test-taking ability.

To use this book to its best advantage, read Chapters 1 through 10. Then answer the questions in Chapter 11. Be sure to study the rationales because this information will review and reinforce the material you are learning in your fundamentals of nursing course. To maximize learning, it is suggested that you answer the questions in the specific categories in Chapter 11 after you have learned the content in class. Then take the Comprehensive Course Exit Exam I on the disk. Immediately after taking the exam evaluate your performance using the tools presented in Chapter 10, Analyze Your Test Performance. This analysis will help you diagnose information processing errors, identify knowledge deficits, and provide suggestions for corrective action. After you have followed your individualized Corrective Action Plan to maximize your strengths and minimize your weaknesses, take the Comprehensive Course Exit Exam II on the disk. Again, evaluate your performance using the self-assessment tools in Chapter 10. By this time you should have expanded your knowledge and abilities and your performance should have improved. Although it is suggested that you take Exam I and Exam II in sequence, the order in which you take them does not matter. Finally, take the Comprehensive Final Book Exam in Chapter 12. Again, evaluate your performance using the self-assessment tools in Chapter 10 and use the corrective action plan to focus your study. The self-assessment tools Identify Information-Processing Errors, Identify Knowledge Deficits, and the Corrective Action Guide for Information Processing Errors should be used not only in conjunction with this book but should be used to analyze your performance after every test you take in your nursing course.

You should be commended for your efforts to achieve success. It is hard work to take responsibility for your own learning. The magnitude of your learning will be in direct proportion to the amount of energy you are willing to expend in the effort to improve your skills. You will become a more successful test taker when you:

- Function from a position of strength
- Think critically
- Manage your time

- Study more effectively
- Become test wise
- Are able to apply the nursing process to determine what the question is asking
- Analyze your test performance

MUCH SUCCESS ON YOUR NURSING EXAMINATIONS!

Empowerment

Develop a Positive Mental Attitude

A positive mental attitude can help you control test anxiety by limiting anxious responses so that you can be a more successful test taker. A positive mental attitude requires you to function from a position of strength. This does not imply that you have to be powerful, manipulative, or dominant. What it does require is that you develop techniques that put you in control of your own thoughts and behavior. To be in control of yourself, you need to operate from a position of positive self-worth with a feeling of empowerment. This begins with self-assessment.

You have both strengths and weaknesses. Both must be identified to maximize your potential. Strengths are easy to focus on because you feel safe and nonthreatened. Weaknesses are more difficult to focus on because you may feel inadequate and uncomfortable. When performing a self-assessment, be honest with yourself. You must separate your ego from your assessment. Only you will know the result. Remember, few people are perfect! Have the courage to be honest with yourself and recognize your imperfections. You can have weaknesses and imperfections and still have a positive self-concept.

To develop self-worth, you must be willing to look within yourself and recognize that you are valuable. Acting from a position of strength requires you to start saying and believing that you are worthwhile. Self-worth increases when you believe down to your very bones that you are important.

A feeling of empowerment arises when you are able to use all your available resources and learned strategies to achieve your goals. To achieve empowerment, you need to develop techniques and skills that not only make you feel in control but actually position you in control. When you are in control, you function from a position of strength.

To achieve a sense of self-worth and a feeling of empowerment that will help you succeed in test taking, you must learn various techniques that must be practiced before taking the test. These techniques will help you to control stressful situations, reduce anxious responses, and enhance concentration, thereby improving your analytical and problem-solving abilities and strengthening your test performance. By learning and practicing the following techniques, you will have a foundation on which to operate from a position of strength.

ESTABLISH A POSITIVE INTERNAL LOCUS OF CONTROL

Henry Ford once said, "Whether you think you can, or think you can't . . . you're right." In other words, what you think can be a self-fulfilling prophecy. It is important to recognize that the way you talk to yourself influences the way you think about yourself. The content of what you say indicates how you feel about the control of your behavior and your life. "I was lucky to pass that test." "I couldn't help failing because the teacher is hard." "I got test anxiety and I just became paralyzed during the test." Each of these internal dialogues indicates that you see yourself as powerless. When you say these things, you fail to take responsibility.

Identify your pattern of talking to yourself. Do you blame others, attribute failure to external causes, and use the words "I couldn't," "I should," "I need," or "I have to?" If you do, you are using language that places you in a position of impotence, dependence, defenselessness, and hopelessness. YOU MUST ESTABLISH A POSITIVE INTERNAL LOCUS OF CONTROL. You do this by replacing this language with language that reflects control and strength. You must say, "I want," "I can," and "I will." When you use these words, you imply that you are committed to a task until you succeed. Place index cards around your environment with "I WANT," "I CAN," and "I WILL" on them to cue you into a positive pattern of talking to yourself.

CHALLENGE NEGATIVE THOUGHTS

Your value as an individual should not be linked to how well you do on an examination. Your self-worth and your test score are distinctly isolated entities. If you believe that you are good when you do well on a test and bad when you do poorly, you must alter your thinking. You need to work at recognizing that this is illogical thinking. Illogical or negative thinking is self-destructive. Negative thoughts must be changed into positive thoughts to build confidence and self-worth. As confidence and self-worth rise, anxiety can be controlled and minimized.

Positive thinking focuses your attention on your desired outcomes. If you think you can do well on a test, you are more likely to fulfill this prophecy. It is critical that you control negative thoughts by developing a positive mental attitude. When you say to yourself, "This is going to be a hard test. I'll never pass," CHALLENGE THIS STATEMENT. Instead say to yourself, "This is a ridiculous statement: of course I can pass it. All I have to do is study hard to pass this test!" It is crucial that you challenge negative thoughts with optimistic thoughts. Optimistic thoughts are valuable because they can be converted into positive actions and feelings, which place you in a position of control.

For this technique to work, you must first be able to stop negative thoughts. To use the technique called ARREST NEGATIVE THOUGHTS, you must first identity the pattern of negative thinking that you use to defend yourself. Envision a police car with flashing lights that signifies ARREST NEGATIVE THOUGHTS. You can even place pictures of police cars around your environment to cue you to ARREST NEGATIVE THOUGHTS. After you identify negative thoughts, handcuff them and lock them away so that they will no longer be a threat. Actually envision negative thoughts locked up in a cell with bars and yourself throwing away the key.

After you stop a negative thought, replace it with a POSITIVE THOUGHT. If you have difficulty identifying a positive thought, praise yourself or give yourself a compliment. Tell yourself, "Wow! I am really working hard to pass this test." "Congratulations! I was able to arrest that negative thought and to be in control." To increase your control, make an inventory of the things you can do, the things you want to achieve, and the feelings you want to feel that contribute to a positive mental attitude. Throughout the day take an "attitude inventory." Identify the status of your mental attitude. If it is not consistent with your list of the feelings you want to feel or the positive image you have of yourself, CHALLENGE YOUR ATTITUDE. Compose statements that support the feelings that you want to feel and read them over and over. Such statements might include "I can pass this test!" or "I am in control of my attitudes, and my attitudes are positive!" Make sure that you end the day with a positive thought, and even identify something that you want to accomplish the next day. Forecasting positive events establishes a positive direction in which you can focus your attention.

USE CONTROLLED BREATHING (DIAPHRAGMATIC BREATHING)

An excellent way to reduce feelings of anxiety is to use the technique of controlled breathing. When you control your breathing, you can break the pattern of shallow short breaths associated with anxious feelings. Deep abdominal or diaphragmatic breathing enhances the relaxation response. When a person exhales, tense muscles tend to relax. You probably do this now unconsciously. Most people take a deep breath and exhale (sigh) several times an hour. When you "sigh," it is a form of diaphragmatic breathing. Diaphragmatic breathing causes the diaphragm to flatten and the abdomen to enlarge on inspiration. On exhalation, the abdominal muscles contract. As you slowly let out this deep breath, the other muscles of the body tend to "let go" and relax. This technique enables you to breathe more deeply than if you just expand your chest on inspiration. Controlled breathing can be helpful to reduce anxious responses that occur at the beginning of a test, when you are stumped by a tough question, or when you are nearing the end of the test. During these critical times you can use controlled breathing to induce the relaxation response.

When practicing diaphragmatic breathing, place your hands lightly over the front of the lower ribs and upper abdomen so that you can monitor the movement you are trying to achieve. As you become accomplished in this technique, you will not need to position your hands on your body. Practice the following steps:

1. Gently position your hands over the front of your lower ribs and upper abdomen.
2. Exhale gently and fully. Feel your ribs and abdomen sink inward toward the middle of your body.
3. Slowly inhale, taking a deep breath through your nose and expanding your abdomen first and then your chest. Do this as you slowly count to four.
4. Hold your breath at the height of inhalation as you count to four.
5. Exhale fully by contracting your abdominal muscles and then your chest. Let out all the air slowly and smoothly through your mouth as you count to eight.

Monitor the pace of your breathing. Notice how your muscles relax each time you exhale. You may feel warm, tingly, and relaxed. Enjoy the feeling as you breathe deeply and evenly. You should practice this technique so that controlled breathing automatically induces the relaxation response after several breaths. After you are able to induce the relaxation response with controlled breathing, you can effectively draw on this strategy when you need to be in control.

It is important not to do this exercise too forcefully or too rapidly because it can cause you to hyperventilate. Hyperventilation may cause dizziness and lightheadedness. If either of these occurs, cup your hands over your nose and mouth and slowly rebreathe your exhaled air. These symptoms should subside. Then you can continue the exercise less vigorously. Always monitor your responses throughout the exercise.

DESENSITIZE YOURSELF TO THE FEAR RESPONSE

Individuals generally connect a certain feeling with a specific situation. To learn to control your feelings, you must first recognize how you consider and visualize events. It is not uncommon to connect a feeling of fear with an event. In a testing situation, the examination is the event and the response of fear is the feeling. If this happens to you, you need to interrupt this fear response. You have the ability to control how you respond to fear. When you are able to sever the event from the feeling, you will establish control and become empowered. However, establishing control does not happen automatically. You need to desensitize yourself to the event to control the fear response.

Desensitization involves repeatedly exposing yourself to the identified emotionally distressing event in a limited and/or controlled setting until the event no longer precipitates the feeling of fear. Desensitization is dependent on associating relaxation with the fear response. To achieve this response, you need to practice the following routine:

First, you must practice a relaxation response. Controlled breathing, an excellent relaxation technique, has already been described. After you are comfortable with the technique of controlled breathing, you can use it in the desensitization routine.

Second, you should make a list of five events associated with a testing situation that cause fear, and rank them starting with the one that causes the most anxiety and progressing to the one that causes the least anxiety. The following is an example:

1. Taking an important examination on difficult material
2. Taking an important examination on material you know well
3. Taking a small quiz on difficult material
4. Taking a small quiz on material you know well
5. Taking a practice test that does not count

Event number 5 should evoke the least amount of fear.

4

Third, you should practice the following routine:

1. Practice controlled breathing and become relaxed.
2. Now imagine event number 5. If you feel fearful, turn off the scene and go back to controlled breathing for about 30 seconds.
3. After you are relaxed, again imagine scene number 5. Try to visualize the event for 30 seconds without becoming uncomfortable.
4. After you have accomplished the previous step, move up the list of events until you are able to imagine event number 1 without feeling uncomfortable.

When you are successful in controlling the fear response in an imagined situation, you can attempt to accomplish the same success in simulated tests at home. After you are successful in controlling the fear response in simulated tests at home, you can take some simulated tests in a classroom setting. Continue practicing desensitization until you have a feeling of control in an actual testing situation. This may take practice. It will not be accomplished in one practice session.

Another way you can use the concept of desensitization is to practice positive dialogue within yourself. For example, imagine the following internal dialogue within yourself:

"How am I feeling about the examination today?" "A little uncomfortable and fearful."

"Do I want to feel this way?" "Absolutely not!"

"How do I want to feel?" "I want to feel calm, in control, and effective."

"What am I going to do to achieve that feeling?" "I am going to practice relaxation and controlled breathing."

You might be saying to yourself, "I don't see myself doing this. This is silly." The resilient and tenacious individual who is flexible and willing to try new techniques is in a position of control. If your goal is to be empowered, you have only to be open and willing to learn.

PERFORM MUSCLE RELAXATION

This technique involves learning how to tense and relax each muscle group of your body until all of your muscle groups are relaxed. This technique requires practice. The basic technique involves assuming a comfortable position and then sequentially contracting and relaxing each muscle group in your body from your head to your toes. When a muscle group is tensed and then released, the muscle smooths out and relaxes. It is not a technique that can be quickly described in a short paragraph. However, the following brief exercise is included as an example:

Find a comfortable chair in a quiet place. Close your eyes and use diaphragmatic breathing, taking several deep breaths to relax. You are now ready to begin progressive muscle relaxation. Sequentially move from one muscle group in the body to another, contracting and relaxing each in an even manner. Contract and relax each muscle group for 10 seconds. After each muscle group is tensed and then relaxed, take a deep, slow breath using diaphragmatic breathing. As you are relaxing, observe how you feel. Experience the sensation. You may want to reinforce the feeling of relaxation by saying, "My muscles are relaxing. I can feel the tension flowing out of my muscles." Remember not to breathe too forcefully to avoid hyperventilation. The following is a sample of muscle groups that should be included in a progressive muscle relaxation routine:

1. Bend your head and try to rest your right ear as close as you can to your right shoulder. Count to 10. Assume normal alignment, relax, and take a deep breath.
2. Bend your head and try to rest your left ear as close as you can to your left shoulder. Count to 10. Assume normal alignment, relax, and take a deep breath.
3. Flex your head and try to touch your chin to your chest. Count to 10. Assume normal alignment, relax, and take a deep breath.
4. Make a fist and tense your right forearm. Count to 10. Relax and take a deep breath.
5. Make a fist and tense your left forearm. Count to 10. Relax and take a deep breath.
6. Tense your right biceps by tightly bending (flexing) the right arm at the elbow. Count to 10. Relax and take a deep breath.

Continue moving from the head to the arms, trunk, and legs by contracting and relaxing each of the muscle groups within these areas of your body. You can understand and master this technique by obtaining a product that is designed to direct and instruct you through the entire routine of tensing and relaxing each muscle group. This technique should be practiced every day until it becomes natural. After you have mastered this technique, you can use a shortened version of progressive relaxation along with controlled breathing at critical times during a test.

USE IMAGERY

Using imagery can help you to establish a state of relaxation. When we remember a fearful event, our heart and respiratory rates increase just as they did when the event occurred. Similarly, when we recall a happy, relaxing period, we can regenerate and recreate the atmosphere and feeling that we had during that pleasant event. This is not a difficult technique to master. Just let go and enjoy the experience.

Position yourself in a comfortable chair, close your eyes, and construct an image in your mind of a place that makes you feel calm, happy, and relaxed. It may be at the seashore or in a field of wild flowers. Let your mind picture what is happening. Observe the colors of the landscape. Notice the soothing sounds of the environment. Notice the smells in the air, the shapes of objects, and movement about you. Recall the positive feelings that flow over you when you are in that scene and relax. You can now open your eyes relaxed, refreshed, and calm.

At critical times during a test, you can take a few minutes to use imagery to induce the relaxation response. To successfully reduce stress, you must position yourself in control. When you are in control, your test performance generally improves.

OVERPREPARE FOR A TEST

One of the best ways to reduce text anxiety is to be overprepared. The more prepared you are to take the test, the more confident you will be. The more confident you are, the more able you are to challenge the fear of being unprepared. Study the textbook, read your notes, take practice tests, and prepare with other students in a study group. Even when you think that you know the information, study the same information again to reinforce your learning. For this technique to be successful, you need to plan a significant amount of time for studying. Although it is time-consuming, it does build confidence and reduce anxiety. No one has said that learning is easy. Any worthwhile goal deserves the effort necessary to achieve success. Being overprepared is the BEST way to place yourself in a position of strength.

Consider the following scenario: a student was not doing well in school and asked what she could do to improve her performance. The concept of being overprepared was discussed, and she worked out a study schedule of 2 hours a day for 2 weeks before the next test. After the test, the student said that she thought she did well because the test was easy. It had to be pointed out that she perceived the test as easy because she had attained the knowledge that enabled her to answer the questions correctly. Her eyes lit up as if someone had turned on a light bulb in her head! When you recognize that you have the opportunity to be in control and take responsibility for your own learning, you become all that you can be.

EXERCISE REGULARLY

Exercising regularly helps you to expend nervous energy. Walking, aerobics, swimming, bike riding, or running at least 3 times a week for 20 minutes is an effective way to maintain or improve your physical and mental status. The most important thing to remember about regular exercise is to slowly increase the degree and duration of the exercise. Your exercise program should not be so rigorous that it leaves you exhausted. It should serve to clear your mind and make you mentally alert and better able to cope with the challenge of a test. Exercise should not be performed just before going to bed because it can interfere with sleep. Regular exercise should become a routine activity in your weekly schedule, not just a response to the tension of an upcoming test. After you establish a regular exercise program, you should experience physical and psychological benefits.

6   Establish Control Before and During the Test

It is important to maximize your opportunities to feel in control in the testing situation. Additional techniques you can use to establish a tranquil and composed atmosphere require you to take control of your testing equipment, your activities before and during a test, and your immediate physical space. Techniques to help create this atmosphere are reinforced in Chapter 7, Test-Taking Techniques. However, they are also discussed here because they can be used to reduce anxiety and promote empowerment.

MANAGE YOUR DAILY ROUTINE BEFORE THE TEST

It is important to maintain your usual daily routine the day before the test. Eat what you usually eat, but avoid food and beverages with caffeine. Caffeine can lessen your attention span and reduce your concentration by overstimulating your metabolism. Avoid the urge to stay up late the night before a test. If you are tired when taking a test, your ability to concentrate and problem-solve may be limited. Go to bed at your regular time. Following your usual routines can be relaxing and can contribute to a feeling of control.

MANAGE YOUR STUDY HABITS BEFORE THE TEST

Do not stay up late studying the night before the big test. Squeezing in last-minute studying may increase anxiety and contribute to feelings of powerlessness and helplessness. DO NOT CRAM. If you have implemented a study routine in preparation for the test, you should have confidence in what you have learned. Establish control by saying to yourself, "I have studied hard for this test and I am well prepared. I can relax tonight because I know the material for the test tomorrow and I will do well." Avoid giving in to the desire to cram. Instead, use the various techniques discussed earlier in this chapter to maintain a positive mental attitude.

MANAGE YOUR TRAVEL THE DAY OF THE TEST

Plan to arrive early the day of the test. It is important to plan for potential events that could delay you, such as traffic jams or a flat tire. The more important the test, the more time you should schedule for travel. If you live a substantial distance from the testing site, you might ask another student who lives closer to allow you to sleep over the night before the test. The midterm or final examination for a course may be held in a different location than the regularly scheduled classroom used for the lecture. If you are unfamiliar with the examination room, make a practice run to locate where it is and note how long it takes to get there. Nothing produces more anxiety than rushing to a test or arriving after the start of a test. A feeling of control reduces tension and the fear response. You can be in control if you manage your travel time with time to spare.

MANAGE THE SUPPLIES YOU NEED FOR THE TEST

The more variables you have control over, the more calm and relaxed you will feel. Compose a list of the items to bring with you to the test. Sometimes the supplies that can be used are stipulated by the institution giving the test. They may include pencils, pens, scrap paper, erasers, a ruler, a watch, and even a lucky charm. It is suggested that you collect the items the day before the test. This eliminates a task that you do not have to perform on the day of the test and contributes to your sense of control.

MANAGE YOUR PERSONAL COMFORT

Maslow's Hierarchy of Needs specifies that basic physiologic needs must be met before you attempt to meet higher-level needs. Be aware of your own basic needs relating to factors such as nutrition, elimination, and physical comfort. Meet these basic needs before the test because unfulfilled needs will compete for your attention. For example, arrive early so that you can visit the restroom, wear layers of clothing so that you can adjust to various environmental temperatures, and eat a light, balanced meal to maintain your blood glucose. After these basic needs are met, you can progress up the ladder of needs to self-actualization.

MANAGE THE TEST ENVIRONMENT

When you arrive early, you generally have the choice of where to sit in the room. This contributes to a feeling of control because you are able to sit where you are most comfortable. You might prefer to sit by a window, near a heat source, or in the back of the room. Generally, it helps to sit near the administrator of the test. Directions may be heard more clearly, and the administrator's attention may be gained more easily if you need to ask a question. It is wise to avoid sitting by a door. The commotion made by people entering or exiting the room can be a distraction and interfere with your ability to concentrate. Take every opportunity to control your environment. Measures that help you feel in control contribute to a positive mental attitude.

MAINTAIN A POSITIVE MENTAL ATTITUDE

Remind yourself of how hard you worked and how well prepared you are to take this test. ESTABLISH CONTROL by arresting negative thoughts and focusing on the positive. Say to yourself, "I am ready for this test! I will do well on this test! I can get an A on this test!" These statements support a positive mental attitude and enhance a feeling of control.

MANAGE YOUR PHYSICAL AND EMOTIONAL RESPONSES

At critical times during the test, you may feel nervous, your breathing may become rapid and shallow, or you may draw a blank on a question. Stop and take a minibreak. Use controlled breathing to induce the relaxation response. You may also use a shortened version of progressive relaxation exercises to induce the relaxation response. Daily practice of breathing and relaxation exercises will enable you to quickly induce the relaxation response during times of stress. After these techniques are implemented, you should again feel empowered.

Summary

The techniques described in this chapter are designed to increase your mastery over the stress of the testing situation. When you feel positive about yourself and have a strong self-image and a feeling of self-worth, you will develop a sense of control. When you are able to draw on various techniques that empower you to respond to the testing situation with a sense of calm, you will improve your effectiveness. Use these techniques along with the other skills suggested in this book, practice the questions, and take the simulated practice tests as instructed in the section "How to Use This Book to Maximize Success" at the beginning of the text. These activities will support your self-worth, provide you with a feeling of control, and increase your effectiveness in the testing situation.

Critical Thinking

If your ultimate goal is to become a competent nurse, first you have to recognize what knowledge base and skills are needed to achieve this goal. Study skills, critical-thinking skills, and problem-solving skills are essential to achieve success as a learner. Your goal should be to develop skills that support your ability to use reasoning and not just react by rote (a fixed, routine, mechanical way of doing something). Several chapters in this book are designed to assist you in the journey toward this goal. General and specific study skills are addressed in Chapter 4; the nursing process as a problem-solving process is addressed in Chapter 6; and critical-thinking skills are addressed in this chapter. No one would argue with the statement that a nurse needs to be a safe, qualified, and technically proficient practitioner. Consumers of nursing care are most aware of the actions (psychomotor skills) that nurses engage in and generally rate the quality of nursing care in relation to the degree to which their expectations are satisfied. However, the quality of nursing care is based on more than just what the nurse does. It is also based on how the nurse thinks (cognitive skills) in relation to how conclusions are drawn, decisions are made, and problems are resolved.

> *Thinking is the hardest work there is, which is the probable reason why so few engage in it.*
> HENRY FORD

The thinking skills that rarely are recognized by the consumer, such as reflecting, clarifying, analyzing, and reasoning, are crucial to the development of a competent nurse. Historically, critical thinking in nursing has been associated with the nursing process (assessment, analysis/diagnosis, planning, implementation, and evaluation). This theoretical framework, which is used to identify and attain solutions to complex problems, has been the foundation for nursing education, practice, and research. It is a systematic, orderly, step-by-step progression with a beginning and an end (linear format). Problem solving in relation to the nursing process produces a nursing care plan or "product." Chapter 6 addresses the steps in the nursing process and provides many sample items that demonstrate application of information within the context of the nursing process.

Because nursing entails more than just the solving of problems, the concept of critical thinking as a "process" is receiving increasing attention. Various researchers believe that critical thinking in nursing is more than just a behavioral, task-oriented, linear approach demonstrated in problem solving and that critical thinking should be based on an emancipatory model. Emancipatory models embrace the concept of empowerment and autonomous action stemming from critical insights. Emancipatory models stress critical thinking as a process rather than just a method of producing a product or solution.

Definition of Critical Thinking

Leaders in the field of nursing do not agree on any one definition of critical thinking. However, the following excerpts may enhance your understanding of the concept. Chaffee (2003) defined critical thinking as "making sense of our world by carefully examining the thinking process in order to clarify and improve our understanding." Alfaro-LeFevre (2004) summarized that critical thinking:

- Entails purposeful, goal-directed thinking
- Aims to make judgments based on evidence (fact) rather than conjecture (guesswork)
- Is based on principles of science and scientific method
- Requires strategies that maximize *human potential* and compensate for problems caused by *human nature*

The Delphi Research Project characterized the ideal critical thinker as one who is habitually inquisitive, well informed, trustful of reason, open minded in evaluation, honest in facing personal biases, prudent in making judgments, willing to reconsider, clear about issues, orderly in complex matters, diligent in seeking relevant information, reasonable in the selection of criteria, focused in inquiry, and persistent in seeking results that are as precise as the subject and the circumstances of inquiry permit (American Philosophical Association, 1990).

Brookfield (1991) described four components of critical thinking: identifying and challenging assumptions, becoming aware of the importance of context in creating meaning, imagining and exploring alternatives, and cultivating a reflective skepticism.

Pless (1993) identified these critical-thinking cognitive skills and subskills as essential for critical thinking:

- Interpretation—categorization, decoding significance, and clarifying meaning
- Analysis—examining ideas, identifying arguments, and analyzing arguments
- Evaluation—assessing claims and assessing arguments
- Inference—querying evidence, conjecturing alternatives, and drawing conclusions
- Explanation—stating results, justifying procedures, and presenting arguments
- Self-Regulation—self-examination and self-correction

Critical Thinking in Nursing

Nursing requires not only the learning of facts and procedures but also the ability to evaluate each unique patient situation. In Chapter 4, Study Techniques, a section titled "Cognitive Levels of Nursing Questions" addresses the variety of thinking processes—knowledge, comprehension, application, and analysis—that the nurse uses when managing data and identifying and meeting a patient's needs.

Because these thinking processes are important to both the process and product inherent in nursing care, multiple-choice questions in Chapter 4 are designed to test your knowledge base, comprehension of information, application of theory and principles, and analytical ability. In all but knowledge-type questions, intellectual skills that involve more than just the recall of information are required. In comprehension-type questions, you are required to translate, interpret, and determine the implications, consequences, and corollaries of the effects of information. In application-type questions you are required to use information in a new situation. In analysis-type questions you are required to interpret a variety of data and recognize the commonalities, differences, and interrelationships among the ideas presented. Numerous sample items in Chapter 4 challenge your analytical abilities, address the cognitive domains, and demonstrate the concepts being presented.

An understanding of the nursing process and the cognitive domains is important; however, critical-thinking skills must be developed if you are going to be a successful thinker and ultimately an expert nurse. The first step is to build a foundation of knowledge and information that can eventually be applied in clinical situations.

> *Both minds and fountain pens will work when filled. But minds, like fountain pens, must first be filled.*
> ARTHUR GUITERMAN

Before you can apply knowledge, you need to know what needs to be known and how the knowledge can be applied. To do this, you need to ask yourself serious questions such as: "What do I know?" "What do I need to know?" "What do I have to do to know it?" This is a new activity for some students. It can be threatening and even anxiety producing. It is not easy to acknowledge the degree of your own lack of knowledge or ignorance, and it can be a sobering experience.

> *The more I know I know, I know the less.*
> ROBERT OWEN

Therefore, to fill voids in your knowledge you need to study. Avoid the pitfall of being a superficial thinker. This type of thinker devotes excessive time to memorization and rote learning. Become a deep thinker.

> *Many bring rakes but few shovels.*
> FRANK C. BROWN

A deep thinker develops a thorough understanding of the material studied. Chapter 4, Study Techniques, discusses strategies that will help you answer some of the previous questions, and study more effectively and efficiently.

After you know basic information, you are better able to recognize the significance of cue data. Nursing questions are carefully designed to test your knowledge and comprehension of information regarding key concepts and your ability to analyze and apply this information in various situations. As you move from being a neophyte to a more experienced student, you are more able to recognize the significance of cues and respond readily in all situations, whether in a laboratory setting, computer simulation, clinical setting, or on a test. In nursing questions, you must recognize the key words and concepts being tested in the question. They require that you ask, "What is happening?" and "What should I do?" Before you can answer these questions, it is helpful to identify the information processing style that you use when confronted with a situation that requires a response.

LEFT-BRAIN AND RIGHT-BRAIN HEMISPHERE INFORMATION PROCESSING

Taggart and Torrance (1984) explored left-brain and right-brain hemisphere information processing. They found that individuals who used **left-brain hemisphere information processing functions** used rational problem-solving strategies and logical sequencing to problem-solve. Rational learners break down situations into components and look for universal rules and approaches that can be applied in all situations. Individuals who used **right-brain hemisphere information processing functions** looked for main ideas to establish relationships that could be abstracted as the foundation for intuitive problem solving. The intuitive learner first learns from context and experience and then applies and analyzes principles. Additional research in this area demonstrates that, although both the novice and the expert use logical and rational problem-solving strategies, it is the expert who uses a broad range of thinking skills that integrate both logical and intuitive thinking to address facts and feelings to achieve accurate decision making.

CLINICAL JUDGMENTS

The ability to build a foundation of data, inferences, and hypotheses for nursing decision making is dependent on your ability to use several types of clinical judgments. **Perceptual judgments** are judgments that you make regarding the data you need to collect and the validation of the importance of the data you collect within the context of the situation. **Inferential judgments** are judgments that you make when you determine which data are significant, eliminate data that are insignificant, and identify the relationship that exists among the data collected. **Diagnostic judgments** are judgments that you make when you link clusters of data with patterns affiliated with a specific nursing diagnosis.

LEVELS OF CRITICAL THINKING

As your knowledge of theory and experience increases, you will be constructing a scientific foundation to support critical thinking and clinical decision making. When developing critical thinking skills, you will advance through three levels of competence: basic, complex, and expert. As a student, you are a basic-level critical thinker. As a **basic-level critical thinker,** you are building a novice's database of information and experiential knowledge. When you are confronted with a situation, initially your response is based on recall and rote memory. You tend to guide your responses by rules and procedures and seek concrete actions. You reduce situations to their distinct and independent parts. For example, when performing a simple dry sterile dressing for an abdominal wound with approximated edges (healing by primary intention), you may use a procedure book and follow each step as outlined. As you acquire more knowledge and experience, you will advance from a basic-level thinker to a complex-level thinker. As a **complex-level thinker,** you will be guided by the need to explore options based on principles and patterns and an understanding of commonalities and differences. Your response will begin to be based on the ability to identify cue data, analyze clustered information, sort and choose the most appropriate action, and evaluate the client's response. For example, when performing a sterile dressing for an open wound where the edges are not readily approximated (healing by secondary intention), you may need to modify the procedure. Depending on the situation, you may need to reposition the patient, use additional sterile equipment, or irrigate the wound. The more knowledge and experience you gain, the more solid the connections between your knowledge base and the application of that knowledge will become. You are now becoming an expert critical thinker. As an **expert critical thinker,** you will develop reasoning based on models, patterns, and standards associated with the "uniqueness" and "wholeness" of each situation. For example, when performing a sterile dressing on a large, gaping wound that has been purposely left open (healing by tertiary intention), your critical thinking will require a higher level of sophistication. You will need to consider concepts such as dehiscence, evisceration, fistula formation, sinus tracking, undermining, presence of infection, necrosis, factors that impair or facilitate wound healing, and dressing alternatives. The expert looks at the situation from an entire perspective that can be accomplished only with a broad and deep knowledge base and experience.

All critical thinkers should be asking, "What is wrong?" "Why?" "How?" "What else?" "What if?" and even "So what!" However, at each successive level of critical thinking, the degree of sophistication needed to explore these questions increases. These questions need to be asked when studying, when faced with a clinical situation (whether simulated or real), and when challenged by a test question. As a beginning nursing student, you are a novice, not an expert! Nursing school is several years long for a purpose. Be realistic with your self-expectations. It takes time to acquire and integrate the knowledge and experience necessary to be an expert critical thinker.

Practice Critical Thinking

You first learned how to turn over, crawl, stand, walk, and then run by practicing balance and building strength and endurance. You also must learn and practice critical-thinking and problem-solving skills until you are proficient in using these skills and can respond accurately and achieve your goal of being an expert critical thinker. To be able to tap your critical-thinking skills when taking an examination, these skills must be well entrenched in your approach to all professional endeavors.

STRATEGIES TO EMPLOY IN CRITICAL THINKING

When challenged by any patient situation, you should employ these strategies:

- Identify assumptions.
- Use a method to collect and organize information.
- Validate the accuracy and reliability of collected information.
- Determine the significance of collected information.
- Determine inconsistencies in collected information.
- Identify commonalities and differences.
- Identify patterns of patient responses.
- Identify stressors and common adaptations to stressors.
- Identify discrepancies or gaps in information.
- Cluster information to determine relationships.
- Make inferences based on collected information.
- Identify actual problems and patients who may be at risk for problems.

- Establish priorities (Maslow's hierarchy is an excellent model to use to achieve this goal).
- Formulate specific, patient-centered, realistic, measurable goals with a time frame.
- Identify appropriate nursing actions.
- Evaluate outcomes.
- Evaluate and modify critical-thinking activities.

This list of strategies reflects sophisticated, deep thinking. Critical thinking is a type of highly developed thinking and a learned skill. The learner has to be actively involved in the learning process. Critical thinking cannot be memorized; it must be practiced.

> *Knowledge is a treasure, but practice is the key to it.*
> THOMAS FULLER

ACTIVITIES TO IMPROVE CRITICAL THINKING

To help you develop or refine thinking that can become more critical, it is suggested that you engage in the following activities while incorporating the strategies previously listed.

THINKING ALOUD   The proficient thinker verbalizes thought processes and rationales. The actual expression of thoughts in words helps to clarify and solidify thinking. This strategy can be used while you are engaged in an activity or later when you review your performance. Clinical postconferences and individual mentoring experiences in which information is exchanged promote critical thinking.

REVIEW OF PATIENT SCENARIOS   Chart review, grand rounds, and case study approaches when performed in a group provide interdisciplinary exchanges, a variety of different thinking perspectives, and learning from role models. These approaches require a verbal exchange that includes reasoning, interpreting, identifying evidence, deducing, and concluding. In these situations you can examine your viewpoint in relation to the viewpoints of others. This exchange promotes learning and stimulates critical thinking.

WRITTEN ASSIGNMENTS   Written assignments are not just "busy work." Journal writing is an activity that requires you to log and respond to important and meaningful events and situations. Faculty review of your journal (with comments) and periodic study and review of it by you will enable you to identify your progress and growth. Journal writing involves you in the process of learning. It encourages you to use abstract thinking and to conceptualize, elaborate, generalize, and interpret, all of which promote critical thinking. When you write a term paper, you are involved not only in the process of writing but in the development of a product. When this product is reviewed by the instructor, conclusions can be drawn regarding your command of the information and your ability to convey your knowledge to others. Written assignments require organizing, prioritizing, integrating, persuading, proving, and summarizing, all of which require *critical thinking*.

COMPUTER-ASSISTED LEARNING   Computers provide an environment that enhances and challenges critical-thinking skills. Software offers a variety of critical-thinking programs, from a simple lesson presenting content using an interactive linear approach to programs in which the learner is challenged to seek solutions to complex problems following a branching design. Computers allow for thinking and learning in a nonthreatening and safe environment. Refer to Chapter 9, Computer Applications in Education and Evaluation, for more details regarding the valuable use of computers to increase learning.

VIDEOTAPING   Videotaping can be used to record role-playing scenarios or the performance of a skill. Videotaping allows you to engage in an activity and then be able to review your performance. During this review, you, as well as others, can examine, analyze, rationalize, justify, and correct your performance, which can support critical thinking.

CLINICAL PROCESS RECORDS   A clinical process record is a focused writing assignment, similar to a case study, that centers on a simulated or specific patient experience. It requires you to use the problem-solving process, examine the scientific reasons for health-care interventions, assess outcomes, and evaluate and modify the plan of care, which all contribute to critical thinking.

EXAMINATIONS   Examinations must be approached as learning opportunities. All examinations should be thoughtfully reviewed. Small groups of four or five students should review and discuss each question. Group members help one another to recognize the key concepts being tested and how to best answer the questions "What is happening?" and "What should I do?" When reviewing examination questions, be willing to listen to other people's interpretation of the question. If all of your energy is spent defending your response, your mind is not open to different perspectives, which limits your learning. Reviewing examinations requires you to integrate information, apply theory and principles, analyze content, compare and contrast information, and rationalize your response, all of which contribute to critical thinking.

Apply Critical Thinking to Multiple-Choice Questions

Case (1994) explored the concept of critical thinking as a journey, not a destination. Case stated, "We cannot stand in the same river twice, because water rushes away as new water takes its place and the rushing water changes the river bed. The decisions we make today may not fit circumstances that change tomorrow." This concept applies to clinical situations as well as nursing test questions. Just as no clinical situation will be exactly like a previous experience, no test question will be exactly like a previous question. One different factor in a situation can change the entire landscape of the situation. One different word in a question can change what the question is asking. Practicing critical thinking when answering questions will improve your ability to think critically and be more successful when taking a test.

IDENTIFY THE KEY CONCEPT BEING TESTED

Each question scenario is different and requires you to identify the key concept being tested and to answer the questions "What is happening?" and "What should I do?" Reframe, critique, and evaluate the stem of each question. Then, try to construct the correct answer before looking at the options. When assessing the options in a multiple-choice question, manipulate the information by cognitive activities such as organizing, correlating, differentiating, reasoning, and evaluating against standards of practice, criteria, and critical elements. Review the following sample item.

SAMPLE ITEM 2–1

A patient has just returned from the operating room with a urinary retention (Foley) catheter, an IV, and an oral airway, and is still unresponsive. Which nursing assessment should be made first?

    (1) Check the surgical dressing to ensure that it is intact.

    (2) Confirm the placement of the oral airway.

    (3) Examine the IV site for infiltration.

    (4) Observe the Foley for drainage.

First, you need to identify the key concept being tested in the question. The key concept in this question is the **priority care for the unresponsive postoperative patient.** The key words in the question that ask "What is happening?" are **postoperative patient, oral airway,** and **unresponsive.** The key words in the question that ask "What should I do?" are **assessment** and **should be made first.** The question being asked is: **What assessment takes priority when caring for an unresponsive postoperative patient with an oral airway?** Although the IV, the retention catheter, and surgical dressing are important and must be assessed, it is ensuring the correct placement of the oral airway that takes priority.

To answer this question you need to know:

- The normal anatomy and physiology associated with the respiratory system and the body's essential need for a continuous exchange of oxygen and carbon dioxide
- That a patent airway is essential to the exchange of oxygen and carbon dioxide
- The ABCs of life support, which refer to Airway, Breathing, and Circulation, and make the connection that maintaining an airway takes priority
- That a common response to anesthesia is lack of a gag reflex
- That a correctly placed oral airway will contribute to maintaining an open airway

Another critical-thinking study technique when answering multiple-choice questions is to explore the consequences of each nursing action presented in the alternatives. You can ask many different questions: "Is the action safe or unsafe?" "Is the statement true or false?" "Is it fact or inference?"

AVOID READING INTO THE QUESTION

Highly discriminating questions are questions that are answered correctly by the test taker who scored in the top percent of the class versus the test taker who answered the question incorrectly and scored in the bottom percent of the class on the same examination. It is believed that the student who answers a highly discriminating question correctly generally is responding to subtle cues based on more highly developed critical-thinking skills. However, students who come to the testing situation with an in-depth perspective sometimes will "read into" the question because of the "context" they bring to the test item. It is often frustrating for students who are sophisticated, deep thinkers to accept lost points on an examination because they "read into" the question. Analyze questions you answer incorrectly and determine "why" by asking questions such as: "Did I add information to the stem?" "Did I have difficulty deciding among the options presented because I would have done something completely different?" "Did I delete an option because my experience was different from the patient situation presented?" "Did I view the question in light of a more sophisticated level of curricular content than that being tested?" "Did I view the patient scenario in more depth and breadth than was necessary?" Multiple-choice questions provide all the data necessary to permit you to answer the question. Your job is to use critical thinking to answer the question, not rewrite the question. For additional information see Chapter 10, Analyze Your Test Performance.

STUDY THE RATIONALES FOR THE RIGHT AND WRONG ANSWERS

Every nursing action is based on a standard of practice that has a scientific foundation. When practicing test taking, in your own words, identify the reason why the option you chose is correct and why the options you considered incorrect are wrong. Now compare your rationales with the rationales presented. When you answered a question correctly review the rationales several times to reinforce your knowledge. When you answered a question incorrectly identify your faulty thinking by comparing your rationale to the presented rationale. When you identify content that you did not know or could not apply, review this content in your nursing text book. An excellent study technique associated with principles is to identify other situations in which the same principle applies and situations in which it is different. See Chapter 10, Analyze Your Test Performance, to design a corrective action plan.

CHANGE THE FOCUS OF THE QUESTION

A great way to explore additional situations using multiple-choice questions is to change one of the key facts in the stem of a question to alter the focus of the question (Sample Items 2–2 and 2–3). Also, in a question that expects you to set a priority, you can eliminate the option that is the correct answer (Sample Items 2–4 and 2–5). This requires you to identify the next best option that answers the question. When the context of the question is altered even slightly, the contour or territory around it changes, which may significantly rearrange the internal structure of the entire question. When a question is altered, the meaning of the situation may require a distinctly different nursing assessment or action.

SAMPLE ITEM 2-2

Which is associated with a physiologic need of a patient with a colostomy?
  (1) Disturbance in body image
  (2) Inadequate nutrition
  (3) Lack of knowledge
  (4) Skin breakdown

The correct answer is option 4. The word "physiologic" modifies the word "need" and is a clue in the stem. For study purposes, you can change the focus of this question by changing the word "physiologic" to "psychologic" in the stem. Now answer this question from this new perspective.

SAMPLE ITEM 2–3

Which is associated with a psychologic need of a patient with a colostomy?

(1) Disturbance in body image

(2) Inadequate nutrition

(3) Lack of knowledge

(4) Skin breakdown

The correct answer is option 1. The entire focus of this question has changed. The focus has moved from "physiologic" to "psychologic." Now the clue in the stem is the word "psychologic." By using this technique, you can apply critical thinking to multiple-choice questions and maximize opportunities for learning. This is an effective strategy either when working alone or when working with a study group.

SAMPLE ITEM 2–4

A preoperative patient talks about being afraid of pain because of a previous experience with painful surgery. What should the nurse do *first* to help the patient cope with this fear?

(1) Encourage the patient not to be afraid

(2) Teach the patient relaxation techniques

(3) Listen to the patient's concerns about pain

(4) Inform the patient that medication is available

The correct answer is option 3. The word "*first*" is asking you to set a priority. For study purposes, you can change the focus of the question by eliminating the correct answer as a choice and then attempting to answer the question from the remaining three options. Now answer the question from this new perspective.

SAMPLE ITEM 2–5

A preoperative patient talks about being afraid of pain because of a previous experience with painful surgery. What should the nurse do *first* to help the patient cope with this fear?

(1) Encourage the patient not to be afraid

(2) Teach the patient relaxation techniques

(3) Inform the patient that medication is available

The correct answer is option 2. The technique of eliminating the correct answer and attempting to select the next best action requires you to rank the options presented in order of importance. This strategy works only with questions that require you to set a priority. Key words such as "initially," "first," "best," "priority," and "most" should alert you that the question is a priority question. By using this strategy, you increase opportunities to sharpen your critical-thinking skills.

STUDY IN A SMALL GROUP

Studying in groups contributes to building a body of knowledge that increases your perspective and context when you are faced with seeking a solution to a highly discriminating question. This technique is particularly helpful because different people bring different perspectives and thinking styles to the sharing that enrich the learning experience. More perspectives produce a variety of views of the problem and generate more approaches to selecting the most accurate response.

> *Where all think alike, no one thinks very much.*
> WALTER LIPPMANN

Summary

With our informational society, there is no way you can know or experience everything. With the explosion of knowledge and technology and changes in the role of the nurse within a fluid health-care delivery environment, what is learned today may be obsolete tomorrow. Consequently, an integral part of your continuing education is the development and refinement of critical-thinking skills. To be a critical thinker, you must be intellectually humble, able to listen, dissatisfied with the status quo, creative, flexible, self-confident but aware of your limitations, and willing to change. Take time to cultivate your critical-thinking skills because they will be the ultimate tool you bring to patient-care situations—the therapeutic use of self. When you can think critically, you are empowered to maximize your abilities to meet patient needs.

18 Answers and Rationales for Sample Items in Chapter 2

2-1 ① Although checking the surgical dressing is important, it does not involve a life-threatening situation.

② **Confirming the placement of the oral airway ensures a patent air passage. An oral airway displaces the tongue and prevents obstruction of the trachea, permitting free passage of air to and from the lungs. Oxygen is essential for life, and this action takes priority.**

③ Although examining the IV site is important, an infiltration can be tolerated for a few minutes while higher priority assessments are made.

④ Although observing the Foley for drainage is important, urinary output at this time is less critical than assessing airway, breathing, and circulation.

2-2 ① Concern about body image is a psychologic, not physiologic, concern.

② Although inadequate nutrition is a physiologic problem, it is not specific to a patient with a colostomy.

③ A knowledge deficit is a cognitive/perceptual problem, not a physiologic problem.

④ **Skin breakdown is a common physiologic problem associated with the presence of a colostomy because of the digestive enzymes present in feces.**

2-3 ① **Concern about body image is a psychologic problem often encountered when a person has surgery that alters the body's structure or function.**

② Nutrition is a physiologic, not a psychologic, problem.

③ Knowledge deficit is a cognitive/perceptual problem, not a psychologic problem.

④ Skin breakdown is a physiologic, not a psychologic, problem.

2-4 ① This denies the patient's fears.

② Although relaxation techniques may be taught eventually, it is not the priority at this time.

③ **This supports the patient's need to verbalize fears.**

④ Although medication may be available, this is false reassurance and cuts off communication.

2-5 ① This denies the patient's fears.

② **Depending on the relaxation technique used, it can reduce muscle tension, distract the person from the stimulus, and/or limit the physiologic response to *fight or flight*, thus reducing pain.**

③ This is false reassurance and cuts off communication.

Time Management

3

Time Management Equals Self-Management

Time is an elusive concept that has been recognized in countless wise sayings. Time is of the essence! Where did the time go? It's now or never! Never put off until tomorrow what you can do today! Time flies when you are having fun! Time is money! A stitch in time saves nine! Time is on your side! And, finally, the most significant saying, You are the only one who can waste your time!

To achieve your goal to be a nurse, you must progress from being a beginning nursing student (HERE) to graduating and passing a licensing examination (THERE). The major difference between HERE and THERE is the letter T. This T represents Time Management, which equals self-management. How you use your time will reflect directly on how successfully you manage the efforts that will ultimately help you attain your goal. The purpose of this chapter is to help you identify personal values and behaviors that relate to time management and learn ways to maximize your productivity through time management strategies.

Take the Time to Assess Your Time Management Abilities

Today many people, particularly students, are attempting to function in a society that stresses the concept of "24/7." They are not running out of time; they are running into it! They are like horses on a merry-go-round that is going faster and faster, and they cannot get off. If you can relate to these people, it is time to take the time to think about time management! The first step in developing a time management program is to know yourself. It is important to identify how you actually spend your time, identify your personal values, and identify your personal barriers to productivity. Take the time to perform the following three self-assessment tools: Assessment of Inconsistencies Between Values and Behavior, Personal Time/Activity Journal, and Self-Assessment of Barriers to Productivity.

ASSESSMENT OF INCONSISTENCIES BETWEEN VALUES AND BEHAVIOR

Values are enduring beliefs or attitudes about the worth of a person, object, idea, or action. A **value system** is the organized set of values that has been internalized by a person. **Values clarification** is a complex process in which you identify, examine, and develop your own individual values. It is impossible to attempt this process here. However, a simple method will be presented for you to identify inconsistencies (i.e., agreement or disagreement, congruencies or discrepancies) between what you consider important and how you behave in relation to the delegation of your time.

20

Make a list of those areas in your life that you value and next to it identify the total percent of time during the day (including travel time) you believe you should allocate to each. After you have completed your Personal Time/Activity Journal, compare the amount of time you devoted to activities related to the areas you identified as important. Evaluate whether or not your behavior reflected what you stated you believe is important. When your behavior reflects your values (attitudes and beliefs), you are in harmony. When your behavior does not reflect your values, you are in "value imbalance," and eventually you will experience emotional and physical consequences. Often, when people have a value imbalance, they are reluctant to create change; but change is necessary to promote harmony intrapersonally (within yourself) and interpersonally (with others). Seeking balance is a challenge. However, the challenge can be manageable because it does not have to be outside your value system, nor does it have to be permanent. Adjustments may be necessary just during an academic semester. A colleague of ours used to say, "You can do anything for 16 weeks!" Following is an example of an assessment tool to identify inconsistencies between values and behavior. Modify the areas in your life that you value accordingly to meet your needs.

Assessment of Inconsistencies Between Values and Behavior		
Areas in My Life That I Value	Desired Percent of Time	Actual Percent of Time
Self-care (eating, sleeping, grooming)		
Work		
Relationships (family, friends)		
Leisure		
School/Studying		
Community activities		
Religion/Spiritual		

PERSONAL TIME/ACTIVITY JOURNAL

Financial consultants who advise on money management recommend to their clients that, for 1 week, they write down every penny they spend. At the end of the week, the information is examined to determine where all the money went. The big difference between time and money is that money can be saved but time cannot. How you spend your minutes and hours can make a difference. Therefore, keep track of what you are doing every hour in a journal. At the end of the week, review what you did, and next to each entry identify whether it is something that you must do, want to do, or do not need to do. The results of this personal time/activity journal should be compared to the areas you have identified as important in your life. Those activities that do not relate to the necessary activities of daily living or your priorities in life should be curtailed, delegated, or eliminated. The following is an example of an activity journal. Modify it to meet your needs.

Personal Time/Activity Journal				
Time	Activity	Must Do	Want to Do	No Need to Do
6-7 A.M.				
7-8 A.M.				
8-9 A.M.				
9-10 A.M.				
10-11 A.M.				
11-12 A.M.				
12-1 P.M.				
1-2 P.M.				
2-3 P.M.				
3-4 P.M.				

Personal Time/Activity Journal				
Time	Activity	Must Do	Want to Do	No Need to Do
4-5 P.M.				
5-6 P.M.				
6-7 P.M.				
7-8 P.M.				
8-9 P.M.				
9-10 P.M.				
10-11 P.M.				

SELF-ASSESSMENT OF BARRIERS TO PRODUCTIVITY

Productivity reflects the amount and quality of outcomes that result from labor. Inherent in this definition are two concepts: outcomes can be numerous and outcomes can be fruitful. These concepts can be related to studying nursing content in a textbook. If you spend 1 hour studying a chapter in a nursing textbook and at the end of the hour you can define all the significant words, you have many concrete results from your studying. Your outcome has been prolific and numerous. If you spend 1 hour studying arterial blood gases and at the end of the hour you are able to understand the interrelationship of the components of acid-base balance, you understand a limited concept. However, you have a quality outcome because this topic is complex. Your effort has been constructive and fruitful!

There are many internal and external factors that can affect your productivity. However, they are not as overwhelming as you may think because most people are creatures of habit and there is a pattern to their behavioral responses and performance. With a little honesty and soul-searching, you should be able to identify some of the barriers to your productivity by taking the Self-Assessment of Barriers to Productivity tool that follows. Read each self-assessment statement in relation to yourself and check either the Yes or No column. After you have completed the self-assessment tool, compare your results to the Corrective Action Plan to Maximize Your Productivity.

Self-Assessment of Barriers to Productivity		
Self-Assessment Statement	Yes	No
1. I tend to procrastinate.		
2. I expect little help from members of my family.		
3. I lack organization.		
4. I flutter from one task to another.		
5. I tend to be obsessive/compulsive.		
6. I tend to socialize when I should be studying.		
7. I fall behind in my responsibilities.		
8. I have difficulty delegating tasks.		
9. I tend to feel overwhelmed.		
10. I have too many conflicting deadlines.		
11. I set high standards for myself.		
12. I attempt to do too much.		

You have just completed the Self-Assessment of Barriers to Productivity tool. Now look at how you answered each question in the tool. Match each number to which you answered "Yes" to its corresponding number in the Corrective Action Plan to Maximize Your Productivity tool. If your response to one or both of the related questions was a "Yes," review the strategies that relate to the factor that may be interfering with or limiting your productivity.

Corrective Action Plan to Maximize Your Productivity

Question Number*	Self-Assessment Statement	Corrective Action Plan
4	I flutter from one task to another.	Identify Goals, page 22
10	I have too many conflicting deadlines.	Set Priorities, page 23
3	I lack organization.	Get Organized,
9	I tend to feel overwhelmed.	page 24
6	I tend to socialize when I should be studying.	Develop Self-Discipline,
12	I attempt to do too much.	page 25
5	I tend to be obsessive/compulsive.	Achieve a Personal Balance,
11	I set high standards for myself.	page 29
2	I expect little help from members of my family.	Delegate,
8	I have difficulty delegating tasks.	page 30
1	I tend to procrastinate.	Overcome Procrastination,
7	I fall behind in my responsibilities.	page 31

* From: Self-Assessment of Barriers to Productivity on page 21.

Maximize Your Productivity

Now that you have given some thought to what is important to you, how you spend your time, and your barriers to productivity, you need to devise a proactive plan to achieve your goals. To maximize productivity, you need to manage your attitudes and behaviors to use time in a constructive manner to achieve your goals.

IDENTIFY GOALS

A **goal** is an object or aim you want to attain. Goals can be long term, intermediate, or short term.

Long-term goals usually are related to lifelong journeys that frequently include career aspirations or ambitions. Long-term goals generally address desired outcomes 5 or more years in the future. Two examples of long-term goals might be: "I will earn a bachelor's degree in nursing by the time my children enter high school." "I will be a nurse manager in an acute care setting within 10 years after graduation from nursing school."

Intermediate goals are related to aims you want to achieve within 1 to 5 years. Appropriately set intermediate goals are the keys to successfully reaching long-term goals. Two examples of intermediate goals are: "I will complete my science prerequisites for the nursing program within 2 years." "I will attend all of my child's soccer games this year."

Short-term goals generally address desired results that take hours, days, weeks, or months to attain. Some people consider them objectives that must be met to reach intermediate and long-term goals. When short-term goals reflect immediate outcomes, they may end up being just a "To Do" list. Examples of short-term goals are: "I will earn a minimum grade of B in my Fundamentals of Nursing course this semester." "I will cook 12 meals this weekend and put them in the freezer."

When setting goals, remember that they must contain certain elements to be effective. They must be specific, measurable, realistic, and have a time frame. A goal that is **specific** identifies precisely what is to be attained. A goal that is **measurable** sets a minimum satisfactory level of performance. A goal that is **realistic** has a reasonable chance of being attained. A goal that has a **time frame** states the length of time it will take to attain the goal. Compare these criteria to the goals stated previously and to each goal that you write in the future. Work tends to expand in length when there are no guidelines for its performance. Goals are a major way to prevent wasting time in this manner because you know your destination before you begin and you have a time frame in which to get there. There is an old saying that goes something like this: "If you want to get something done, give it to the busiest person you know." Effective busy people understand the need to set specific, measurable, realistic goals that can be achieved within a specific time frame.

Most students understand the importance of goals but do not understand how to set them because of the complexity of their lives. One way to begin goal setting is to identify your roles in life. How you identify your roles depends on your frame of reference. For example, you may decide you want to look at your roles in relation to how you relate to people (individual, spouse, parent, friend, co-worker) or you may decide you want to look at your roles in relation to what you do (housekeeper, cook, family support person, nurse's aide, Girl Scout leader, Sunday School teacher). After you have defined your roles, identify one or more goals that you want to achieve in each role. They can be short-term, intermediate, or long-term goals, depending on what is important to you. When setting goals, ensure that you take into account the various areas in your life that you considered important when you completed the tool Assessment of Inconsistencies Between Values and Behavior. Your goals need to be in harmony with your values (attitudes and beliefs).

Involve your family when writing a goal. They will have a vested interest in your attaining your goal when they understand the rationales for the goal. For example, when you earn your license as a Registered Nurse, you can quit your second job, earn more money for vacations, or work the night shift, all of which will allow you to spend more time with them. These are the rewards for attaining your goal. Family-centered goals should be like a pebble dropped in a lake—the ripples of pleasurable rewards should affect all members of the family. Put your goals in writing. It makes them more tangible, and you can review them routinely to remain focused. Share your goals with everyone who will listen. A goal that exists only in your mind is a dream or fantasy and is less likely to become reality. Telling people your goals can be motivating because you create additional emphasis on the need to perform. When you attain goals, reward yourself and family members when appropriate. This will motivate you and recognize the significant others in your life who are helping you to attain your goals.

Goals need to be revisited. In our fast-paced society, our roles, responsibilities, and relationships change over time. You need to be flexible enough to revise, eliminate, or reset a goal, depending on the factors that change in your life. For example, after taking 12 college credits in one academic semester while working full time, you realize that you are overwhelmed. You may revise your goal of attaining a bachelor's degree in nursing by prolonging the time frame in which to attain this goal. If you get pregnant and have twins while in school, you may decide that taking one course a semester is more realistic than taking three courses a semester. Revising your goals is not a sign of failure, but rather a mature recognition of reasonable expectations, which requires you to reset your goals accordingly.

SET PRIORITIES

After students identify their goals, they often ask, "Now what?" Well, now is the time to set priorities! **Setting priorities** is the process of identifying the preferential order of doing something. In other words, what requires your attention first? It is helpful to have criteria for classifying activities so that you can prioritize with less difficulty. For example, you can classify things to do into four categories:

1. **Pressing/Important Tasks**—Tasks that are pressing and important insist on your immediate attention and relate to activities that you consider vital or valuable. Examples are reviewing class notes for an examination the next day, taking care of a sick child, finishing writing an assignment that has to be submitted tomorrow, and making dinner for the family.
2. **Not Pressing/Important Tasks**—Tasks that are not pressing but are important relate to activities that you consider vital and valuable. However, they require you to be self-directed and proactive to take the initiative to complete them. Examples are planning a weekly calendar, playing with your children, reading the textbook for an examination in 2 weeks, and doing laundry.
3. **Pressing/Not Important Tasks**—Tasks that are pressing but are not important compete for your immediate attention, but they relate to activities you do not consider vital or important. Examples are listening to a telephone call from a telemarketer, watching a specific program on television, and doing something that someone else thinks you should do.
4. **Not Pressing/Not Important Tasks**—Tasks that are not urgent and not important are small, minor, insignificant, trivial activities. They are not competing for your immediate attention, nor do you consider them important. Examples are cleaning the sock drawer, sharpening all the pencils in your desk, and socializing with uninvited visitors.

The examples provided may not reflect your values. Obviously, you need to identify those activities that are important and pressing to you. Important activities relate to your values and your stated goals. Pressing activities relate to tasks that have to be accomplished in the short term, hours or days. These activities belong in the pressing/important category and must be tackled first. We all have urgent or unexpected activities that must be addressed, but this should not become a standard method of functioning. If you put most of your activities in this category, you are in a crisis management mode because you are dealing with emergencies, problems, or last minute deadlines. When you constantly function in this mode, you will be anxious, over-worked, overwhelmed, and speeding toward burnout.

Activities that are important but have several days or weeks before they need to be completed can be placed in the not pressing/important category. Most of your life's activities, including academically related tasks, can be placed in this category. Have the self-discipline to tackle these tasks while you have the luxury of time. If you put most of your activities in this category, you are probably self-directed and an effective manager of your time. However, if you delay or ignore activities in this category, the pressure to accomplish the task increases until it must be reclassified into the pressing/important category. Attention to details in this category is like preventive maintenance on a car. It gets accomplished before the car breaks down and it becomes a crisis. When you function in this category, you are in control and anxiety is kept to a minimum.

When setting priorities, you need to limit activities in the pressing/not important category because they are not important. If most of your activities are in this category, reacting and responding are your modes of action rather than being proactive. You are responding to urgent stimuli, but more often than not the urgency and importance of the activity are based on the expectations of others. You are meeting other people's needs, not your own.

Finally, when setting priorities, you need to limit or eliminate activities in the not pressing/not important category. Why get involved with tasks that are insignificant and unimportant? Why waste your time? If you put most of your activities into this category, you may be overwhelmed and trying to escape from the pressing problems or activities in the pressing/important category. Escape may be your only way to obtain relief.

When setting priorities, you are the only person who can decide if something is important. You can make choices that are in harmony with your values and goals. Unfortunately, you may or may not have control over time frames. Emergencies arise that need immediate attention; due dates for school assignments may be indicated weeks in advance; and some deadlines are self-imposed. Some deadlines cannot be altered, but others may be extended without giving up your goals. The ability to set priorities puts you in a position of control because you are the one making the decisions.

GET ORGANIZED

When you look at your life, do you feel like a juggler attempting to keep multiple balls aloft all at the same time while walking on a bed of fire? If so, you are on overload. You may be a mother, daughter, father, son, brother, sister, wife, husband, friend, employee, student, social advocate, etc. Each role has its related responsibilities and stresses. As a result, you may have multi-role overload! In our world, and especially in nursing, the volume of new information is expanding dramatically. Years ago a nursing fundamentals textbook was several hundred pages long. Today a fundamentals textbook is over a thousand pages long. As a result, you may have information overload! Today corporations are focusing on increasing productivity. Your place of business may be reorganizing to maximize your work effort. As a result, you may have work overload! In the last few years, the explosion in technology has produced fax machines, voicemail, call forwarding, beepers, answering machines, e-mail, and cell phones. You are connected and accessible "24/7." As a result, you may have access overload! When overloaded for any length of time, you can spiral toward an overload crisis. You must be organized to regain control of the situation.

Being on overload is a problem, and time management may be the solution. There are many ways to manage time, but a simple, concrete method is the use of calendars. If your goal is to graduate from an associate degree nursing program in 2 years, you should make a 2-year master calendar listing the courses you must take each semester to successfully meet the curriculum requirements for graduation. Next, you may need more detailed calendars, such as monthly, weekly, or daily, to provide additional structure. Also, calendars help you to plan for short- and long-range assignments, provide consistency with a regular schedule, identify priorities, and reduce anxiety.

Monthly calendars help control mental clutter. Make monthly calendars for every month within a semester and insert important personal events (such as social engagements, doctor's appointments) and school-related requirements (such as first and last days of the semester, examinations, special projects, due dates for written assignments). Also, insert school holidays and vacation periods. These reminders provide a broad overview of your monthly activities. After you insert important events in the calendar do not use mental energy to keep that information in the forefront of your mind. You just need to check your calendar to verify when an event will take place.

Weekly calendars provide an overview of the week and achieve consistency concerning your day-to-day schedule. They should be constructed just before beginning a new week. Block in all of your required commitments on your weekly calendar. Include time for activities of daily living (such as sleeping, grooming, food preparation, eating, doing laundry), children-related activities, work, scheduled classes, religious services, etc. Allocate additional time to those commitments that require travel. After all your required tasks are inserted into the calendar, you can begin deciding how to carve up the remaining time. Factors that must be considered include: setting consistent times to study each day, scheduling breaks within study periods, ensuring recreational activities, determining the time of day when you are most productive, deciding how much time you need to study, and so on. There is an old formula that states that you should study 1 to 2 hours a week for every hour you are in class. For example, if you are in school 12 hours a week, you should be studying 12 to 24 hours a week outside of class. Although this is often true, it is a generality. Only you can decide from your past and present performance how much time you need to study or prepare written assignments outside of class to be successful. In addition, when developing a weekly calendar it is essential to establish consistency in activities from one day to the next because it creates a routine that is familiar, and familiarity reduces anxiety. Also, it reduces the need to expend energy to make decisions. You made the decision once at the beginning of the week to study from 7 to 9 PM Monday through Friday. Your job now is to implement the plan without the need to use energy to explore the pros and cons of studying or overcome your own objections to studying. You made a commitment to yourself to study, and you need to have the integrity to keep your commitment.

Daily calendars organize your activities so that you can achieve your daily goals efficiently and effectively. Design the calendar in the evening for the next day. This helps to reduce anxiety because you have organized your thoughts, identified your goals, and planned a time to accomplish them. Plan a calendar that is simple. Start by slotting in all the personal and school-related special events for the day that appear on your weekly calendar. Do not include routine tasks such as class time, work, or personal activities such as eating, sleeping, etc. Now make a list of all the academic and nonacademic activities that you want to accomplish. Be as specific as you can. Many people call this a "To Do List." Rank each activity on the list in order of priority; that is, items that must get done first, then those that should get done, and finally those you would like to get done. Plot these activities (particularly the tasks that must get done) around your standard tasks and coordinate the scheduling of activities to take advantage of blocks of available time that are appropriate for the tasks. Also, combine activities so that you can accomplish more than one task at a time. For example, shop at stores that have multiple departments so that school supplies and food for dinner can be bought at one stop; study flash cards while performing a chore, or use a similar topic for assignments in two different courses so that one search of the literature can be used for both assignments. Welcome to "multitasking," a necessity when maintaining a busy schedule! Although you may have a full schedule, every minute of every day does not have to be accounted for. Tasks may take longer than planned and unexpected situations may occur. Some tasks may not be accomplished by the end of the day, preferably the lower-priority activities. If you have tasks left over, you may have to revise your future daily lists with a more realistic attitude, move an uncompleted task to the next day, delegate the task, or eliminate it entirely.

Obviously, everyone's calendar will be different, depending on family, school, and work-related commitments. Although individualized, calendars should all be simple, realistic, and flexible. They should not be so complex that they become an additional chore. The course of study to become a nurse is demanding and takes time and energy. Energy can be conserved if time is used efficiently. Many people say they do not have the time to design calendars, but a well-thought-out plan that is followed promotes the efficient use of time, resulting in more available time. You need to spend time to save time!

DEVELOP SELF-DISCIPLINE

When you feel overwhelmed, have you ever said to yourself, "If only there were 25 hours in a day I would get all my work done." If the truth be told, you probably still would not get your work done if you had 26 hours in a day. The reality is there are only 24 hours in a day and only 168 hours in a week. How you manage yourself in relation to that time is the key to feeling in control rather than feeling overwhelmed.

You start by setting your goals and priorities. If you are to be successful and graduate from nursing school, school must be a priority. If you work full time or several days a week, manage a home with children, and are involved in community activities, the demands on your time and energy may be excessive. Only you can decide what you are capable of doing. Setting realistic demands on your time and energy is difficult. You may be able to do anything you want, but you may not be able to do everything you want. Rarely in life can you have it all. Therefore, to manage your time and responsibilities efficiently and fairly, you may have to make hard decisions. Reducing work hours, sharing household chores, hiring a babysitter, or limiting your social life may be necessary strategies to help you manage your responsibilities in relation to your school work. You may even decide to delay your goal by taking fewer credits per semester or deciding that this is not the best time to be going to school. Sacrifices in and of themselves should not be viewed negatively. Often these sacrifices will promote growth in you and your family.

After you and your family have set your goals and priorities, you must get their help in establishing your weekly calendar. This calendar should set "firm boundaries" for your future behavior, recognizing that it must be flexible to "bend" with emerging or unexpected priorities. With this calendar, you have made a commitment to yourself and others to achieve certain goals within a time frame. In other words, you have made a promise. Now you must keep it! Keeping promises expands your basic habits of personal effectiveness and builds character, but it requires self-discipline.

Self-discipline is orderly conduct in relation to self-imposed constraints. Self-discipline is an internal factor that is influenced only by what you bring to a situation. Self-discipline involves three important abilities: the ability to say "NO," the ability to avoid time traps, and the ability to self-motivate.

Saying "NO"

The word "NO" is a short word that can have a big impact on your ability to manage your life. If you are similar to others who enter the helping professions, you usually use the word YES more often than you use the word NO. You want to help and give of yourself, and as a result put the needs of others before your own. However, when you are going to school, it is the time to make your needs a priority. Learn to say "NO." When asked to do something by someone else, you have to ask yourself questions such as:

- Is this consistent with my identified goal/priorities?
- Is this something I must do?
- Is this something I want to do?
- Is this something I have no need to do?
- Is this person able to do this by himself or herself?
- Is there anyone else who can do this task?

Based on your response to these self-directed questions you can respond with a YES or NO to the person who is asking you to do something. If you are undecided, buy yourself some time with a response such as, "That sounds interesting, but let me think about it overnight and I will get back to you tomorrow." This response allows you an opportunity to consider how much time the activity will demand and to make a decision that is within your value system. If your answer is "NO" it gives you time to construct a response.

The most common consequence of saying "NO" is the feeling of guilt. Guilt is a self-imposed feeling that occurs when your conscience identifies that something you have done or not done is unacceptable; only you can make yourself feel guilty. You waste energy when you feel guilty; therefore, use the energy of guilt to prevent guilty feelings. You can deal with guilt in several ways:

- Recognize that you may never eliminate feelings of guilt because you are human. However, you can limit feelings of guilt.
- Understand that there is "good guilt" and there is "bad guilt." **Good guilt** is feeling bad about something you have done or not done that you have based on what you identify as ethically or morally correct. Use the energy of good guilt to reestablish your goals, priorities, and calendars. For example: "I will schedule time in my calendar to spend an hour a day in the evening playing with my children." **Bad guilt** is feeling bad about something over which you have no control. Do not waste energy on bad guilt because it is irrational and physically and emotionally draining. For example: "I am a single parent and I must work to put food on the table and a roof over our heads. I am going to school so that I will be able to reach my goals of being a nurse and earning a better living. While I am in school I must spend more time with my studies and less time with my children."

- You can change the belief on which your guilty feelings are based. For example: "It is appropriate for me to meet my needs before someone else's needs; I am not a bad person if I decide not to do whatever someone else expects of me."
- You can make a weekly calendar that respects your goals and priorities. When studying, you should not feel guilty about not spending time with the family because you have scheduled time to address family needs.
- You can compensate for your behavior. Compensation is repaying yourself or someone else when something is done or not done as expected. It is used when unexpected priorities arise. However, if you are constantly using compensation, you need to revisit your goals, priorities, and calendars. For example: "I want to watch the ball game on TV tonight, so I will study 2 hours more on the weekend." "We had fast food three times this week, so tonight I will make a great home-cooked meal."

Use feelings of guilt to your advantage. This is an opportunity for personal change and growth.

Avoiding Time Traps

Time traps are interruptions that interfere with your ability to use your time effectively to be productive. Earlier in this chapter you were advised to complete a personal time/activity journal. A review of your journal should reveal to you how you spent your time and whether it was productive or you got caught in time traps. You were also asked to perform a self-assessment to identify your barriers to productivity, which included procrastination, difficulty with delegation, lack of organization, an inability to set goals and priorities, perfectionism, and lack of self-discipline. Each of these barriers to productivity has time-trap elements, and corrective actions for each are addressed in this chapter. This section will help you identify seemingly unavoidable events that interfere with your use of time. Do not dribble away time when you are out of control or when others control you. Some time traps cannot be completely avoided. However, awareness of how events are interfering with your use of time and then effective management can help you address most of them. First, you must recognize when you are caught in a time trap and realize how much time is wasted. Second, you need to set limits on yourself and others and regain control of your time. Some events over which you may believe you have little control are:

- Unwanted phone calls or phone calls that involve unimportant conversations (small talk)
- Long-winded conversations that do not get to the point
- Arrival of unwanted guests
- A crowded library or store
- Waiting for others
- Rush-hour traffic
- Excessively researching a topic
- Too much socializing
- Unnecessary meetings
- Assuming the role of listener or counselor to meet the emotional needs of friends

Many of these occur because you are unaware of how much time they waste; you have not organized your day; or you have not set limits on yourself or others. You are not powerless to control these events. However, to limit or eliminate time traps, you must be proactive. Suggested solutions are as follows:

Manage accessibility:

- Turn off your cell phone or use it only for outgoing calls.
- Indicate on your voicemail that you are available only during certain times.
- Make your home phone unlisted.
- Give your e-mail address only to selected individuals.
- Use caller ID to screen phone calls.
- Turn off the ringer or unplug the phone when studying.
- Block out time for study when you absolutely cannot be interrupted.
- Learn to say, "It's nice to hear from you, but I really can't talk right now. I'll catch up with you next week." This generally works. If the other person is persistent, say, "I'm sorry, I really have to go." And then close the door or hang up.

- Put a "Do Not Disturb" sign on your door. I used this approach when I had a newborn and I put a picture of a sleeping baby on the sign.
- Give family members instructions to interrupt you when you are studying only if there is an emergency.

Manage waiting time:

- Set limits on the amount of time you are willing to wait.
- Capture moments of time and study flash cards or notes.
- Use captured moments of time to get small tasks accomplished. For example, while waiting for an appointment, write a thank-you note for a gift, make out your meal plan and grocery list for the week, review your weekly schedule, write a check and prepare a bill to be mailed, or brainstorm how you are going to tackle an upcoming assignment.
- Make appointments with health-care providers the first or last appointment of the day. Call to ensure that the provider is on schedule.

Avoid wasting time:

- Keep a list of what has been done and what still needs to be done so that if you stop in the middle of a project you can pick up where you left off.
- Multitask your errands. Go one-stop shopping. For example, some stores carry food, hardware, clothes, and so forth.
- Simplify shopping. Reduce trips to the store, keep a shopping list, and maintain a full pantry.
- Simplify meals. Cook one-dish meals.
- Cook double the amount for your family and freeze half for another day.
- Eat out or take-out when short on time.
- Avoid travel during rush hour. Leave earlier or later and use the saved time to your best advantage. Truck stops are filled with trucks during rush hour. Professional drivers use this time to eat and sleep rather than spend time in "gridlock." Do the same.
- Simplify gift giving. For example, books are a great gift and all your holiday shopping can be done in one store. Each book can be personalized by topic and a personal message inscribed on the inside cover.
- Avoid meetings unless they are absolutely necessary, such as a parent/teacher conference. If a meeting is necessary, set a time limit on each subject to be discussed and the amount of time each person can speak and stick to it. This requires participants to be concise and focused.
- Food shop when the stores open in the morning or late at night, preferably on a Wednesday, because these are the least crowded times.
- Avoid using the library just before midterms and finals. Using the library at these times is generally the sign of a procrastinator.

Manage your own emotions:

- Lower your expectations. For example, you do not have to prepare four-course meals every day, or you do not have to research every project beyond what is necessary to meet the criteria of the assignment. Perfection is not necessary to pass a nursing course.
- Recognize when you are experiencing "good guilt" versus "bad guilt" and act accordingly. For more information, see the section on self-discipline in this chapter.
- Avoid accepting the role of counselor for your friends. Listening to other people's problems is a time-consuming and emotionally exhausting process. Listen for a few minutes and then say, "I'm not a counselor. I think you need to talk to someone who is trained to help you with this problem."

Motivating Yourself

Motivation is the driving force that encourages you to do something. It is an incentive or bribe that induces you to action. Motivation can come from within. Learning something new, attaining a goal, and being impressed with your performance are examples of internal motivation. You have to be future oriented to use internal motivation to stimulate yourself toward the achievement of a long-term goal. For example, visualize yourself walking up to receive your diploma, wearing your nurse's uniform, or receiving your first paycheck for being a nurse. This can be difficult because you have to delay gratification in the present for a future abstract goal.

Motivation can also come from without. Earning a high grade, obtaining respect from others, and receiving a reward are examples of external motivation. To deal with the present, a break from studying, a candy bar, a walk around the block, a cold drink, or just sitting down and getting started may be motivating.

Each person's motivator is individual. Think about the tasks that you accomplish every day. What payoff do you receive for completing them? When you are able to identify what really spurs you to action, then you can use these same incentives for accomplishing school-related activities. For a further discussion about motivation, see Balance Sacrifices and Rewards in Chapter 4, Study Techniques.

ACHIEVE A PERSONAL BALANCE

Do you write and rewrite an assignment until it is perfect? Do you always have to get an A on every test? Do you think that no one can do as good a job on a particular project as you can? Do you like others to have an image of you that you are superman or superwoman? Do you study constantly to the detriment of your other personal needs? Do you think that you can be all things to all people? Do you think that the office/committee/family will collapse without you? If you answered "Yes" to several of these questions, you may be a perfectionist.

A **perfectionist** is a person who compulsively strives to attain a degree of excellence according to a given standard. In other words, you think you are perfect. Also, a perfectionist tends to have an idealized self-image. That is, he or she displays to the world a self that is expected to be admired, respected, and loved by others. Unfortunately, if you are a perfectionist, you are striving for the impossible. It is humanly impossible to be perfect, and attempting to maintain an idealized image is irrational, impractical, and self-destructive.

Perfectionism can be physically and emotionally debilitating. Because you can never really achieve perfection, you set yourself up for not performing according to your own imaginary standard of perfection. When this happens, emotionally you shatter your self-image, which can at best be demoralizing and unmotivating and at worst promote feelings of failure. Also, attempting to complete every role (spouse, parent, worker, student) to perfection can take its toll on your body. A little stress keeps you alert, helps to motivate, and promotes concentration. However, excessive stress taxes the endocrine, neurologic, and cardiovascular systems, which eventually results in physical depletion and exhaustion. Perfectionism, although considered a noble trait by some, can be emotionally and physically self-destructive and needs to be brought under control.

To conquer obsessive/compulsive, perfectionistic thinking, you must achieve a sense of personal balance. There is a big difference between expecting perfection and striving for excellence! First, you need to recognize that no one, including you, is perfect. Then you must alter your frame of reference. You do this by putting the new set of circumstances into the present situation. Examples of some questions you may ask yourself are:

- Will I still graduate if I earn less than an A in my nursing courses?
- Is a grade of A on a written assignment worth not going to a child's sporting event?
- Will what it takes to earn an A in a nursing course negatively affect the other things I think are important in my life?
- Does this task require perfect effort?
- Does dinner really have to be on the table at 6:00?
- Can I afford to have my lawn cut rather than cut it myself?
- Does dust provide a protective barrier for the surface of furniture?

Individualize the questions you ask yourself to reflect your personal and family responsibilities. We are not suggesting that you lower your standards on those things that are most important to you. You can still strive for excellence and give 100 percent, but you are doing so in light of your present circumstance. If you are adding a huge commitment into your life (e.g., nursing school), something else in your life has to give. A student once told us that although she picked up around the house every day, she dusted only every other week. One day she saw the following note from her husband written in the dust on a table top. "I love you!" Underneath the note she wrote back, "Ditto!" She said they had a good laugh over the exchange, but she also demonstrated to him that the dust was not one of her priorities and she was not going to be pressured into dusting. One of our male students indicated that he never studied on Saturday night. He and his girlfriend always had a standing date so that they could spend time together. At graduation several graduates have an opportunity to talk to the convocation. Usually at least one graduate will make reference to the fact that there will be more home-cooked meals and less pizza and Chinese food now that they have graduated. One of the examples presented reflects a behavior that may result in a lower grade but addresses an important value (spending time with a significant other). Other examples demonstrate a relaxation of standards of perfection (a dust-free house and home-cooked meals).

Controlling perfectionism and relaxing an idealized self-image is not an easy task. However, you must remain true to yourself in light of your values and goals. Seek growth and development, not perfection, as you seek balance in your personal life.

DELEGATE

If you look up the word "delegate" in a dictionary, you will find words such as "surrender," "relinquish," "renounce," and "give up" used to explain its meaning. Unfortunately, this is why many people have difficulty delegating tasks to others. They look at delegation as a loss, giving something up, or yielding control. Delegation does the exact opposite. When you delegate, you transfer a task to another person and you gain, not lose, something. You gain more time! For delegation to achieve desired results and positive feelings for both people involved, you must follow the guidelines in the following paragraphs.

Identify the personal qualities of the people to whom you can delegate. Before you delegate a task to another person you must identify, alone or in conjunction with the other person, whether the person has the capacity to complete the task. Does the person have the appropriate intellectual, physical, and/or attitudinal ability to be successful at the task? The focus here is not on whether or not this person has ever done this task before, but whether or not the person has the potential to do the task and is the appropriate person for the task. For example, it is inappropriate to expect 5-year-old children to clean a house, but it is appropriate to expect them to pick up their own toys.

Identify the outcomes of the task to be accomplished. Explore with the other person the expected result. You should both have a clear, concise, mutual understanding of what is to be accomplished. The focus here is not on how the task will be done, but rather on the product or conclusion. For example, if you delegate doing the laundry, the outcome may be that clothing will be clean, dried, and folded every 2 days. You are not focusing on how the clothing got washed or what cleaning products were used.

Identify the resources that are necessary to accomplish the task. For a task to be accomplished, you must consider the human, economic, technical, or organizational resources that may be necessary for the person to accomplish the desired outcome. There may be necessary information or skills that must be practiced for the person to be successful in performing a new task. The focus here is not on excessive detail, but rather on flexibility in the extent of support. For example, to cook dinner, one person may draw on past experiences; another may need a cookbook; and another may require a demonstration with supervised practice.

Relinquish accountability for the task. Accountability exists when a person assumes responsibility for something. When you delegate in your personal life, you transfer the responsibility for the task to another person, and that person assumes ownership of their actions and the results of those actions. You will not feel free from the burden of a task unless you relinquish accountability for the task. The focus here is not on authoritarian supervision or consequences for tasks not accomplished, but rather on the concept of trust. For example, you cannot hover over, breathe down the neck of, or micromanage another person when he or she is working on a delegated task. You must allow the person room to explore, practice, and grow. Occasionally you may have to wear pink underwear, tolerate dusty baseboards, or eat tasteless meals. Initially, less than perfect outcomes go with the territory of delegation.

Delegation does not occur in isolation. Communicate your needs to family and friends. Have a family meeting and explore what tasks need to be done, what people would like to do, and what skills need to be learned. When family members are involved in the decision-making process, there is ownership, which increases the probability of success. This is an opportunity for both you and family members to grow. You will learn the art of delegation, share your needs, recognize that you are interdependent, and reinforce that you must trust in others. Family members, even children, will learn new skills, feel important, develop confidence, and gain independence. Finally, routinely review the plan and evaluate how it is working. Ask questions such as: Are people accountable? Do tasks need to be rotated? Do people need additional resources? Is someone ready to learn a new skill? Are priorities being met? Change the plan as necessary. Delegation plans must be flexible to meet the needs of both the family as a whole and the individuals within it.

OVERCOME PROCRASTINATION

Procrastination is putting off or postponing something until a future time. It is a protective mechanism to delay having to deal with something that we would rather not deal with. We procrastinate because in the short term it reduces anxiety. However, in the long term procrastination will waste time and increase anxiety. We all procrastinate to some degree, but when taken to an extreme, it can interfere with our ability to complete tasks for which we are responsible. When delaying a project, have you ever said to yourself:

- This is boring.
- This is too hard.
- I do not know where to begin.
- I am not in the mood.
- I am too tired.
- I am angry/annoyed/frustrated that I have to do this.
- I have more important things to do.
- I can do it tomorrow.
- I have plenty of time.
- I work better under pressure.

These are just a few of the ways in which we rationalize our behavior. **Rationalization** is giving socially acceptable reasons or explanations for our behaviors. When used in relation to why we did not do something we were expected to do, usually it is an excuse! Sometimes our excuses are so believable that we convince ourselves. To overcome procrastination, you must first realize that you are procrastinating, stop the procrastinating behavior, and then take constructive action to overcome the procrastination.

Breaking the cycle of procrastination requires a new mindset. When we delay tasks, it is often because we look at them as "chores," routine activities or responsibilities that we may consider demanding or unpleasant. The word "chores" has a negative undertone. Therefore, tasks associated with schoolwork must never be viewed as chores but placed within a positive frame of reference. They are tasks that must be accomplished to reach your goal of becoming a nurse. Now, take the reason that you stated why something should be postponed and challenge the statement with logic or motivating strategies. For example:

- This is boring. "This is not dull and unexciting because it will help prepare me to be a nurse. It has to get done sooner or later and it might as well be now."
- This is too hard. "I can do this! It may be difficult, but I did not get this far in my education without being able to do what I have to do to pass a course."
- I do not know where to begin. "Yes, I do! I need to review the requirements related to this assignment. I will make an outline on how I should move forward. I will focus on just a small part of the assignment. I will discuss what I finish today with my instructor tomorrow."
- I am not in the mood. "I will never be in the mood to do this assignment. I can divide the assignment into several parts and reward myself when I finish each part."
- I am too tired. "I am always tired. I will break down the job into sections and at least I can do one section today."
- I am angry/annoyed/frustrated that I have to do this. "I am feeling this way because . . . , but my feelings are standing in the way of my completing this task. I need to *get a grip*. I will deal with my feelings in more depth after finishing what I have to do now."
- I have more important things to do. "Oh, really! Let me list the other things I have to do and I will put them in order of importance. Which of these things can I eliminate or delegate? This is the most important thing I have to do now."
- I can do it tomorrow. "No, I will think about it right now. I should not put off until tomorrow what I can do today!"
- I have plenty of time. "I never have plenty of time. There is no time like the present!"
- I work better under pressure. "Who am I kidding? When I leave it to the last minute, I get it done because I have no other choice. I can do a much better job now if I give myself enough time to do it right."

These examples of self-challenge statements are not universal responses. Make your own statements. However, each statement should follow these simple guidelines: identify that you are procrastinating, challenge the procrastination with a direct opposing thought, and justify your challenging statement with a logical explanation. Sometimes the explanations to challenge procrastination involve larger changes such as modifying your priorities or restructuring your activities of daily living. However, more often than not, it involves smaller changes such as using strategies of motivation. You can motivate yourself by setting short-term goals, providing rewards for finished tasks, using positive self-talk, or being a firm self-taskmaster. Procrastination is a behavior that is initiated from within. When you know and manage yourself, you will be in control of your learning instead of the other way around.

Summary

Controlling the use of time to your best advantage depends on your desire and effort to identify and correct negative patterns that waste time. You need to be proactive in the control of your time. To be proactive you need to implement the tools presented in this chapter to identify barriers to productivity, identify common time traps, and implement suggested corrective actions. If successful, you will have more time to tackle the tasks that are not pressing but important. When addressing tasks in this category, you will feel more in control and productive and less overwhelmed and anxious. With a little effort and a desire to change, you can be a master of your own time! Using your time productively can maximize the time you have for studying for nursing examinations.

Study Techniques

4

Learning is the activity by which knowledge, attitudes, and/or skills are acquired. Learning is a complex activity that is influenced by various factors such as genetic endowment, level of maturation, experiential background, effectiveness of formal instruction, self-image, readiness to learn, level of motivation, and extent of self-study. Although some of these factors are unchangeable, others you can control.

Learning is an active process that takes place within the learner. Therefore, the role of the learner is to participate in or initiate activities that promote learning. Like test taking, learning is a learned skill. This chapter presents both general and specific study techniques that should increase your ability to learn. The general study techniques presented include skills that facilitate learning regardless of the topic being studied. The specific study techniques are presented in relation to levels of thinking processes that are required to answer questions in nursing: knowledge, comprehension, application, and analysis. Use of these techniques when studying will help you to comprehend more of what you have studied and retain the information for a longer period of time. This information should increase your success in answering test questions.

General Study Techniques

There are general techniques to improve study skills that can be applied to any subject and a few specific techniques particularly applicable to studying for nursing examinations. We discuss both here.

ESTABLISH A ROUTINE

Set aside a regular time to study. Learning requires consistency, repetition, and practice. Deciding to sit down to study is the most difficult part of studying. We tend to procrastinate and think of a variety of things we must do instead of studying. By committing yourself to a regular routine, you eliminate the repetitive need to make the decision to study. If you decide that every night from 7:00 PM to 8:30 PM you are going to study, you are using your internal locus of control and establishing an internal readiness to learn. You must be motivated to learn.

Your study schedule must be reasonable and realistic. Shorter, more frequent study periods are more effective than long study periods. For most people, 1- to 3-hour study periods with a 10-minute break each hour are most effective. Periods of learning must be balanced with adequate rest periods because energy, attention, and endurance decrease over time and limit learning efficiency. Physical and emotional rest make you more alert and receptive to new information.

When planning a schedule, involve significant family members in the decision making. Because a family is an open system, the action of one family member will influence the other family members. If they are involved in the decision making, they will have a vested interest and probably be more supportive of your need to study.

SET SHORT- AND LONG-TERM GOALS

A goal is an outcome that a person attempts to attain, and it may be long term or short term. A long-term goal is the eventual desired outcome. A short-term goal is a desired outcome that can be achieved along the path leading to the long-term goal. In other words, a long-term goal is your destination, whereas each short-term goal is an objective that must be attained to help you eventually reach your destination. Each long-term goal may have one or more short-term goals. Goals should be formulated to promote learning that is purposeful, to serve as guides for planning action, and to establish standards so that learning can be evaluated. Goals must be specific, measurable, and realistic, and must have a time frame. A specific goal states exactly what is to be accomplished. A measurable goal sets a minimum acceptable level of performance. A realistic goal must be potentially achievable. A goal with a time frame states the time parameters in which the goal will be achieved.

A typical long-term goal would be to correctly answer 90 percent of the study questions at the end of Chapter 1 in a fundamentals of nursing textbook within 7 hours. Typical short-term goals might be to read and highlight important information in Chapter 1 within 2 hours, to list the principles presented in Chapter 1 within 1 hour, and to compare and contrast information in your class notes with information in the textbook within 2 hours. Each of these short-term goals can be achieved as a step toward attaining the long-term goal. It is wise to break a big task into small, manageable tasks because it is easier to learn small bits of information than large blocks of information. The most effective learning is goal-directed learning because it is planned learning with a purpose. In addition, when goals are attained, they increase self-esteem and motivation.

SIMULATE A SCHOOL ENVIRONMENT

The familiar generally is less stressful than the unfamiliar. Therefore, your posture, surroundings, and equipment should be similar to those in the school or testing environment. Study at a desk or table and chair. Avoid the temptation to study in a reclining chair, on the couch, or in bed. If you are too comfortable, you may become too relaxed or even fall asleep. Gather all the necessary equipment for studying, such as your textbook, class notes, paper, pens, a highlighter, a dictionary, and so on. When simulating test taking, use the same tools you plan to use when you take your examinations. Control other factors that reflect the testing environment such as ensuring adequate light and avoiding eating while you are studying. The study environment should be comfortable enough to promote learning but strict enough to keep you alert and focused.

CONTROL INTERNAL AND EXTERNAL DISTRACTORS

Stimuli, both internal and external, must be controlled to eliminate distractions. External stimuli are environmental happenings that interrupt your thinking and should be limited. Select a place to study where you will not be interrupted by family members, phone calls, the doorbell, or family pets. Do not study while watching television or listening to the radio. These stimuli compete for your attention when you need to be focusing on your work. Internal stimuli are your inner thoughts, feelings, or concerns that interfere with your ability to study. Internal stimuli are often more difficult to control than external stimuli because they involve attitudes. Review the techniques in Chapter 1 that promote a positive mental attitude. By limiting or eliminating internal and external distractors, you should improve your ability to concentrate.

PREPARE FOR CLASS

To prepare adequately for class, you need to know the content that will be addressed. Look at the course outline or ask your instructor. "If you don't know where you're going, you can't get there!" After you know the topic, identify the appropriate content in your textbook. To pre-**pare** for class you must pare down the written information in your textbook. To **pare** means to cut, clip, shave, or whittle away. When reviewing textbook material before class, it is not always necessary to read every word.

- **First,** read the chapter headings. This will give you an overview of the topic presented.
- **Second,** look at tables and figures and read their captions. These provide visual cues.
- **Third,** skim the chapter content but read information that is CAPITALIZED, **boldfaced,** or *italicized.* These formats indicate important information; use a highlighting marker to accentuate these and other meaningful content.
- **Fourth,** list the questions you may want to ask in class. You are now minimally prepared for class. Finally, to be well prepared, read the chapter thoroughly to gain an in-depth understanding of the content.

TAKE CLASS NOTES

Taking notes in class is critical. Class notes are valuable because they provide you with a blueprint for study when preparing for an examination. The following are note-taking tips:

- **Stay focused on the topic being presented.** Generally, instructors present material that they believe is important. Compare this information to the material you highlighted in your textbook.
- **Use your notebook creatively.** Open your notebook so that you have facing sheets. Use the page on the left side for class notes. Save the page on the right side for adding information from the textbook or other sources that clarify the class notes.
- **Use an outline format and abbreviations.** There is no way that you can write down every word that comes out of your instructor's mouth. Focus on concepts because you can expand on the content later. For example, if an instructor is talking about abnormal respiratory rates such as apnea, bradypnea, and tachypnea, write these words down and listen to the instructor's presentation. The definitions can be added at a later time to the page on the right side of your notebook.
- **Ask questions to clarify information.** Your goal is not to be a stenographer. Your goal is to understand the information. Ask questions that you have prepared before class or that you may have as a result of the discussion in class. If you have a question, there are probably other students who have the same question. Have the courage to ask questions. Some of the roles of the instructor are to make the information more understandable and clarify misconceptions. Your tuition pays the instructor's salary, so get your money's worth!
- **Review your notes after class.** You should review your notes within 48 hours after class. Reviewing, reorganizing, and rewriting class notes are techniques of reinforcement. Repetition helps commit information to memory. Some instructors allow you to use a tape recorder in class. Reviewing class tapes is particularly helpful to students who are auditory learners, those who have difficulty grasping complex material the first time, and those for whom English is a second language.

IDENTIFY LEARNING DOMAINS

How we learn is never identical for two different people, nor is it identical for one person in different situations. Over the years you have developed a learning style with which you feel comfortable and that has proved successful. It is in your best interest, however, to be open to a variety of learning approaches.

Learning is the process by which you attain new information (cognitive domain), acquire new physical skills (psychomotor domain), or form new attitudes (affective domain).

Cognitive Domain

Cognitive learning is concerned with understanding that advances from the simple to the complex. It involves acquiring and developing thoughts, ideas, and concepts and progresses from knowing and comprehending information to applying and analyzing information.

New information usually is learned through symbols such as words or pictures. We read them, see them, or hear them. Use all your senses to acquire new information. The more routes information takes to travel to your brain, the greater are the chances that you will learn the information. For example, when reading information about positioning patients, learning is reinforced by viewing pictures of patients in the various positions.

Psychomotor Domain

Psychomotor learning is concerned with the development of motor skills. It involves perceptual abilities as well as physical abilities related to endurance, strength, flexibility, and agility. Integrated body movements progress from reflexive movements, to basic fundamental movements, to skilled movements.

New skills involve the physical application of information. It is possible for a person to understand all the goals and steps of a procedure and yet not be able to perform the procedure. For information to get from the head to the hands, the learner must do more than read a book, look at pictures, view a video, or watch other people. The learner must become actively involved. Physical skills are not learned by osmosis or diffusion; they are learned by doing. For example, when learning how to change a sterile dressing, the learner can read a book and look at a video, but it is essential that the learner actually practice changing a sterile dressing.

Affective Domain

Affective learning is concerned with the development of attitudes, which includes interests, appreciations, feelings, and values; it progresses from an awareness to an increasing internalization or commitment to the attitude.

Learning new attitudes is the most difficult type of learning because attitudes result from lifelong experiences and tend to be well entrenched. For example, a student may know and understand the theory concerning why a person should be nonjudgmental and yet in clinical situations be judgmental toward the patient. The development of new attitudes is best learned in an atmosphere of acceptance by exploring feelings, becoming involved in group discussions, and observing appropriate role models. For example, before providing physical hygiene for a patient for the first time, it is beneficial to explore feelings about invading a patient's personal space.

CAPTURE MOMENTS OF TIME

Using your spare moments for reviewing information is a method of maximizing your time for constructive study. We all have periods during the day that are less productive than others, such as waiting at a red light or standing in line at a store. Also, there are times when you engage in repetitive tasks such as vacuuming a rug or raking the leaves. Capture these moments of time and use them to study. Carry flash cards, a vocabulary list, or categories of information that you can review when you have unexpected time. These captured moments should be in addition to, rather than a replacement for, your regularly scheduled study periods. There is an old saying that states, "Time is on your side." Capture spare moments of time and use them to your advantage. For additional information about time management, review Chapter 3, Time Management.

USE APPROPRIATE RESOURCES

The theories and principles of nursing practice are complex. They draw from a variety of disciplines (psychology, sociology, anatomy and physiology, microbiology, and so on), use new terminology, and require unique applications to clinical practice. When you study, you will find that your learning will not proceed in a straight line, moving progressively forward. You may experience plateaus, remissions, and/or periods of confusion when dealing with complex material. When your forward progress is slowed, identify your needs and immediately seek help. Your instructor, another student, a study group, or a tutor may be beneficial. When studying with another student, make sure that the person is a source of correct information. When studying in groups, three to five students are ideal because a group of more than five people becomes a "party." The group should be heterogeneous; that is, there should be a variety of academic abilities, attitudes, skills, and perspectives among the members. This variety should enrich the learning experience and provide checks and balances for the sharing of correct information. Remember, you learn not only from the instructor but also from yourself and your classmates.

Generally, people do not like to admit that they have learning difficulties because they think it makes them look inadequate in the eyes of others. For this reason, people may be embarrassed to ask for help. This can be self-destructive because it denies people the opportunity to use resources that support growth. Be careful that you do not fall into this trap! To obtain access to the appropriate resources, you must be willing to be open to yourself and others. Resources (e.g., extra help sessions; computer labs; reading, writing, and math centers; psychologic counseling; and availability of faculty during office hours) are there to be used. Have the courage to acknowledge to yourself and others that you need help. Seeking help is a sign of maturity rather than a sign of weakness. When you ask for help, you are in control because you are solving problems to meet your own needs.

BALANCE SACRIFICES AND REWARDS

When you decided to enter nursing school, no one promised you a rose garden. Your commitment to become a nurse requires sacrifice. Your time and energy are being diverted from your usual activities related to a job, family members, friends, and pleasurable pastimes. Rigorous activity, whether physical or mental, requires concentration and endurance. However, too much work hinders productivity. You must establish a balance between energy expenditure and rewards for your efforts. Rewards can be internal or external. Internal rewards are stimulated from within the learner and relate to feelings associated with meaningful achievement. Learning something new, achieving a goal, or increasing self-respect are examples of internal rewards. External rewards arise from outside the learner. A grade of 100 percent, respect and appreciation from others, or a present for achieving a goal are examples of external rewards.

Unfortunately, the rewards for studying usually are not immediate but in the extended future. Graduating from nursing school, passing the NCLEX, earning a paycheck, and enjoying the prestige of being a nurse are future-oriented rewards. Therefore, you should be the one to provide immediate rewards for yourself for studying. During study breaks or at the completion of studying, reward yourself by thinking about how much you have learned, reflecting on the good feelings you have about your accomplishments, relaxing with a significant other, having a cup of coffee, watching a favorite television show, calling a friend on the telephone, or taking a weekend off. Short-term rewards promote a positive mental attitude, reinforce motivation, and provide a respite from studying.

Specific Study Techniques Related to Cognitive Levels of Nursing Questions

The nurse uses a variety of thinking processes when caring for patients. Therefore, nursing examinations must reflect these thinking processes to effectively evaluate the safe practice of nursing. There are four types of thinking processes that may be required to answer questions concerning the delivery of nursing care: **knowledge, comprehension, application,** and **analysis (including synthesis and evaluation).** These thinking processes are within the cognitive domain and are ordered according to complexity. That is, a knowledge question requires the lowest level of thinking (recalling information), whereas an analysis question requires the highest level of thinking (comparing and contrasting information).

In this section of the book each cognitive level is discussed and sample multiple-choice items are presented to illustrate the thinking processes involved in answering the item. In addition, specific study techniques are presented to help you to strengthen your critical-thinking abilities.

The correct answers for the sample items in this chapter and the rationales for all the options are at the end of this chapter.

KNOWLEDGE QUESTIONS

Knowledge questions require you to **recall or remember information.** To answer a knowledge question, you need to commit facts to memory. Knowledge questions expect you to know terminology, specific facts, trends, sequences, classifications, categories, criteria, structures, principles, generalizations, and theories. This basic information is necessary before you can think critically.

SAMPLE ITEM 4–1

Hospice care lies in which level of prevention?
   (1) Secondary prevention
   (2) Morbidity prevention
   (3) Tertiary prevention
   (4) Primary prevention

To answer this question you need to know the definitions of the various types of prevention as well as what service hospice provides.

SAMPLE ITEM 4–2

The nurse is aware that the first step of the procedure for making an unoccupied bed is:
   (1) Pulling the curtain
   (2) Washing your hands
   (3) Collecting the clean linen
   (4) Placing the bottom sheet

To correctly answer this question, you need to know the sequence of steps in the procedure of making an unoccupied bed or the basic principle that your hands must be washed before all procedures.

SAMPLE ITEM 4–3

What is the expected range of a radial pulse in an adult?
   (1) 50 to 65
   (2) 70 to 85
   (3) 90 to 105
   (4) 110 to 125

To answer this question correctly, you have to know the expected range of a radial pulse for an adult.

Study Techniques to Increase Your Knowledge

Repetition/Memorization

Through repetition, information is committed to the brain for recall at a later date. Repeatedly studying information by reciting it out loud, reviewing it in your mind, or writing it down increases your chances of remembering the information because a variety of senses are used. Memorization can be facilitated by using lists of related facts, flash cards, or learning wheels. For example:

- On an index card you can list the steps of a procedure. This can be carried with you to study when you capture moments of time.
- On the front of an index card you can write a word and on the back define the word. An entire deck of cards can be developed for the terminology within a unit of study. Again, use the flash cards when you have unexpected time to study.
- To make a learning wheel, cut a piece of cardboard into a circle and draw pie-shaped wedges on the front and back. On a front wedge write a unit of measure, such as 30 mL, and on the corresponding back wedge write its conversion to another unit of measure, such as 1 ounce. Then, on individual spring clothespins, write each of the units of measure that appear on the back of the wheel. When you want to study approximate equivalents, mix up the clothespins and attempt to match each one to its

corresponding unit of measure. You can turn the wheel over and evaluate your success by determining if the clothespin you attached to the wheel matches the unit of measure on the back of the wheel.

Alphabet Cues

The memorization of information can be facilitated if the information is associated with letters of the alphabet. Each letter serves as a cue that stimulates the recall of information. The most effective alphabet cues are those you make up yourself. They meet a self-identified need, and you must review the information before you can design the alphabet cue. You can use any combination of letters as long as they have meaning for you and your learning. Examples of alphabet cues include:

- The **ABCs** of cardiopulmonary resuscitation are: **A**irway—clear the airway; **B**reathing—initiate artificial breathing; **C**irculation—initiate cardiac compression.
- Identify patients at risk for injury through the letters **A, B, C, D, E, F, G**:
  Age—the young and very old; **B**lindness—lack of visual perception; **C**onsciousness—decreased level of consciousness; **D**eafness—lack of auditory perception; **E**motional state—reduced perceptual awareness; **F**requency of accidents—previous history of accidents; and **G**ait—impaired mobility.
- The **Three Ps** for the cardinal signs of diabetes mellitus are: **P**olyuria, **P**olydipsia, and **P**olyphagia.

Acronyms

An acronym is a word formed from the first letters of a series of statements or facts. Each part of the acronym relates to the information it represents. It is useful to learning because each letter of the word jolts the memory to recall information. An acronym is a technique used to retrieve previously learned information. Examples of acronyms include the following:

- The American Cancer Society teaches the early warning signs of cancer through the acronym of **CAUTION.**

  Change in bowel and bladder habits

  A sore that does not heal

  Unusual bleeding or discharge

  Thickening or a lump

  Indigestion or difficulty in swallowing

  Obvious change in a wart or mole

  Nagging cough or hoarseness

- When assessing a patient for adaptations indicating the presence of infection, remember the acronym **INFECT.**

  Increased pulse, respirations, and white blood cell count

  Nodes enlarged

  Function impaired

  Erythema, Edema, Exudate

  Complaints of discomfort or pain

  Temperature—local and/or systemic

Acrostics

An acrostic is a phrase, motto, or verse in which a letter of each word (usually the first letter) prompts the memory to retrieve information. Memorizing information can be difficult and boring. This technique is a creative way to make learning more effective and fun. Examples of acrostics include:

- When studying the fat-soluble vitamins, recall this motto, "**A**ll **D**ieters **E**at **K**ilocalories." This should help you remember that **A, D, E,** and **K** are the fat-soluble vitamins.

- On Old Olympus's Towering Tops, A Finn and a Swedish Girl Viewed Some Hops, which stands for Olfactory, Optic, Oculomotor, Trochlear, Trigeminal, Abducens, Facial, Sensorimotor (vestibulo-cochlear), Glossopharyngeal, Vagus, Spinal accessory, and Hypoglossal nerves.

Mnemonics

A mnemonic, a variation of an acrostic, is a phrase, motto, or verse that jogs the memory. It differs from an acrostic in that not every word is related to a specific piece of content. Mnemonics promote retention by connecting new or difficult information to known or less difficult information using mental associations or visual pictures.

- When studying apothecary and metric equivalents, remember this verse, "There are **15 grains** of sugar in **1 graham (gram)** cracker." This sentence should help you remember that **15 grains** are equivalent to **1 gram.**
- When trying to remember the difference between Low Density Lipoproteins (LDL) and High Density Lipoproteins (HDL) refer to the following mnemonic, **LDH** is **l**ousy cholesterol and **HDL** is **h**appy cholesterol. This sentence should help you remember that elevated LDH levels are associated with athrosclerosis and is undesirable (lousy cholesterol) and HDL promotes excretion of cholesterol from the body (happy cholesterol).

These techniques help increase the retention of information. The information is learned by rote without any in-depth understanding of the information learned. Information learned by repetition uses short-term memory and generally is quickly forgotten unless reinforced through additional study techniques or application in your nursing practice.

COMPREHENSION QUESTIONS

Comprehension questions require you to **understand information.** To answer a comprehension question, you must commit facts to memory as well as translate, interpret, and determine the implications of that information. You demonstrate understanding when you translate or paraphrase information, interpret or summarize information, or determine the implications, consequences, corollaries, or effects of information. Comprehension questions expect you not only to know but also to understand the information being tested. After you understand basic information, you can recognize the significance of data, an initial step in critical thinking.

SAMPLE ITEM 4–4

The nurse administers a cathartic to a patient. To evaluate the therapeutic effect of the cathartic, the nurse should assess the patient for:

(1) Increased urinary output

(2) A decrease in anxiety

(3) A bowel movement

(4) Pain relief

To answer this question, you have to know not only that a cathartic is a potent laxative that stimulates the bowel (knowledge) but also that the increase in peristalsis will result in a bowel movement (comprehension).

SAMPLE ITEM 4–5

When clarifying is used as a therapeutic communication tool, the nurse is:

(1) Summarizing the patient's communication

(2) Verifying what is implied by the patient

(3) Restating what the patient has said

(4) Paraphrasing the patient's message

To answer this question, you not only have to know that clarifying is a therapeutic tool that promotes communication between the patient and nurse (knowledge), but you also must explain why or how this technique facilitates communication (comprehension).

SAMPLE ITEM 4–6

After administering an intramuscular injection, the nurse should massage the needle insertion site to:

(1) Limit infection

(2) Prevent bleeding

(3) Reduce discomfort

(4) Promote absorption

To answer this question, you not only have to know that massage is one step of the procedure for an intramuscular injection (knowledge), but you also must understand the consequence of massaging the needle insertion site after the needle is withdrawn (comprehension).

Study Techniques to Increase Your Comprehension of Information

Explore "Whys" and "Hows"

The difference between knowledge questions and comprehension questions is that you must know facts to answer knowledge questions, but you must understand the significance of the facts to answer comprehension questions. Facts can be understood and retained longer if they are relevant and meaningful to the learner. When studying information, ask yourself **why** or **how** the information is important. For example, when learning that immobility causes pressure ulcers, explore why they occur. Pressure compresses the capillary beds, which interferes with the transport of oxygen and nutrients to tissues, resulting in ischemia and necrosis. When studying a skill such as bathing, explore *how* soap cleans the skin. Soap reduces the surface tension of water and helps remove accumulated oils, perspiration, dead cells, and microorganisms. If you interpret information and identify why or how the information gained is relevant and useful, then the information has value. When information increases in value, it also increases in significance and is less readily forgotten.

Study in Small Groups

After you have studied by yourself, usually it is valuable to study the same information with another person or in a small group. The sharing process promotes your comprehension of information because you listen to the impressions and opinions of others, learn new information from a peer tutor, and reinforce your own learning by teaching others. In addition, the members of the group reinforce your interpretation of information and correct your misunderstanding of information. The value of group work is in the exchange process. Group members must listen, share, evaluate, help, support, reinforce, discuss, and debate to promote learning. There is truth in the saying "One hand washes the other." Not only do you help the other person when you study together, but you also help yourself.

APPLICATION QUESTIONS

The application of information demonstrates a higher level of understanding than just knowing or comprehending information because it requires the learner to **show, solve, modify, change, use, or manipulate information** in a real situation or presented scenario. To answer an application question, you must apply concepts you learned previously to concrete situations. The concepts may be theories, technical principles, rules of procedures, generalizations, or ideas that have to be applied in a presented scenario. Application questions test your ability to use information in a new situation. The making of rational and reflective judgments, which are part of the critical-thinking process, results in a course of action.

SAMPLE ITEM 4–7

An older adult's skin looks dry, thin, and fragile. When providing back care, the nurse should:

(1) Apply a moisturizing body lotion

(2) Wash the back with soap and water

(3) Massage using short, kneading strokes

(4) Leave excess lubricant on the patient's skin

To answer this question, you must know that dry, thin, fragile skin is common in older adults (knowledge) and that moisturizing lotion helps the skin to retain water and become more supple (comprehension). When presented with this patient scenario, you have to apply your knowledge concerning developmental changes in older adults and the consequences of the use of moisturizing lotion (application).

SAMPLE ITEM 4–8

When caring for several patients on bladder-retraining programs, the nurse should understand that an intervention that is always implemented during a bladder-retraining program is toileting:

(1) Every 2 hours when awake

(2) At 8 AM, 2 PM, 8 PM, and 2 AM

(3) Every 4 hours and through the night

(4) When the patient goes to bed at night

To answer this question, you have to know the principle that nursing care should be individualized (knowledge). You also must understand the commonalities within the procedure of bladder retraining (comprehension). When presented with this concrete situation, you have to apply your knowledge about patient-centered care and the theoretic components of bladder-retraining programs (application).

SAMPLE ITEM 4–9

When lifting a heavy patient higher in bed, the nurse can prevent self-injury by:

(1) Keeping the knees and ankles straight

(2) Straightening the knees while bending at the waist

(3) Placing the feet together and keeping the knees bent

(4) Positioning the feet apart with one foot placed forward

To answer this question, you have to know and understand the principles of body mechanics (knowledge and comprehension). You also need to apply these principles in a particular patient-care situation, moving a heavy patient higher in bed (application).

Study Techniques to Increase Your Ability to Apply Information

Relate New Information to Prior Learning

Learning is easier when the information to be learned is associated with what you already know. Therefore, relate new information to your foundation of knowledge, experience, attitudes, and feelings. For example, when studying the principles of body mechanics, review which principles are used when you carry a heavy package, move from a reclining to a standing position, or assist an older person to walk up a flight of stairs.

When studying the principles of surgical asepsis, recall and review the various situations when you performed sterile technique and identify the principles that were the foundation of your actions. Applying concepts, such as principles and theories, in concrete situations reinforces your ability to use them in future circumstances.

Recognize Commonalities

To facilitate learning to apply information, identify commonalities when studying principles and theories that can be used in a variety of situations. A commonality exists when two different situations require the application of the same or similar principle. For example, when studying the principle of gravity, you must understand that it is the force that draws all mass in the earth's sphere toward the center of the earth. Now try to identify situations that employ this principle. As a nurse, you apply this principle when you place a urine collection bag below the level of the bladder, hang an intravenous bag higher than the IV insertion site, raise the head of the bed for a patient with dyspnea, and raise the foot of the bed for a patient with edema of the feet. This study technique is particularly effective when working in small groups because it involves brainstorming. Others in the group may identify situations that you have not considered. Recognizing commonalities reinforces information and maximizes the application of information in patient-care situations.

ANALYSIS QUESTIONS

Analysis questions require you to **interpret a variety of data** and **recognize the commonalities, differences, and interrelationships among presented ideas.** To answer an analysis question, you must identify, examine, dissect, evaluate, or investigate the organization, systematic arrangement, or structure of the information presented in the question. Analysis questions make the assumption that you know, understand, and can apply information. It then requires an ability to examine information, which is a higher thought process than knowing, understanding, or applying information. For example, when studying blood pressure, you first memorize the parameters of a normal blood pressure (knowledge). Then you develop an understanding of what factors influence and produce a normal blood pressure (comprehension). Then you identify a particular patient situation that would necessitate obtaining a blood pressure (application). Finally, you must differentiate among a variety of situations and determine which has the highest priority for assessing the blood pressure (analysis). Analysis questions are difficult because they demand scrutiny of a variety of complex data presented in the stem and options and require a higher-level critical-thinking process.

SAMPLE ITEM 4–10

A patient has dependent edema of the ankles and feet and is obese. Which diet should the nurse expect the physician to order?

    (1) Low in sodium and high in fat

    (2) Low in sodium and low in calories

    (3) High in sodium and high in protein

    (4) High in sodium and low in carbohydrates

To answer this question, you have to know and understand the relationships between salt in the diet and fluid retention, and between obesity and caloric intake (knowledge and comprehension). You must also understand the impact of carbohydrates, proteins, and fats in a diet for a patient with edema and obesity (comprehension). When you answer this question, you must examine the information presented, identify the interrelationships among the elements, and arrive at a conclusion (analysis).

SAMPLE ITEM 4–11

A patient who is undergoing cancer chemotherapy says to the nurse, "This is no way to live." Which response uses reflective technique?

    (1) "Tell me more about what you are thinking."

(2) "You sound discouraged today."

(3) "Life is not worth living?"

(4) "What are you saying?"

To answer this question, you must know and understand the communication techniques of reflection, clarification, and paraphrasing (knowledge and comprehension). Also, you must analyze each statement and identify the communication technique being used. This question requires you to differentiate information presented in the four options to arrive at the correct answer.

SAMPLE ITEM 4–12

The physician orders 500 mg of an antibiotic to be administered via an intramuscular injection. The label on a 1-gram vial of the medication, which needs to be reconstituted, states: Add 2.7 mL of solution to yield 3 mL. How much solution should the nurse administer?

(1) 0.5 mL

(2) 1 mL

(3) 1.5 mL

(4) 2 mL

To answer this question, you must know and understand how to use a formula for ratio and proportion (knowledge and comprehension). This question requires you to identify the various components of the problem, select the appropriate formula required to solve the problem, place the correct elements within the formula, and then do the mathematical calculation to arrive at the answer (analysis).

Study Techniques to Increase Your Ability to Analyze Information

Recognize Differences

To study for complex questions, you cannot just memorize and understand facts or recognize the commonalities among facts; you must learn to discriminate. Analysis questions often require you to use differentiation to determine the significance of information. When studying the causes of an elevated blood pressure, identify the different causes and why they may result in an increased blood pressure. For example, a blood pressure can rise for a variety of reasons: infection causes an increased metabolic rate; fluid retention causes hypervolemia; anxiety causes an autonomic nervous system response that constricts blood vessels. In each situation, the blood pressure increases but for a different reason. Recognizing differences is an effective study technique to broaden the interrelationship and significance of learned information.

Practice Test Taking

Taking practice tests is an excellent way to improve the effectiveness of your learning. Reviewing rationales for the right and wrong answers serves as an effective study technique. It reinforces learning, and it can help you identify areas that require additional study.

As you practice test taking, not only do you increase your knowledge but you also become more emotionally and physically comfortable in the testing situation and better at selecting the correct option when answering a question. It is most effective if you gradually increase the time you spend taking practice tests to 2 to 3 hours. This will help build stamina, enabling you to concentrate more effectively during a shorter test. Marathon runners have long recognized the value of building stamina and the need for practice to achieve a "groove" that enhances performance. Marathon runners also manage their practice so that they "peak" on the day of the big event. The same principles can be applied to the nursing student preparing for an important test. You are at your peak and can achieve a groove when you feel physically, emotionally, and intellectually ready for the important test.

Practicing test taking should assist you to learn by:

- Acquiring new knowledge
- Comprehending information
- Understanding concepts
- Identifying rationales for nursing interventions
- Applying theories and principles
- Identifying commonalities and differences in situations
- Analyzing information
- Reinforcing previous learning
- Applying critical thinking

In addition, practicing test taking should assist you to:

- Use test-taking techniques
- Effectively manage time during a test
- Control your environment
- Control physical and emotional responses
- Feel empowered and in control
- Develop a positive mental attitude

Answers and Rationales For Sample Items in Chapter 4

4-1   ① Secondary prevention refers to strategies for people in whom disease is present. The goal is to halt or reverse the disease process.

        ② There is no category called morbidity prevention. The word "morbidity" refers to illness; "mortality" refers to death.

        ③ **Tertiary prevention uses strategies to assist people to adapt physically, psychologically, and socially to permanent disabilities.**

        ④ Primary prevention refers to strategies used to prevent illness in people who are considered free from disease.

4-2   ① Pulling the curtain is unnecessary when making an unoccupied bed; this is required to provide for privacy when making an occupied bed.

        ② **Washing the hands removes microorganisms that can contaminate clean linen.**

        ③ Collecting the clean linen is done after your hands are washed to prevent contamination of the linen.

        ④ Placing the bottom sheet is done after your hands are washed and you have collected the sheets.

4-3   ① 50 to 65 beats is below the expected range for the pulse in an adult.

        ② **70 to 85 is within the expected range of 60 to 100 beats for the pulse of an adult.**

        ③ Although 90 beats is within the high end of the expected range for the pulse of an adult, 105 beats is above the expected range.

        ④ 110 to 125 beats is above the expected range for the pulse of an adult.

4-4   ① Diuretics, not cathartics, produce an increase in urinary output.

        ② Antianxiety agents (anxiolytics) reduce anxiety.

        ③ **Cathartics stimulate bowel evacuation; therefore, the patient should be assessed for a bowel movement.**

        ④ Analgesics, not cathartics, alter the perception and interpretation of pain.

4-5   ① Summarizing involves reviewing the main points in a discussion; this is useful at the end of an interview or teaching session.

        ② **Verifying (clarifying) is a method of making the patient's message more understandable; it is an attempt to obtain more information without interpreting the original statement.**

        ③ Restating, also called "paraphrasing," is a technique that repeats the patient's basic message in similar words to promote further communication.

        ④ Same as #3.

4-6   ① Using sterile equipment and sterile technique limits infection, not massaging the needle insertion site.

        ② Removing the needle along the line of insertion limits trauma, which prevents bleeding.

        ③ Removing the needle along the line of insertion limits trauma, which reduces discomfort.

        ④ **Massage disperses the medication in the tissues and facilitates its absorption.**

4-7   ① **Moisturizing lotion limits dryness and reduces the friction of the hands against the skin, which prevents skin trauma.**

        ② Soap should be avoided because it can further dry the skin.

        ③ Massaging with short, kneading strokes can cause injury to delicate, thin skin; light, long strokes should be used.

        ④ Excess lubricant on the skin can promote skin maceration, and also it provides a warm, moist environment for the growth of microorganisms, which should be avoided.

4-8   ① This may not be appropriate for all patients.

        ② Same as #1.

        ③ Same as #1.

        ④ **All patients, regardless of the specifics of each individual bladder-retraining program, will be toileted before going to bed at night and after awakening in the morning.**

4-9 ① This places strain on the muscles of the back and should be avoided.
② Same as #1.
③ Keeping the feet together produces a narrow base of support that can result in a fall.
④ **Both actions provide a wide base of support that promotes stability; placing one foot in front of the other facilitates bending at the knees, which permits the muscles of the legs, rather than the back, to bear the patient's weight.**

4-10 ① Although a low-sodium diet is appropriate to limit edema, a diet high in fat should be avoided by an obese individual because fats are high in calories.
② **Sodium promotes fluid retention and increased calories add to body weight; therefore, both should be avoided by an obese patient with edema.**
③ Sodium promotes fluid retention and should be avoided by a patient with edema; protein may or may not be related to this patient's problem.
④ Although carbohydrates may be restricted in an obese individual to facilitate weight loss, a high-sodium diet would promote fluid retention and should be avoided.

4-11 ① This response is using the technique of clarification and asks the patient to expand on the message so that it becomes more understandable.
② **This response is using reflective technique because it attempts to identify feelings in the patient's message.**
③ This response is using the technique of paraphrasing; this response restates the patient's basic message in similar words.
④ Same as #1.

4-12 ① This is less than the ordered dosage of medication.
② Same as #1.
③ **Use ratio and proportion to solve for x by cross-multiplying; 500 mg is equal to 0.5 grams.**

$$\frac{0.5 \text{ g (desired dosage)}}{1.0 \text{ g (supplied dosage)}} = \frac{x \text{ mL}}{3 \text{ mL}}$$

$$1.0\,x = 3 \times 0.5$$
$$x = 1.5 \text{ mL}$$

④ This is more than the ordered dosage of medication.

5

The Multiple-Choice Question

In our society, success is generally measured in relation to levels of achievement. Before you entered a formal institution of learning, your achievement was subjectively appraised by your family and friends. Success was rewarded by smiles, positive statements, and perhaps favors or gifts. Lack of achievement or failure was acknowledged by omission of recognition, verbal corrections, and possibly punishment or scorn. When you entered school, your performance was directly measured against acceptable standards. In an effort to eliminate subjectivity, you were exposed to objective testing. These tests included true/false questions, matching columns, and multiple-choice questions. Achievement was reflected by numerical grades or letter grades. These grades indicated your level of achievement and by themselves provided rewards and punishments.

In nursing education, achievement can be assessed in a variety of ways: a patient's physiologic response (did the patient's condition improve?), a patient's verbal response (did the patient verbalize improvement?), student nurses' clinical performance (did the students do what they were supposed to do?), and student nurses' levels of cognitive competency (did the students know what they were supposed to know?). You must pass the National Council Licensing Examination known as NCLEX-PN to work legally as a Licensed Practical Nurse or NCLEX-RN to work legally as a Registered Nurse. These examinations consist mainly of multiple-choice questions. Consequently, multiple-choice questions frequently are used in schools of nursing to evaluate student progress throughout the nursing curriculum. They also are used because they are objective, time efficient, and can assess comprehensively the understanding of curriculum content that has depth and breadth. Therefore, it is important for you to understand the components and dynamics of multiple-choice questions early in your nursing education.

In the spring of 2003, alternate format items were introduced in nursing licensure examinations. **Alternate format items** require the test taker to select multiple answers to a multiple-choice question, perform a calculation and fill in the blank, place options in priority order, or respond to a question in relation to one or more charts, graphs, or pictures. For information about and examples of alternate format items, review Chapter 8, Testing Formats Other Than Multiple-Choice Questions.

Components of a Multiple-Choice Question

A multiple-choice question is an objective test item. It is objective because the perceptions or opinions of another person do not influence the grade. In a multiple-choice question, a question is asked, three or more potential answers are presented, and only one of the potential answers is correct. The student answers the question either correctly or incorrectly.

The entire multiple-choice question is called an **item.** Each item consists of two parts. The first part is known as the **stem.** The stem is the statement that asks the question. The second part contains the possible responses offered by the item, which are called **options.** One of the options answers the question posed in the stem and is the **correct answer.** The remaining options are the incorrect answers and are called **distractors.** They are referred to as "distractors" because they are designed to distract you from the correct answer.

The correct answers and the rationales for all the options of the sample items in this chapter are at the end of the chapter. Test yourself and see if you can correctly answer the sample items.

SAMPLE ITEM 5–1

What should the nurse do immediately before performing any procedure?	STEM
(1) Shut the door DISTRACTOR	
(2) Wash the hands CORRECT ANSWER	OPTION
(3) Close the curtain DISTRACTOR	
(4) Drape the patient DISTRACTOR	

(ITEM)

SAMPLE ITEM 5–2

When providing care to a patient with a nasogastric tube, the nurse understands that the tube goes into the:	STEM
(1) Stomach CORRECT ANSWER	
(2) Bronchi DISTRACTOR	OPTION
(3) Trachea DISTRACTOR	
(4) Duodenum DISTRACTOR	

(ITEM)

SAMPLE ITEM 5–3

A man describes his son as being difficult to get along with and concerned about what his friends think about him. How old is the son?	STEM
(1) 3 years old DISTRACTOR	
(2) 7 years old DISTRACTOR	OPTION
(3) 14 years old CORRECT ANSWER	
(4) 22 years old DISTRACTOR	

(ITEM)

The Stem

The stem is the initial part of a multiple-choice item. The purpose of the stem is to present a problem in a clear and concise manner. The stem should contain all the details necessary to answer the question.

The stem of an item can be a complete sentence that asks a question. It also can be presented as an incomplete sentence that becomes a complete sentence when it is combined with one of the options of the item.

In addition to sentence structure, a characteristic of a stem that must be considered is its polarity. The polarity of the stem can be formulated in either a positive or negative context. A stem with a positive polarity asks the question in relation to what is true, whereas a stem with negative polarity asks the question in relation to what is false.

THE MULTIPLE-CHOICE QUESTION

THE STEM THAT IS A COMPLETE SENTENCE

A complete sentence is a group of words that is capable of standing independently. When a stem is a complete sentence, it will pose a question and end with a question mark (?). It should clearly and concisely formulate a problem that can be answered before reading the options.

SAMPLE ITEM 5–4

What should be the first action of the nurse when a fire alarm rings in a health-care facility?
(1) Close doors on the unit.
(2) Take an extinguisher to the fire scene.
(3) Move patients laterally toward the stairs.
(4) Determine if it is a fire drill or a real fire.

SAMPLE ITEM 5–5

What is the most common reason why older adults become incontinent of urine?
(1) The muscles that control urination become weak.
(2) They tend to drink less fluid than younger patients.
(3) Their increase in weight places pressure on the bladder.
(4) They use incontinence to manipulate and control others.

SAMPLE ITEM 5–6

What part of the body requires special hygiene when a patient has a nasogastric feeding tube?
(1) Rectum
(2) Abdomen
(3) Oral cavity
(4) Perineal area

THE STEM THAT IS AN INCOMPLETE SENTENCE

When a stem is an incomplete sentence, it is a group of words that forms the beginning portion of a sentence. The sentence becomes complete when it is combined with one of the options in the item. Some tests will have a period at the completion of each option and others will not. Whether there is a period or not, each option should complete the sentence with grammatical accuracy. However, the answer is the only option that correctly completes the sentence in relation to the informational content. When reading a stem that is an incomplete sentence, usually it is necessary to read the options before the question can be answered.

SAMPLE ITEM 5–7

To best understand what a patient is saying, the nurse should:
(1) Demonstrate interest
(2) Listen carefully
(3) Remain silent
(4) Employ touch

SAMPLE ITEM 5–8

The most important reason why nurses should teach people not to smoke in bed is because it can:

    (1) Result in a fire

    (2) Upset a family member

    (3) Trigger a smoke alarm

    (4) Precipitate lung cancer

SAMPLE ITEM 5–9

When assisting a female patient with dementia to groom her hair, the nurse should:

    (1) Offer constant support and encouragement

    (2) Set time aside for a long teaching session

    (3) Alternate using a brush and a comb

    (4) Teach her how to braid her hair

THE STEM WITH POSITIVE POLARITY

The stem with positive polarity is concerned with truth. It asks the question with a positive statement. The correct answer is accurately related to the statement. It is in accord with a fact or principle, or it is an action that should be implemented. A positively worded stem attempts to determine if you are able to understand, apply, or differentiate correct information.

SAMPLE ITEM 5–10

An older adult who is dying starts to cry and says, "I was always concerned about myself first, and I hurt many people during my life." What is the underlying feeling being expressed by the patient?

    (1) Ambivalence

    (2) Sadness

    (3) Anger

    (4) Guilt

SAMPLE ITEM 5–11

Which intervention most accurately supports the concept of informed consent?

    (1) Obtaining the patient's signature

    (2) Explaining what is being done and why

    (3) Involving the family in the teaching plan

    (4) Teaching preoperative deep breathing and coughing

SAMPLE ITEM 5–12

What should the nurse do when a patient appears to be asleep but does not react when called by name?

    (1) Loudly say, "Are you awake?"

    (2) Say to the patient, "Can you squeeze my hand?"

(3) Inform the nurse manager in charge immediately.

(4) Gently touch the patient's arm and say the patient's name.

THE STEM WITH NEGATIVE POLARITY

The stem with negative polarity is concerned with what is false. It asks the question with a negative statement. The stem usually incorporates words such as "except," "not," or "never." These words are obvious. However, sometimes the words that are used are more obscure, for example, "contraindicated," "further," "unacceptable," "least," and "avoid." When a negative term is used, it may be emphasized by an underline (<u>except</u>), italics (*least*), dark type (**not**), or capitals (NEVER). A negatively worded stem requires you to recognize exceptions, detect errors, or identify interventions that are unacceptable or contraindicated. NCLEX-RN does not emphasize the negative word when used in a stem, and many nursing examinations do not have questions with negative polarity. However, this information has been included in the event that you may be challenged by questions with negative polarity.

SAMPLE ITEM 5-13

On what part of the body should the nurse avoid using soap when bathing a patient?

(1) Eyes

(2) Back

(3) Under the breasts

(4) Glans of the penis

SAMPLE ITEM 5-14

The nurse determines that range-of-motion (ROM) exercises should NOT be done:

(1) For comatose patients

(2) On limbs that are paralyzed

(3) Beyond the point of resistance

(4) For patients with chronic joint disease

SAMPLE ITEM 5-15

Which suggestion by the nurse is the least therapeutic when teaching the patient about promoting personal energy?

(1) Eat breakfast every day.

(2) Exercise three times a week.

(3) Get adequate sleep each night.

(4) Drink a cup of coffee each morning.

SAMPLE ITEM 5-16

Which position is contraindicated for the patient who has dyspnea?

(1) Supine

(2) Contour

(3) Fowler's

(4) Orthopneic

SAMPLE ITEM 5-17

Which action by the nurse is unacceptable during a bed bath?
1. Uncovering the area being washed
2. Using long, firm strokes toward the heart
3. Washing from the rectum toward the pubis
4. Replacing the top sheets with a cotton blanket

The Options

All of the possible answers offered within an item are called "options." One of the options is the best response and is therefore the correct answer. The other options are incorrect and distract you from selecting the correct answer. These options are called "distractors." An item must have a minimum of three options to be considered a multiple-choice item, but the actual number varies among tests. The typical number of options is four or five responses, which reduces the probability of guessing the correct answer while limiting the amount of reading to a sensible level. Options are usually listed by number (1, 2, 3, and 4), lowercase letters (a, b, c, and d), or upper-case letters (A, B, C, and D). The grammatical presentation of options can appear in four different formats. An option can be: a sentence, complete the sentence begun in the stem, an incomplete sentence, or a single word.

THE OPTION THAT IS A SENTENCE

A sentence is a unit of language that contains a stated or implied subject and verb. It is a statement that contains an entire thought and stands alone. Options can appear as complete sentences. Some tests have a period at the end of these options and others do not. Whether there is a period or not, each option should be grammatically correct. When the option is a verbal response, it should be grammatically correct and incorporate the appropriate punctuation, such as quotation marks (" "), comma (,) exclamation point (!), question mark (?), or period (.).

SAMPLE ITEM 5-18

Before performing a procedure, what should the nurse do first?
1. Raise the patient's bed to its highest position.
2. Collect the equipment for the procedure.
3. Position the patient for the procedure.
4. Explain the procedure to the patient.

SAMPLE ITEM 5-19

A Catholic patient tells the nurse, "Before being hospitalized I went to Mass and received Communion every morning." What should the nurse do to meet this patient's spiritual needs?
1. Encourage the patient to say the rosary every day.
2. Make arrangements for the patient to receive Communion.
3. Transfer the patient to a room with another Catholic patient.
4. Have a priest administer the Sacrament of Annointing of the Sick to the patient.

SAMPLE ITEM 5-20

A male patient is crying, and the only word the nurse understands is "wife." What should the nurse say?
1. "I'm sure that your wife is fine."

(2) "You are concerned about your wife?"

(3) "What did your wife do to upset you?"

(4) "Your wife will be visiting later today."

THE OPTION THAT COMPLETES THE SENTENCE BEGUN IN THE STEM

When the option completes the sentence begun in the stem, the stem and the option together should form a sentence. Some tests have correct punctuation at the end of these options and others do not. Whether or not there is a period, each option should complete the stem in a manner that is grammatically accurate.

SAMPLE ITEM 5-21

The nurse understands that the primary etiology of obesity is a:

(1) Lack of balance in the variety of nutrients

(2) Glandular disorder that prevents weight loss

(3) Caloric intake that exceeds metabolic needs

(4) Psychologic problem that causes overeating

SAMPLE ITEM 5-22

The nurse can best prevent the patient from getting a chill during a bed bath by:

(1) Rubbing briskly to cause vasodilation

(2) Exposing only the area being washed

(3) Giving a hot drink before the bath

(4) Pulling the curtain around the bed

SAMPLE ITEM 5-23

The nurse is to assist a patient with a bed bath; however, the patient has just returned from x-ray, is in pain, and refuses the bath. The nurse should:

(1) Cancel the bath today.

(2) Delay the bath until later.

(3) Give a partial bath quickly.

(4) Encourage a shower instead.

THE OPTION THAT IS AN INCOMPLETE SENTENCE

When an option is an incomplete sentence, it does not contain all the parts of speech (e.g., subject and verb) necessary to construct a complete, autonomous statement. The option that is an incomplete sentence usually is a phrase or group of related words. Although not a complete sentence, it conveys a unit of thought, an idea, or a concept.

SAMPLE ITEM 5-24

Which nursing intervention is common when caring for all patients with infections?

(1) Donning a mask

(2) Wearing a gown

(3) Washing the hands

(4) Discouraging visitors

SAMPLE ITEM 5–25

When should the nurse administer mouth care to an unconscious patient?

(1) Whenever necessary

(2) Every four hours

(3) Once a shift

(4) Twice a day

SAMPLE ITEM 5–26

Which action by the nurse helps meet a patient's basic need for security and safety?

(1) Addressing the patient by name

(2) Explaining what is going to be done

(3) Accepting a patient's angry behavior

(4) Ensuring the patient gets adequate nutrition

THE OPTION THAT IS A WORD

A word is a series of letters that form a term. It is the most basic unit of language and is capable of communicating a message. The option that is a single word can be almost any part of speech (e.g., noun, pronoun, verb, or adverb) as long as it conveys information.

SAMPLE ITEM 5–27

Which is a primary source for obtaining information related to the independent functions of a nurse?

(1) Chart

(2) Patient

(3) Physician

(4) Supervisor

SAMPLE ITEM 5–28

A patient's husband just died. What approach should be used by the nurse when caring for this grieving patient?

(1) Confronting

(2) Supporting

(3) Avoiding

(4) Limiting

SAMPLE ITEM 5–29

What is the nurse doing when formulating a nursing diagnosis?

(1) Planning

(2) Assessing

(3) Analyzing

(4) Implementing

SAMPLE ITEM 5–30

Which word best describes feelings associated with a child in Erikson's stage of autonomy versus shame and doubt?

(1) Hers

(2) Mine

(3) Theirs

(4) Nobody's

58   Answers and Rationales for Sample Items in Chapter 5

5-1   ① This should be done before washing the hands.
         ② **Before touching the patient, the nurse should wash his or her hands to remove microorganisms.**
         ③ Same as #1.
         ④ This is done after handwashing.

5-2   ① **The tube enters the nose, passes through the posterior nasopharynx and esophagus, and enters the stomach through the cardiac sphincter.**
         ② The bronchi are passages between the trachea and bronchioles and are part of the respiratory system.
         ③ The trachea is a passage between the posterior nasopharynx and bronchi and is part of the respiratory system.
         ④ The duodenum is distal to the stomach and is the first portion of the small intestine; a nasogastric tube is designed to be advanced into the stomach, not the duodenum.

5-3   ① Toddlers are concerned about themselves and their autonomy, not others.
         ② School-age children are easy to get along with and are concerned about performing and achieving.
         ③ **Adolescents are concerned about their identity, independence, and peer relationships; this causes tension between them and their parents.**
         ④ Young adults are developing intimate relationships and becoming socially responsible.

5-4   ① **This should be the initial action. A closed door provides for patient safety.**
         ② The location of the fire must be identified before an extinguisher can be taken to the scene.
         ③ Patients should be moved only if they are in danger.
         ④ Whenever the fire alarm rings, it should always be considered an indication of a real fire.

5-5   ① **Muscles, particularly the perineal muscles, tend to lose strength as people age.**
         ② Incontinence is unrelated to fluid intake.
         ③ Older adults do not necessarily gain weight; many lose weight because of the loss of subcutaneous fat associated with aging. Body weight does not influence incontinence.
         ④ This is untrue; most people want to be independent and in control of their bodily functions.

5-6   ① Special care of this area of the body is unnecessary; care provided during a routine bed bath is adequate.
         ② Same as #1.
         ③ **A nasogastric tube feeding generally negates the need to chew; with lack of chewing, salivation decreases, which causes the mucous membranes to become dry.**
         ④ Same as #1.

5-7   ① Although this may indicate acceptance and encourage ventilation of feelings, it does nothing to promote understanding.
         ② **Attentive listening is important so that the nurse can pick up key words and identify emotional themes within the message.**
         ③ Same as #1.
         ④ Touch is used to communicate a message, not to receive, understand, or interpret a message from another person.

5-8   ① **Confused, weak, or lethargic individuals may drop lighted cigarettes or ashes, which can ignite bed linens.**
         ② Although smoking can physically and emotionally disturb a family member, it is not the priority.
         ③ Smoke from a cigarette will not trigger a smoke alarm.
         ④ Although smoking may precipitate lung cancer, safety is the priority.

5-9   ① **People with dementia become confused easily and need support and encouragement to stay focused and motivated.**
         ② People with dementia cannot concentrate long enough for a prolonged teaching session; learning occurs best with short, frequent teaching sessions.

(3) Alternating a brush and a comb could promote confusion; patients with dementia need consistency.

(4) Braiding the hair involves cognitive and psychomotor skills that the patient with dementia probably does not possess.

5-10 (1) Ambivalence demonstrates two simultaneous conflicting feelings.

(2) Although the patient may be unhappy about past behaviors, it is the underlying thoughts about hurting others that precipitated the patient's statement.

(3) Anger is a feeling of displeasure caused by opposition or mistreatment and is demonstrated by the words or gestures used by the patient in an effort to fight back at the cause of the feeling.

(4) **Guilt is a painful feeling of self-reproach resulting from the belief that one has done something wrong.**

5-11 (1) Although obtaining the patient's signature is part of consent, the signature by itself does not imply that the patient understands.

(2) **The patient's knowledge and understanding of what is going to be done, why it is being done, and what the outcomes will be is what constitutes being informed before giving consent.**

(3) Although the family may be involved, it is the patient who must sign the informed consent.

(4) Preoperative teaching is necessary only if the patient consents to surgery.

5-12 (1) Speaking loudly could frighten the patient; one of the patient's other senses should be stimulated because the patient previously has not responded to a verbal intervention.

(2) The nurse must get the patient's attention before giving a direction.

(3) The nurse needs to assess the patient further before informing the nurse in charge.

(4) **This action is the first step to further assess this patient. Touch and sound stimulate two senses, and using the patient's name is individualizing care.**

5-13 (1) **Soaps usually contain sodium or potassium salts of fatty acids, which are irritating and can injure the sensitive tissues of the eyes.**

(2) The back needs soap and water to remove perspiration that collects on the skin.

(3) Body surface areas that touch are dark, warm, and moist areas and must be washed with soap and water to limit the growth of microorganisms.

(4) The glans of the penis needs soap and water to remove perspiration, urine, and smegma.

5-14 (1) ROM should be performed for unconscious patients because they usually are immobile and are at risk for developing contractures.

(2) Paralyzed limbs must be moved through full ROM by the nurse to prevent loss of range secondary to inactivity.

(3) **Resistance indicates that there is strain on the muscles or joints; continuing ROM beyond the point of resistance can cause injury.**

(4) People with chronic joint disease usually need gentle ROM to keep the joints mobile.

5-15 (1) Food contains nutrients and calories, which provide energy.

(2) Exercise promotes muscle tone and energy.

(3) Sleep is restful and restorative.

(4) **Caffeine, although a stimulant, can be harmful to the body.**

5-16 (1) **In the supine position, the abdominal contents press against the diaphragm, impeding expansion of the lungs.**

(2) This position is desirable because the abdominal contents drop by gravity, permitting efficient contraction of the diaphragm and expansion of the thoracic cavity.

(3) Same as #2.

(4) Same as #2.

5-17 (1) Only the area being washed should be exposed, to permit adequate bathing and inspection.

(2) Using long, firm strokes toward the heart is desirable because it promotes venous return.

(3) **This will contaminate the urinary meatus with microorganisms from the perianal area.**

(4) Using a cotton blanket is desirable; it absorbs moisture, provides warmth, and promotes privacy.

5-18
(1) This may be frightening if the patient does not know why the action is being done; this also is unsafe.
(2) Collecting equipment should be done after the patient agrees to the procedure.
(3) Same as #1.
(4) **Explaining the procedure meets the patient's right to know why and how care will be provided.**

5-19
(1) This focuses on a different ritual and denies the patient's concerns about missing Mass and not receiving Communion.
(2) **This helps to meet the patient's spiritual needs and is easily accomplished in a hospital setting.**
(3) The nurse, not other patients, must assist the patient to meet spiritual needs.
(4) Same as #1.

5-20
(1) This statement offers false reassurance and draws a conclusion based on insufficient information.
(2) **This response encourages further communication, which is necessary to obtain more information about what is upsetting the patient.**
(3) This is a judgmental statement that is not based on fact.
(4) This is not an open-ended question that allows the patient to express concerns; this is a statement that may or may not be true.

5-21
(1) A lack of balance in nutrients can result in malnutrition, not necessarily obesity; it also can result in weight loss.
(2) Although glandular disorders such as hypothyroidism may result in obesity, they are not the primary causes of obesity.
(3) **If more calories are ingested than the body requires for energy, they will be converted to adipose tissue, which causes weight gain.**
(4) A psychologic problem is just one of many factors that influence overeating; it is not the primary etiology of obesity.

5-22
(1) Vasodilation promotes heat loss.
(2) **Exposing only the area being washed limits the evaporation of fluids on the skin and radiation of heat from the body, which prevents the patient from getting a chill.**
(3) A hot drink will not prevent a chill.
(4) Although this may prevent drafts, it will not prevent the patient's getting a chill from the environmental temperature, excessive exposure, or evaporation of water from the skin.

5-23
(1) The bath may eventually be canceled, but it should be delayed first.
(2) **Delaying the bath accepts the patient's present refusal to bathe; rest and pain reduction may make the patient more amenable to hygiene later in the day.**
(3) This ignores the patient's right to refuse care and the fact that the patient is in pain.
(4) Same as #3.

5-24
(1) This personal protective equipment is not necessary for all Standard and Transmission-Based Precautions.
(2) Same as #1.
(3) **Washing the hands before and after patient care and whenever contaminated is the most important action for preventing the spread of microorganisms.**
(4) After they have been taught how to use Standard and Transmission-Based Precautions, people are permitted to visit patients with infections.

5-25
(1) **Unconscious patients usually have dry mucous membranes of the oral cavity because they frequently breathe through the mouth, are not drinking fluids, and may be receiving oxygen; oral hygiene is required whenever necessary, which usually is at least every 2 hours.**
(2) This is too long; drying, sordes, and lesions of the mucous membranes can occur.
(3) Same as #2.
(4) Same as #2.

5-26 (1) This action meets the patient's need for self-esteem.
(2) **Knowing what will happen and why provides for the patient's security needs; also, it is a patient's right. The unknown can be frightening.**
(3) Same as #1.
(4) This action meets the patient's basic physiologic need for adequate nutrients for body processes.

5-27 (1) The chart is a secondary source; it also contains physicians' orders, which are dependent functions of the nurse.
(2) **The primary and most important source for obtaining information referring to the patient is the patient. The independent functions of the nurse include interventions that relate to human responses, which are identified by direct contact with the patient.**
(3) The physician is a secondary source of information; when the nurse follows a physician's order, it is a dependent function of the nurse.
(4) The supervisor is a secondary source; independent functions of the nurse can be performed independently of others.

5-28 (1) A confrontation may take away the patient's current coping mechanisms and leave the patient defenseless.
(2) **A patient who is grieving is using defenses to deal with the crisis; these defenses should be supported.**
(3) Avoiding the patient is a form of abandonment; the nurse should be present to provide support.
(4) Setting limits may take away the patient's coping mechanisms and leave the patient defenseless.

5-29 (1) Planning occurs after the assessment and analysis phases of the nursing process.
(2) Assessing involves collecting data, which must be gathered before it can be analyzed and nursing diagnoses formulated.
(3) **Data must be clustered and interpreted to identify human responses that indicate potential or actual health problems that can be treated by the nurse; statements that indicate actual or potential health problems treatable by the nurse are nursing diagnoses. These actions require analysis.**
(4) Implementation is putting the plan of care into action, which occurs after assessment, analysis, and planning.

5-30 (1) This word is associated with others rather than the self or self-interests.
(2) **Toddlers are developing a sense of autonomy and are discovering the difference between independence and dependence; they are concerned about themselves and their mastery over their environment.**
(3) Same as #1.
(4) Same as #1.

The Nursing Process

Problem solving is a process that provides a framework for identifying solutions to complex problems. It is a step-by-step process that uses a systematic approach. One might say that problem solving is a "blueprint" that can be followed to identify and solve problems. The concept of problem solving is not used exclusively by nurses. It is used by other professionals to find solutions within the context of their own job responsibilities. Nurses use the problem-solving process to identify human responses and to plan, implement, and evaluate nursing care. When scientific problem solving is used within the context of nursing, it is known as the nursing process. The nursing process contains five steps: **assessment, analysis/nursing diagnosis, planning, implementation,** and **evaluation.**

Because the nursing process incorporates critical thinking used by nurses to meet patients' needs, items on nursing examinations are designed to test the use of this process. Test items are not written haphazardly. They are carefully designed to test your knowledge of a specific concept, skill, theory, or fact, from the perspective of one of the five steps of the nursing process. When reading an item, being able to identify its place within the nursing process should contribute to your ability to recognize what the test item is asking. To do this, you must focus on the critical words within the item.

This chapter explores the five steps of the nursing process: assessment, analysis, planning, implementation, and evaluation. Sample items are presented to demonstrate item construction as it relates to each step. Critical words associated with each step of the nursing process are illustrated within the sample items. Attempt to identify variations of critical words within the sample items indicating activities associated with each step of the nursing process. Practice answering the questions. The better you understand the focus of the item you are reading, the better you will be at identifying what is being asked and the greater your chances of identifying the correct answer. The correct answers and the rationales for all the options of the sample items in this chapter are at the end of the chapter.

Assessment

During assessment, data must be accurately collected, verified, and communicated. Assessment items are designed to test your knowledge of information, theories, principles, and skills related to the assessment of the patient. This establishes the foundation on which nurses base the subsequent steps in the nursing process. Assessment questions ask you to:

- Obtain vital statistics
- Perform a physical assessment

6

- Collect specimens
- Identify patient adaptations that are objective or subjective
- Identify patient adaptations that are verbal or nonverbal
- Identify adaptations that are expected (normal) or unexpected (abnormal)
- Use various data collection methods
- Identify sources of data
- Verify critical findings
- Identify commonalities and differences in response to illness
- Communicate information about assessments to appropriate members of the health team

The critical words within a test item that indicate that the item is focused on assessment include these: *inspect, identify, verify, observe, determine, notify, check, inform, question, communicate, verbal and nonverbal, signs and symptoms, stressors, adaptations, sources, perceptions,* and *assess.* See whether you can identify variations of these critical words in the sample items in this chapter.

Most testing errors that occur on assessment items occur because options are selected that:

- Collect insufficient data
- Have data that are inaccurately collected
- Use unscientific methods of data collection
- Rely on a secondary source rather than the primary source, the patient
- Contain irrelevant data
- Fail to verify data
- Reflect bias or prejudice
- Fail to accurately communicate data

COLLECT DATA

Methods of Data Collection

Collecting data is the first part of assessment. The nurse collects data through specific **methods of data collection,** such as performing a physical examination, interviewing, and reviewing records.

A **physical examination** includes the assessment techniques of inspection, palpation, auscultation, and percussion. Also, it includes obtaining the vital signs and recognizing acceptable and unacceptable parameters of obtained values.

Interviewing collects data using a formal approach (e.g., obtaining a health history) or an informal approach (e.g., exploring feelings while providing other nursing care).

Review of records includes consideration of reports such as the results of laboratory tests, diagnostic procedures, and assessments or consultations by other members of the health team.

SAMPLE ITEM 6-1

While making rounds, the nurse finds a patient on the floor in the hall. What should be the nurse's initial response?

(1) Inspect the patient for injury

(2) Transfer the patient back to bed

(3) Move the patient to the closest chair

(4) Report the incident to the nursing supervisor

This item tests your ability to recognize that, in an emergency situation, the nurse must first assess (inspect) the condition of the patient. This principle is basic to any emergency response by a nurse. Moving a patient before an assessment could worsen an injury. This item demonstrates how a basic concept related to assessment can be tested.

SAMPLE ITEM 6-2

What should the nurse do to avoid patient accidents?

(1) Keep an overbed table in front of a sitting patient

(2) Determine the strength of a patient before walking

(3) Provide a cane for ambulation if the patient is weak

(4) Apply a vest restraint when a patient uses a wheelchair

This item tests your ability to recognize the concept that the nurse must assess a patient before implementing care. The three distractors are all concerned with implementing care. This question also tests your ability to recognize physical examination as a method of collecting data about the status of a patient.

SAMPLE ITEM 6-3

Which assessment by the nurse most likely indicates that a patient is having difficulty breathing?

(1) 18 breaths per minute and inhaled through the mouth

(2) 20 breaths per minute and shallow in character

(3) 16 breaths per minute and deep in character

(4) 28 breaths per minute and noisy

This item tests your ability to identify the option that reflects a respiratory rate and characteristic that is outside expected parameters. To successfully answer this question, you need to know the rate and characteristics of acceptable and unacceptable respirations.

SAMPLE ITEM 6-4

What should the nurse always do when taking a rectal temperature?

(1) Allow the patient to insert the thermometer.

(2) Position the patient on the left side.

(3) Use an electronic thermometer.

(4) Lubricate the thermometer.

Option 4 identifies what must be done (a critical element) to safely take a rectal temperature. The three distractors may or may not be done when obtaining a rectal temperature. Although this appears to be an implementation question because it involves an action, it is actually an assessment question because it is concerned with collecting data.

SAMPLE ITEM 6-5

When the nurse determines if a person's body weight is ideal, it is also important to assess the person's:

(1) Body height

(2) Daily intake

(3) Clothing size

(4) Food preferences

This item tests your ability to recognize that, to calculate the patient's ideal body weight, the nurse must also know the patient's height. The ideal body weight is the measurement that reflects the range of weight that is considered appropriate in relation to the patient's height. The ideal body weight is the measurement against which the patient's present weight is compared to determine if the patient is underweight or obese. Although the question does not address these concepts, the nurse also must know the patient's age and extent of bone structure.

Sources of Data

Data can be gathered not only by different methods but also from different sources. **Sources of data** available to the nurse include those that are primary, secondary, and tertiary. There is only one **primary source,** the patient. The patient is the most valuable source of information because the data collected are the most current and specific to the patient.

A **secondary source** produces information from someplace other than the patient. A family member is a secondary source who can contribute information about the patient's likes and dislikes, ethnic and cultural background, similarities and differences in behavior, and functioning before and during the health problem. The patient's medical record (chart) is another example of a secondary source. It is a legal document containing information that concerns the patient's physical, psychosocial, religious, and economic history and documents the patient's physical and emotional adaptations. Controversy surrounds the labeling of diagnostic test results in a chart as being from either primary or secondary sources. Although the chart itself is a secondary source, diagnostic test results are direct objective measurements of the patient's status and therefore are considered by some health-care providers to be a primary source. The nurse must remember that the information in a chart is history and does not reflect the current status of the patient because the patient is dynamic and constantly changing. Secondary sources are valuable for gathering supplementary information about a patient.

A **tertiary source** provides information from outside the specific patient's frame of reference. Examples of tertiary sources include textbooks, the nurse's experience, and accepted commonalities among patients with similar adaptations. The nurse's or other health team members' responses to the patient are tertiary sources of patient data.

SAMPLE ITEM 6–6

The nurse asks a patient's wife specific questions about the patient's health complaints before admission. When collecting this information, the nurse is seeking information from a:

(1) Primary source

(2) Tertiary source

(3) Subjective source

(4) Secondary source

This item tests your ability to recognize that a family member is a secondary source of information. Secondary sources provide information that is supplemental to the information collected from the patient.

Types of Data

The **types of data** collected when assessing a patient can be objective or subjective, verbal or nonverbal.

Objective data are measurable assessments collected when the nurse uses sight, touch, smell, or hearing to acquire information. Examples of objective data include an excoriated perineal area, diaphoresis, ammonia odor of urine, crackles, and vital signs. **Subjective data** can be collected only when the patient shares feelings, perceptions, thoughts, and sensations about a health problem or concern. Examples of subjective data include patient statements about pain, shortness of breath, or feeling depressed.

SAMPLE ITEM 6–7

The nurse is performing a physical assessment of a newly admitted patient. Which patient statement communicates subjective data?

(1) "I have sores between my toes."

(2) "I dye my hair but it is really grey."

(3) "My left leg drags on the floor when I walk."

(4) "My joints hurt when I get up in the morning."

This item tests your ability to differentiate between subjective and objective data. The nurse should know the types of data collected for the purposes of future clustering and determining their significance. Any information that the patient shares regarding feelings, thoughts, and concerns is subjective. Any information that the nurse verifies using the senses (e.g., vision, hearing, smell, and touch) or via some form of instrumentation (e.g., thermometer, pulse oximetry, laboratory data) is objective.

Communication can be verbal or nonverbal. **Verbal data** are collected via the spoken or written word. For example, statements made to the nurse by the patient are verbal data. **Nonverbal data** are collected via transmission of a message without words. Crying, a fearful facial expression, the appearance of the patient, and gestures are all examples of nonverbal data.

SAMPLE ITEM 6–8

What is an example of nonverbal communication?

(1) A letter

(2) Holding hands

(3) Noise in the room

(4) A telephone message

This item tests your ability to recognize that holding hands is a form of nonverbal communication. Nonverbal communication does not use words. Touch, gestures, posture, and facial expressions are examples of nonverbal communication.

VERIFY DATA

After data are collected, they must be verified. To **verify data** is to confirm information by collecting additional data, questioning orders, obtaining judgments and/or conclusions from other team members when appropriate, and by collecting data oneself rather than relying on technology. Verifying data ensures authenticity and accuracy. For example, when a vital statistic is outside the expected range, the nurse must substantiate the results first by collecting the data again and then collecting additional data to supplement the original information.

SAMPLE ITEM 6–9

The nurse takes the patient's blood pressure and records a diastolic pressure of 120. What should the nurse do first?

(1) Retake the blood pressure

(2) Take the other vital signs

(3) Notify the nurse in charge

(4) Notify the physician

This item tests your ability to identify that you need to verify data when they are unexpectedly outside the acceptable range. Your first action should be to wait a minute and then retake the blood pressure. An error may have been made when taking the blood pressure.

COMMUNICATE INFORMATION ABOUT ASSESSMENTS

The last component of assessment includes the nurse's ability to communicate information obtained from assessment activities. Sharing vital information about a patient is essential if members of the health team are to be alerted to the most current status of the patient. Communication methods vary (e.g., progress notes, verbal notification, flow sheets); however, they all share the need to be accurate, concise, thorough, current, organized, and confidential.

SAMPLE ITEM 6–10

> When assessing a patient with a fluid volume deficit, which assessment should the nurse document on the patient's record?
>
> (1) Thready radial pulse and straw-colored urine
>
> (2) Straw-colored urine and decreased skin turgor
>
> (3) Urine specific gravity of 1.015 and thready radial pulse
>
> (4) Decreased skin turgor and a urine specific gravity of 1.035
>
> This item tests your ability to assess for patient adaptations related to a fluid volume deficit and document these adaptations on the patient's record so that they can be communicated to other health team members.

Analysis/Nursing Diagnosis

Analysis, the second step of the nursing process, is the most difficult component. Analysis requires that data be validated and clustered and that their significance be determined. To analyze data, you need a strong foundation in scientific principles related to nursing theory, social sciences, and physical sciences. You need to know the commonalities and differences in patients' responses to various stresses. You need to use reasoning to apply your knowledge and experience when answering analysis items. After the initial analysis of data, sometimes additional data need to be collected and analyzed. Only after all the data have been analyzed should a nursing diagnosis be made. Analysis questions ask you to:

- Validate interrelationship of data
- Cluster data
- Identify clustered data as meaningful
- Interpret validated and clustered data
- Identify when additional data are needed to further validate clustered data
- Identify nursing diagnoses
- Communicate nursing diagnoses to others

The critical words within a test item that indicate that the item is focused on analysis/nursing diagnosis include these: *valid, organize, categorize, cluster, reexamine, pattern, formulate, nursing diagnosis, reflect, relate, problem, interpret, contribute, relevant, decision, significant, deduction, statement,* and *analysis.* See whether you can identify variations of these critical words in the sample items in this chapter.

Testing errors occur on analysis items when options are selected that:

- Omit data
- Cluster data prematurely
- Make a nursing diagnosis before all significant data have been clustered
- Force the nursing diagnosis to fit the signs and symptoms collected

CLUSTER DATA

Clustering data groups related information together. Information is more meaningful when its relationship to other data is established. Clustering enables the nurse to organize data; eliminate that which is insignificant, irrelevant, or redundant; and reduce the data into manageable categories. First data must be organized into general categories such as physical, sociocultural, psychologic, and spiritual. Then data can be grouped into specific categories such as nutrition, mobility, and elimination. Data can be obvious and easy to cluster or obscure and difficult to cluster. Some data are clustered easily because the information collected is clearly related to only one system of the body. For example, hard stool, a feeling of rectal fullness, and straining on defecation all relate to intestinal elimination. These adaptations are easy to group and lead to the interpretation that the patient may be constipated. Other data are more difficult to cluster because the patient's adaptations may involve a variety of systems of the body. A weak, thready pulse; weight loss; hypotension; and dry mucous membranes can be grouped together. At first, this information may not appear to be related because the adaptations cross several body systems. However, with a thorough analysis the nurse should recognize that the data are interrelated and interpret that the patient may be dehydrated. Established frameworks such as Marjory Gordon's Functional Health Patterns (1994) and Abraham Maslow's Hierarchy of Human Needs (1970) provide structures for organizing and clustering data.

SAMPLE ITEM 6–11

A patient had a stroke (brain attack) that resulted in paralysis of the right side. When clustering data, the nurse grouped the following data together: drooling of saliva and slurred speech. Which information is most significant to include with this clustered data?

(1) Receptive aphasia

(2) Difficulty swallowing

(3) Inability to perform ADLs

(4) Incontinence of bowel movements

This item tests your ability to recognize a cluster of data that indicates that a patient is at risk for aspiration. Oxygenation is a basic physiologic need. A patient who is drooling saliva and has slurred speech, right-sided paralysis, and difficulty swallowing is at serious risk for aspiration of material into the respiratory tract. Although the other options are all problems that must be addressed by the nurse, they are not data related to oxygenation and have no significance to this specific cluster.

SAMPLE ITEM 6–12

The nurse understands that pressure ulcers are most often associated with patients who:

(1) Are immobilized

(2) Have psychiatric diagnoses

(3) Experience respiratory distress

(4) Need close supervision for safety

This item tests your ability to recognize the relationship between immobility and the formation of pressure ulcers. It is designed to test your knowledge of the fact that prolonged pressure on a site interferes with cellular oxygenation, which causes cell death resulting in a pressure ulcer.

INTERPRET DATA

Interpretation of data is critical in the analysis/nursing diagnosis step of the nursing process. It is associated with the nurse's ability to determine the significance of clustered data. "Significance" in this context refers to some consequence, importance, implication, or gravity connected to the cluster as it relates to the patient's health problem. Finally, the interpretation of the significant clustered data should lead to a conclusion. Conclusions are the opinions, decisions, or inferences that result from the interpretation of data.

SAMPLE ITEM 6–13

The nurse is caring for a dying patient who has a loss of appetite (anorexia), difficulty falling asleep (insomnia), and decreased interest in activities of daily living. Which feeling reflects these adaptations?

(1) Anger

(2) Denial

(3) Depression

(4) Acceptance

This item tests your ability to come to a conclusion based on a cluster of data. The word "reflect" in the stem cues you to the fact that this is an analysis question. You need to draw from your knowledge of commonalities of human behavior and theories of grieving to arrive at the conclusion that the patient probably is depressed.

SAMPLE ITEM 6–14

A patient who is debilitated and unsteady when standing insists on walking to the bathroom without calling for assistance. This behavior best reflects a need to be:

(1) Alone

(2) Accepted

(3) Independent

(4) Manipulative

This item tests your ability to come to a conclusion based on a cluster of data. To answer this question, you must analyze and interpret the information in the stem and come to a conclusion. Your knowledge of human behavior should enable you to select the correct answer.

COLLECT ADDITIONAL DATA

After arriving at an initial conclusion, additional data collection might be indicated to provide more information to support the suspected conclusion. This is done to ensure the relationship among the original data. The nurse continually reassesses the condition of the patient and the presence of needs, recognizing that the patient is dynamic and ever changing throughout all phases of the nursing process.

SAMPLE ITEM 6–15

The nurse assesses that a postoperative patient has a decreased blood pressure and weak, thready pulse and concludes that the patient may be hemorrhaging. The nurse should reassess the patient for the additional sign of:

(1) Pain

(2) Jaundice

(3) Tachycardia

(4) Hyperthermia

This item is designed to test your ability to recognize that the nurse needs to reassess a patient for additional data to reinforce the proposed conclusion that the patient is hemorrhaging. Hypotension; a weak, thready pulse; and tachycardia are related to a decreased blood volume that is associated with postoperative hemorrhage.

IDENTIFY AND COMMUNICATE NURSING DIAGNOSES

Converting a conclusion into a diagnostic statement changes it from a general statement of a problem into a specific statement, or a nursing diagnosis. A nursing diagnosis is a statement of a specific health problem that a nurse is legally permitted to treat. The diagnostic statement should include the problem and the factors that contributed to the development of the problem.

It is necessary to include the contributing factors because, although two patients may have the same problem, it may have been caused by different stresses. This concept is important because the nature of the contributing factors generally drives the choice of interventions being planned. For example, two patients have impaired skin integrity. However, one patient's skin problem is related to incontinence and edema, and the other patient's skin problem is related to immobility and pressure. The interventions may be very different because the factors contributing to the problem are different. This is discussed in more detail in the section in this chapter titled "Planning." Some nurses use the taxonomy of nursing diagnoses developed by the North American Nursing Diagnosis Association (NANDA) as a blueprint. This taxonomy provides for classifying nursing problems, standardizing language, facilitating communication, and focusing on an individualized approach to identifying and meeting a patient's nursing needs. The following are examples of nursing diagnoses:

- Risk for impaired skin integrity, related to incontinence
- Feeding self-care deficit, related to bilateral arm casts
- Ineffective airway clearance, related to excessive secretions

Nurses need to communicate nursing diagnoses to other nurses via a written plan of care. The plan should include the nursing diagnosis, expected outcomes, and planned interventions. The section of this chapter titled "Planning" discusses outcomes and planned nursing interventions in more detail.

SAMPLE ITEM 6–16

The patient has suffered a brain attack (cerebrovascular accident, stroke), has left-sided hemiparesis, and is incontinent. Which is an appropriately worded nursing diagnosis for this patient?

(1) The patient has a need to maintain skin integrity.

(2) The patient has a stroke evidenced by hemiparesis and incontinence.

(3) The patient will be clean and dry and will receive range-of-motion exercises every 4 hours.

(4) The patient is at risk for impaired skin integrity related to left-sided hemiparesis and incontinence.

This item tests your ability to recognize language used by the NANDA taxonomy. To answer this item correctly, you must be able to identify the differences among a patient need, an expected outcome, a nursing intervention, and a properly stated nursing diagnosis associated with a cluster of data.

Planning

Planning is the third step of the nursing process. It involves identifying goals, projecting expected outcomes, setting priorities, identifying interventions, ensuring that the patient's health-care needs will be appropriately met, modifying the plan of care as needed, and collaborating with other health team members. To plan care, you must have a strong foundation of scientific theory, understand the commonalities and differences in response to nursing interventions, and know theories related to establishing priority of needs. You will need to use your knowledge and clinical experience when answering planning questions. Planning questions will ask you to:

- Involve the patient in the planning process
- Set goals
- Establish expected outcomes against which results of care can be compared for the purpose of evaluation
- Plan appropriate interventions based on their effects
- Establish priorities of nursing interventions
- Anticipate patient needs
- Recognize the need to collaborate with others
- Recognize the need to coordinate planned care with other disciplines
- Recognize that plans must be flexible and modified based on changing patient needs

The critical words within a test item that indicate that the item is focused on planning include these: *achieve, desired, plan, effective, desired result, goal, priority, develop, formulate, establish, design, prevent, strategy, select, determine, anticipate, modify, collaborate, arrange, coordinate, expect,* and *outcome.* See whether you can identify variations of these critical words in the sample items in this chapter.

Testing errors occur during the planning phase when options are selected that:

- Do not include the patient in setting goals and priorities
- Are inappropriate goals
- Misidentify priorities
- Reflect goals that are unrealistic
- Reflect goals that are unmeasurable
- Reflect planned interventions that are inappropriate or incomplete
- Fail to include family members and significant others when appropriate
- Fail to coordinate and collaborate with other health team members

IDENTIFY GOALS

Goals are general statements that direct nursing interventions. They provide broad parameters regarding the desired results of nursing care and stimulate motivation. Goals can be long term or short term. A **long-term goal** is one that will take time to achieve (years). A **short-term goal** is one that can be achieved relatively quickly (usually within weeks or months). Goals should be:

- Patient centered
- Specific (measurable)
- Realistic
- Achievable within a time frame

A long-term goal for a patient who has a respiratory tract infection might be, "Mr. Brown will be free of infection within 3 weeks." "Mr. Brown" is the subject of the statement and therefore the goal is patient centered. Being "free of infection" is specific, realistic, and measurable. The phrase "within 3 weeks" indicates the time frame in which the goal should be achieved. Eventually a goal can be further developed to become an expected outcome. An outcome provides a standard of measure that can be used to determine whether the goal has been reached. An expected outcome for the long-term goal listed above might be, "Mr. Brown's sputum culture will be negative within 2 weeks." Outcomes are discussed in more detail next.

SAMPLE ITEM 6–17

The nurse is caring for a patient with a new temporary colostomy. Which is a realistic short-term goal for this patient?

(1) The patient's bowel will function within 2 days.

(2) The patient will have regular bowel elimination.

(3) The patient will be at risk for impaired skin integrity.

(4) The patient's skin will remain intact around the stoma.

This item tests your ability to recognize a short-term goal. To answer this question, you need to know commonalities related to caring for a patient with a new temporary colostomy and be able to identify the differences among short- and long-term goals, a nursing diagnosis, and an outcome statement.

PROJECT EXPECTED OUTCOMES

Expected outcomes are the changes in the patient's condition that are expected in response to care given. Expected outcomes are derived from goal statements, but they are more specific because they describe the behavior to be demonstrated or data to be collected that indicate that the goal is achieved. Expected outcomes are the benchmarks against which the patient's actual outcomes are compared to determine the effectiveness of the interventions provided. To be meaningful, they must be patient centered, realistic, measurable, and within a certain time frame. The process of comparing actual outcomes with expected outcomes occurs in the evaluation phase, which is the last step in the nursing process. Examples of outcomes are: "The patient states a reduction in anxiety in 1 week" and "The patient's diastolic blood pressure is below 90 mm Hg by discharge." Sometimes the nurse may state goals and outcomes together. For example, "The patient will continuously maintain an effective airway clearance as evidenced by expectoration of sputum, clear lung fields, and noiseless breathing." The first part of the statement is the goal and what follows "as evidenced by" are the expected outcomes. The first part of the statement is general and the second part is specific.

SAMPLE ITEM 6–18

A nurse is caring for a patient experiencing loss of appetite (anorexia) and nausea. Which statement includes an expected outcome? The patient's:

(1) Intake will be 50 percent of every meal during the next week

(2) Nutritional intake is less than body requirements

(3) Privacy will be maintained when providing care

(4) Mouth will be cleaned every 4 hours

This item tests your ability to recognize a statement that reflects an expected outcome. To answer this question, you need to know commonalities of caring for a patient with anorexia and nausea. You also need to recognize the differences among a goal, an expected outcome, a nursing diagnosis, and a nursing intervention.

SET PRIORITIES

Setting priorities is an important step in the planning process. After nursing diagnoses and goals are identified, they must be ranked in order of importance. Maslow's Hierarchy of Needs (1970) is helpful in establishing priorities. Basic physiologic needs are ranked first, with the need for safety and security, belonging and love, self-esteem, and self-actualization following in rank order. It is important, however, to recognize that at one point in time any one of Maslow's needs may take priority depending on the needs of the individual patient. Obviously, if someone is choking on food, clearing the airway is the priority. However, there are times when the emergency or immediate need of the patient is in the psychologic dimension. The nurse must be aware of the patient's perceptions and perspective when setting priorities because patients are the center of the health team. When possible, the patient should always be involved in setting priorities.

SAMPLE ITEM 6–19

A patient has just returned from surgery with an IV and does not have a gag reflex. Which planned intervention takes priority?

(1) Observe the dressing for drainage

(2) Ensure adequacy of air exchange

(3) Check for an infiltration

(4) Monitor vital signs

This item tests your ability to prioritize care. All of these planned interventions are important. However, oxygenation is essential to sustain life, and therefore maintaining a patent airway is the priority.

IDENTIFY INTERVENTIONS

After priorities are established, a plan for nursing action must be formulated. To plan appropriately, the nurse must rely on scientific knowledge, clinical judgment, and knowledge about the patient. Relying on this background, the nurse determines what nursing measures are most effective in assisting the patient to achieve a goal or outcome. For example, when caring for a patient with a pressure ulcer, the nurse reasons, "If I turn and reposition the patient and massage around the area with lotion every 2 hours, then circulation will increase and healing will be promoted." When planning care, the nurse must know the scientific rationales for nursing interventions so that the interventions selected are the most appropriate for the patient-care situation. It is not enough to just know how; also you must know why.

When making decisions, the nurse must consider the concepts of "cause and effect," "risk and probability," and "value of the consequence to the patient." The action you plan is the "cause." The patient's response is the "effect." The likelihood of the occurrence of either a positive or negative effect is the "probability." The probability of the patient suffering harm from the action is the "risk." The value of the effect, in relation to its probability of occurring, influences the degree of risk one is willing to take to achieve the effect.

To facilitate this process of problem solving, an **information-processing model of decision making** should be used.

- First, identify all the possible nursing actions (cause) that may help the patient.
- Second, you need to identify all possible positive and negative consequences (effect) associated with each action.
- Third, you need to determine the odds (probability) that each consequence will occur. This includes determining the probability of a negative effect occurring (risk).
- Fourth, you need to arrive at a judgment based on the value of each effect to the patient.
- Fifth, you must choose the action that is "best" for the patient. The "best" action is one that has the lowest risk and the highest probability of helping the patient achieve the expected outcome (effect).

The concept of probability versus risk can be applied to buying a lottery ticket. If you buy one lottery ticket, your chances of winning are small (low probability). If you do not win, your risk will be small because you will lose only one dollar (low risk). On the other hand, if you spend your entire paycheck on lottery tickets, you will not dramatically increase your chances of winning (low probability). However, if you do not win, you will lose your whole paycheck and have no money to pay your bills (high risk). When making clinical decisions, you want to choose an action that has the highest probability of being successful with the lowest risk to the patient.

Also, the appropriateness of clinical decisions depends on the quality of the data collected and the accuracy of the inferences made in the earlier steps of the nursing process. Each step of the nursing process relies on the quality and accuracy of the preceding step.

SAMPLE ITEM 6-20

What is the most effective way that nurses can prevent the spread of microorganisms in a hospital?

    (1) Washing the hands

    (2) Implementing contact precautions

    (3) Administering antibiotics to sick patients

    (4) Using linen hampers with foot-operated covers

This item tests your ability to be aware that handwashing is the single most effective measure to prevent the spread of microorganisms. This is a question that focuses on a specific action that can contribute to the protection of all patients from the risk of infection.

SAMPLE ITEM 6-21

A patient on bed rest needs a complete change of linen. What should the nurse plan to do?

    (1) Make an occupied bed

    (2) Change the draw sheet and top sheet

    (3) Raise the patient with a mechanical lift

    (4) Transfer the patient to a chair during the linen change

This item tests your ability to identify the needs of a patient on bed rest and, therefore, to plan to make an occupied bed. The word "plan" used in the stem is an obvious clue that this is a planning question.

The nurse should make an occupied bed for a patient who is:

(1) Obese

(2) In a cast

(3) Immobile

(4) On bed rest

This item is similar to sample item 6–21; however, the content of the stem and the correct option are reversed. This item is more difficult to identify as a planning item because the word "plan" is not in the stem.

ENSURE THAT HEALTH CARE NEEDS WILL BE MET APPROPRIATELY

The nurse is obligated to take an action that will ensure that appropriate care will be provided. If adequate care cannot be administered because the provider's expertise is unrelated to the patient's needs, the provider is inexperienced for caring for a patient with a particular problem, or there is inadequate staffing, a patient may be placed at risk. This might necessitate rearranging the assignment, or it might require intervention by the nurse supervisor. Once the nurse embarks on a "duty of care," the nurse is obligated to provide a standard of care defined by the Nurse Practice Act in the state in which the nurse works.

SAMPLE ITEM 6–23

The nurse manager arrives on duty and discovers that several staff members have just called in sick. What is the nurse manager's most appropriate response?

(1) Inform the supervisor and ask for additional staff

(2) Identify which patients need care and assign staff accordingly

(3) Explain to patients that when the unit is short staffed, only essential care can be provided

(4) Provide the best care possible, but refuse to accept responsibility for the standard of care delivered

This item tests your ability to recognize your responsibility to ensure that patients' needs are met appropriately. Once the nurse perceives a risk to patient safety, the nurse is obligated to take action that will ensure that appropriate care will be provided.

MODIFY THE PLAN OF CARE AS NEEDED

Planning generally takes place before care is given. However, patient needs sometimes change while the nurse is in the process of implementing care, and a plan must be immediately modified. Modification of the plan of care also may take place after evaluation. The original plan may have been inadequate or inappropriate, or the patient's condition may have improved. It is important to recognize that plans of care are not set in stone but are modified in response to the changing needs of the patient. Because a patient's needs are dynamic, the nursing plan also is dynamic. It must be continually changed to be kept current, substituting new nursing diagnoses, goals, expected outcomes, and planned interventions as indicated by the patient's changing needs.

SAMPLE ITEM 6–24

A patient is diaphoretic and is receiving oxygen by nasal cannula. During a bath, the patient experiences dyspnea and complains of feeling tired. The nurse should plan to:

(1) Give a complete bath quickly

(2) Bathe only the body parts that need bathing

(3) Arrange for several rest periods during the bath

(4) Continue with the bath because dyspnea is unavoidable

This item tests your ability to recognize the need to modify a plan of care based on new data. The words "planning" in the stem and "arrange" in the correct answer are obvious clues that this is a planning question.

COLLABORATE WITH OTHER HEALTH TEAM MEMBERS

Another component of planning is consultation and collaboration with other health team members to brainstorm, seek additional input, and delegate and coordinate the delivery of health services. The nurse is responsible for coordinating the members of the nursing team as well as the entire health team. The nurse manages the members of the nursing team by appropriately delegating and supervising nursing interventions. The plan also identifies and coordinates the services of other health-care professionals. The nurse is responsible for ensuring that services such as laboratory tests, radiologic studies, and physical therapy are performed within the context of the patient's physical and emotional abilities. For example, the nurse may arrange for a patient to go to physical therapy in the morning before the patient tires, or the nurse may consult with the dietitian for help with designing a menu that incorporates a patient's preferences. Effective planning contributes to the delivery of patient care that has continuity and is patient centered, coordinated, and individualized.

SAMPLE ITEM 6–25

A nurse is caring for a patient with a large pressure ulcer that has not responded to common nursing interventions. To best deal with this problem, the nurse should consult with the:

(1) Plastic surgeon

(2) Physical therapist

(3) Attending physician

(4) Clinical nurse specialist

This item is designed to test your ability to recognize that planning nursing care may require the nurse to seek the expertise of a specialist. A clinical nurse specialist is educated and prepared to provide expert advice and lend problem-solving and educational skills to seek solutions to difficult clinical nursing problems. Although the nurse consults with health team members of other disciplines for various reasons, the nurse should consult with a clinical nurse specialist or other resources in nursing for assistance with solving nursing problems.

Implementation

Implementation is the step of the nursing process whereby planned actions are initiated and completed. It includes tasks such as organizing and managing planned care; providing total or partial assistance with activities of daily living (ADLs); counseling and teaching the patient and significant others; providing planned care; supervising, coordinating, and evaluating the process of the delivery of care by the nursing staff (this does not include the actual delegation of care that occurs in planning or the evaluation of the patient's response to care that occurs in evaluation); and recording and sharing data related to the care implemented.

To implement safe nursing care designed to achieve goals and expected outcomes, the nurse must understand and follow the implementation process. In addition, the nurse must have knowledge of scientific rationales for nursing procedures, psychomotor skills to implement procedures safely, and the ability to use different strategies to effectively implement nursing care. Implementation questions will ask you to:

- Recognize steps in the implementation process
- Identify independent, dependent, and interdependent actions of the nurse
- Implement a procedure or treatment
- Respond to common or uncommon outcomes in response to interventions

- Respond to life-threatening or adverse events
- Prepare a patient for a procedure, treatment, or surgery
- Choose an approach that is most appropriate when implementing care
- Identify safe or unsafe practices
- Rationalize a step in a procedure
- Identify or apply concepts associated with teaching
- Identify or apply concepts associated with counseling
- Identify or apply principles associated with motivation
- Identify or apply techniques for therapeutic communication
- Recognize the relationship between a procedure and an expected outcome
- Identify when an intervention must be modified in response to a change in the patient's condition
- Identify when additional assistance is required to provide safe care
- Identify the nurse's responsibility associated with supervising and evaluating care delivered by those to whom interventions have been delegated
- Identify how and when to document or report care given along with the patient's response

The critical words within a test item that indicate that the item is focused on implementation include these: *dependent, independent, interdependent, change, assist, counsel, teach, give, supervise, perform, method, procedure, treatment, instruct, strategy, facilitate, provide, inform, refer, technique, motivate, delegate,* and *implement.* See whether you can identify variations of these words indicating implementation activities in the sample items.

Testing errors occur on implementation items when options are selected that:

- Implement actions outside the definition of nursing practice
- Fail to respond to an adverse or life-threatening situation
- Fail to modify interventions in response to the changing needs of the patient
- Fail to identify when additional assistance is required for the delivery of safe care
- Reflect a lack of knowledge to safely implement interventions
- Do not accurately document the patient's response to the care given
- Fail to supervise and evaluate the delivery of delegated interventions

LEGAL PARAMETERS OF NURSING INTERVENTIONS

Implementation occurs when the nurse uses an intervention to help a patient meet expected outcomes. Nursing interventions can be dependent, independent, or interdependent in nature.

Dependent interventions are interventions that require an order prescribed by a primary care provider such as a physician, nurse practitioner, or physician's assistant. Administering a medication, providing IV fluids, and removing a nasogastric tube are examples of dependent interventions because they all require a legal order. When implementing a dependent intervention, the nurse does not blindly follow the order, but determines whether the order is appropriate. A nurse who does not question and carries out an inappropriate order is contributing to the initial error and will be held accountable.

Independent interventions (nurse prescribed) are those actions that a nurse is legally permitted to implement with no direction or supervision from others. Independent interventions do not require a physician's order. Tasks related to collecting data, providing assistance with ADLs, teaching regarding health, and counseling are in the realm of independent legal nursing practice. Encouraging coughing and deep breathing, encouraging verbalization of fears, teaching principles related to nutrition, and providing a bed bath also are examples of independent nursing interventions.

Interdependent interventions (collaborative) are actions implemented in partnership with other appropriate professionals. An example of an interdependent intervention is implementing actions identified in standing orders or a protocol. These situations delineate the parameters within which the nurse is permitted to administer to the patient. Protocols and standing orders are commonly found in emergency and critical care areas. Another example of an interdependent intervention is when a physician orders, "Out of bed as tolerated." When ambulating this patient, the nurse must assess the patient's response to the activity. Based on the patient's response, the nurse can decide to terminate the activity or to increase the time and/or distance to be ambulated.

The primary nurse assigns a staff nurse to insert an indwelling urinary (Foley) catheter. What is the first thing the staff nurse should do?

(1) Explain the procedure to the patient

(2) Gather equipment at the bedside

(3) Check the physician's order

(4) Wash hands thoroughly

This question is designed to test your ability to recognize that the insertion of a urinary catheter is a dependent nursing intervention that requires a physician's order.

TYPES OF NURSING INTERVENTIONS

Examples of nursing actions associated with the implementation step of the nursing process include:

- **Assisting with Activities of Daily Living (ADLs):** Assisting with ADLs refers to activities associated with eating, dressing, hygiene, grooming, toileting, transfer, and locomotion. Situations associated with needs addressing ADLs can be acute, chronic, temporary, permanent, or related to maintaining or restoring function. ADLs are an integral part of daily life, and therefore their implementation is often tested.

- **Teaching:** To effectively teach in the cognitive (learning new information), psychomotor (learning new skills), and affective (developing new attitudes, values, and beliefs) domains, the nurse must apply teaching/learning principles to motivate patients to learn and grow. Health teaching activities are incorporated throughout the health-illness continuum, in a variety of health-care delivery settings, and across the life span. For these reasons, teaching principles are often incorporated into patient situations in test questions.

- **Responding to Life-Threatening Situations:** Responding to adverse or life-threatening situations requires the use of clinical judgment and decision making. Activities such as stopping the administration of an antibiotic in response to a patient's allergic reaction, initiating cardiopulmonary resuscitation, implementing the abdominal thrust procedure (Heimlich maneuver), and administering emergency medication are examples of measures that can be implemented in life-threatening situations. Most of these interventions address the basic physiologic needs required for survival and are therefore frequently tested.

- **Implementing Preventive Actions:** These actions are activities that help the patient to avoid a health problem. Administering immunizations, applying an allergy bracelet, employing medical and surgical asepsis, ensuring physical safety, and leading a group on weight reduction are examples of preventive measures. Because today's society emphasizes health, wellness, and illness prevention, these topics are often tested.

- **Performing Technical Skills:** The nurse must know how and when to implement a procedure and the expected outcomes of the procedure. Inserting a urinary catheter, providing a tube feeding, administering medication, performing an enema, and preparing a patient for a diagnostic test are examples of procedures implemented by the nurse. Steps, principles, rationales, and expected outcomes associated with procedures are concepts that are often tested in nursing questions.

- **Implementing Interpersonal Interventions:** These activities help the nurse to assist a patient to adapt to changes that are caused by loss, illness, disability, or stress. Emotional care can be provided by activities such as promoting a supportive environment, motivating a patient, providing for privacy, addressing spiritual needs, and accepting feelings. Counseling also is a component of interpersonal interventions. To effectively counsel, the nurse must apply therapeutic communication principles to explore patients' feelings and meet their emotional needs. Another aspect of interpersonal interventions is coordinating health-care activities. When the nurse collaborates with others and coordinates health-care activities, the nurse functions as the patient's advocate. People are complex human beings, and nursing care must address the mental, physical, emotional, spiritual, and legal/ethical realms. Because these realms are so important, associated nursing interventions are often tested in nursing questions.

- **Supervising and Evaluating the Effectiveness of Delegated Interventions:** Occasionally, the nurse who formulates the plan of care delegates all or part of the implementation of the plan to other members of the nursing team. Uncomplicated and basic interventions, particularly those associated with ADLs, are often delegated to a nursing assistant or licensed practical nurse. The nurse who delegates is responsible for the plan of care and is accountable for ensuring that the care is delivered according to standards of the profession. With the changing roles in health-care delivery, the importance of the nurse as manager is increasing and is therefore tested.

- **Reporting and Recording:** After care is given, it is recorded along with an assessment of the patient's response to care. Written communication establishes a permanent document of the care patients receive and their responses. In addition to documenting, the nurse may verbally report to other health team members the care that was provided along with the patients' responses. Also, verbal reports are given at the change of shifts and when responding to an emergency. Because communication and documentation are essential to the provision of quality care, it is often tested.

SAMPLE ITEM 6–27

A patient has an order for a 2-gram sodium diet. What should the nurse teach this patient to avoid?

(1) Salt
(2) Sugar
(3) Liquids
(4) Margarine

This item tests your ability to identify information that needs to be taught to a patient. Teaching is performed by the nurse to assist a patient to meet a health need. Mainly, this question tests your ability to recognize that salt is sodium, and therefore, it should be avoided when a patient is receiving a 2-gram sodium diet.

SAMPLE ITEM 6–28

A patient vomits while in the supine position. What should the nurse do?

(1) Position the patient's head between the knees.
(2) Raise the patient to a low-Fowler's position.
(3) Transfer the patient to the bathroom.
(4) Turn the patient to the side.

This item is designed to test your ability to respond appropriately to an event. To answer this question, you need to recognize that it is important to assist the patient to expectorate the vomitus to avoid aspiration. In addition, you need to know that turning the patient on the side is putting the patient in the best position to facilitate drainage of matter from the mouth. Responding to an event by instituting an action is an implementation question.

SAMPLE ITEM 6–29

A patient complains of nausea. What should the nurse do to provide support for this patient?

(1) Give mouth care every hour
(2) Delay meals until the nausea passes
(3) Position the emesis basin in easy reach
(4) Explain that the nausea will lessen with time

TEST SUCCESS: TEST-TAKING TECHNIQUES

Actions that anticipate an event is a type of implementation. The word "provide" in the stem gives you a clue that this is an implementation question. To answer this question correctly, you need to know that a complaint of nausea is a precursor to vomiting and that providing an emesis basin will support the nauseated patient.

SAMPLE ITEM 6–30

The nurse understands that the underlying rationale for turning a patient every 2 hours is to:

  (1) Relieve pressure

  (2) Assess skin condition

  (3) Ensure that skin is dry

  (4) Provide massage to bony prominences

This item tests your ability to identify the correct rationale for a nursing procedure. Relieving pressure is the rationale for regularly turning a patient. To implement safe and effective care, nurses need to have a strong understanding of the scientific rationales for nursing actions.

SAMPLE ITEM 6–31

When administering medications, the safest way for the nurse to identify a patient is to:

  (1) Ask the patient his or her name

  (2) Check the identification bracelet

  (3) Call the patient's name and observe the response

  (4) Double-check the medication administration record

This test item is designed to see if you can correctly identify a step in a procedure. Although more than one of the options might be an action implemented by the nurse, the question is asking you to choose the best answer from all the options offered. In this set of options, checking the identification bracelet is the most reliable and safest method to verify a patient's identity.

SAMPLE ITEM 6–32

To provide aseptically safe perineal care to all female patients, what should the nurse do?

  (1) Use different parts of the washcloth with each stroke

  (2) Apply deodorant spray to the perineal area

  (3) Sprinkle talcum powder on the perineum

  (4) Cleanse the labia in a circular motion

This item tests your ability to identify a step in a procedure based on a specific scientific principle (asepsis). To answer this question correctly, you need to know that medical asepsis is promoted when the spread of microorganisms is limited. Using one area of the washcloth for each stroke when washing the perineum contributes to aseptically safe perineal care. Identifying a step in a procedure is an implementation question.

SAMPLE ITEM 6–33

The Registered Nurse (RN) delegates the implementation of a nasogastric tube feeding to a Licensed Practical Nurse (LPN). Which statement is accurate in terms of the responsibility of the RN?

  (1) The RN should implement the planned care and not delegate.

(2) The LPN should respectfully refuse to implement this care.

(3) The LPN is accountable for his or her own actions.

(4) The RN is responsible for delegated care.

This item tests your ability to recognize that a nurse who delegates care to another nursing staff member is responsible for supervising and evaluating the delivery of that care. This is an important component of implementation and is a concept that may be tested.

SAMPLE ITEM 6–34

When the nurse signs a turning and positioning schedule form, it indicates that the patient:

(1) Received a backrub with lotion

(2) Was turned at the time initialed

(3) Received range-of-motion exercises

(4) Was encouraged to turn to a different position

This question tests your ability to recognize the purpose of a turning and positioning flow sheet. Documenting the care given is a component of the step of implementation.

Evaluation

Evaluation is the fifth and final step of the nursing process. Evaluation is a process that consists of four steps that must be implemented after care is delivered if the effectiveness of the nursing care is to be determined. The evaluation process includes identifying patient responses to care (actual outcomes), comparing a patient's actual outcomes to the expected outcomes, analyzing the factors that affected the outcomes for the purpose of drawing conclusions about the success or failure of specific nursing interventions, and modifying the nursing plan when necessary. Evaluation questions will ask you to:

- Identify the steps in the evaluation process
- Identify whether an outcome is met or not met
- Identify progress or lack of progress toward a goal and/or expected outcome
- Identify the need to modify the plan of care in response to a change in the status of the patient or a plan that is ineffective
- Understand that the process of evaluation is continuous
- Understand that the nursing process is dynamic and cyclical

The critical words within a test item that indicate that the item is focused on evaluation include these: *expected, met, desired, compared, succeeded, failed, achieved, modified, reassess, ineffective, effective, response,* and *evaluate.* See whether you can identify variations of these words indicating evaluation activities in the sample items. Most testing errors occur on evaluation items when options are selected that:

- Do not thoroughly and accurately reassess the patient after care is implemented
- Fail to appropriately cluster new data
- Fail to determine the significance of new data
- Come to inappropriate or inaccurate conclusions when comparing actual outcomes to expected outcomes
- Fail to modify the plan of care in response to the changing needs of the patient or in response to an ineffective plan

IDENTIFY PATIENT RESPONSES (ACTUAL OUTCOMES)

The process of evaluation begins with a reassessment that collects new information. After nursing care is implemented, the patient is reassessed and new clusters of data are identified and their significance determined. In the nursing literature, the term "evaluation" has often been used interchangeably with the term "assessment," which causes confusion. It is important to remember that assessment is only one component in the process of evaluation. The nurse needs to first reassess to identify the patient's responses (actual outcomes). Actual outcomes are the patient's responses to nursing care. These data are then clustered and their significance determined before the patient's actual outcomes can be compared with expected outcomes.

SAMPLE ITEM 6–35

A patient on a bland diet complains about a reduced appetite. What is the MOST effective way for the nurse to determine whether the patient's nutritional needs have been met?

(1) Institute a three day food intake study

(2) Weigh the patient at the end of the week

(3) Request an order for a dietary assessment

(4) Compare a current weight with the weight history

This item is designed to test your ability to identify a common way to evaluate a patient's nutritional status. In this situation, the results of nutritional care are determined by comparing a current weight assessment with a previous weight assessment in an effort to identify any gain or loss in the patient's weight. After a change in status is identified, a conclusion about the effectiveness of care can be determined from the data.

COMPARE ACTUAL OUTCOMES WITH EXPECTED OUTCOMES TO DETERMINE GOAL ACHIEVEMENT

Expected outcomes and goals are the criteria that are established for the evaluation of nursing care. A comparison is made between the patient's actual outcomes and the expected outcomes to determine the effectiveness of nursing interventions. When reassessing the patient after care and comparing this new data with expected outcomes, it is possible to determine which expected outcomes have been achieved and which have not been achieved. The closer the patient's actual outcomes are to the expected outcomes, the more positive the evaluation. When expected outcomes are achieved, the goal is attained. Negative evaluations reflect situations in which the expected outcomes are not achieved. When expected outcomes are not achieved, the goal is not attained. Negative evaluations indicate that an error occurred in the implementation of the nursing process or that nursing care was ineffective. For example: goal—"The patient will be free of a wound infection when discharged 5 days after abdominal surgery"; outcomes—"as evidenced by the presence of a normal white blood cell count, approximation of wound edges with granulated tissue, and vital signs within expected limits." If the patient's actual outcomes meet these expected outcomes, the goal is achieved. If the patient's actual outcomes indicate elevated vital signs, an increased white blood cell count, the presence of purulent exudate, erythema, and/or unapproximated wound edges, the goal is not achieved.

SAMPLE ITEM 6–36

The nurse identifies that the patient understands the teaching about a 2-gram sodium diet when the patient selects which item from a menu?

(1) Milk

(2) Fruit

(3) Celery

(4) Vegetables

This item is designed to test your ability to recognize that of all the options presented, fruit has the least amount of sodium. In addition, the stem is worded in such a way that it requires the nurse to evaluate the correctness of the patient's response. The action described in the stem is an attempt to evaluate the patient's understanding of the teaching provided.

ANALYZE FACTORS THAT AFFECT ACTUAL OUTCOMES OF CARE

After a determination is made of whether or not care is effective, the nurse must come to some conclusions about the potential factors that contributed to the success or failure of the plan of care. If a plan of care is ineffective, the nurse must examine what contributed to its failure. This requires the nurse to start at step 1 of the nursing process, assessment, and work through the entire process again in an attempt to identify why the plan was ineffective. Questions the nurse must ask include these: "Was the original assessment accurate?" "Was the nursing diagnosis accurate, and did it include all the *related-to* factors?" "Was the goal realistic?" "Were the outcomes measurable?" "Were the interventions consistently implemented?" For example, when plans of care fail because *related-to* factors used in the NANDA terminology were incorrectly identified or omitted, nursing strategies generally were inappropriate or were never implemented.

SAMPLE ITEM 6–37

A patient returns to the clinic after taking a 7-day course of antibiotic therapy and is still exhibiting signs of a urinary tract infection. What should be the nurse's initial action?

(1) Arrange for the physician to order a different antibiotic.

(2) Obtain another urine specimen for a culture and sensitivity.

(3) Determine if the patient took the medication as prescribed.

(4) Make an appointment for the patient to be seen by the physician.

This item is designed to test your ability to recognize that the nurse must analyze the factors that influence outcomes of care. Options 1, 2, and 4 can be eliminated because these actions immediately move to an intervention before collecting more information. They may be unnecessary, depending on the information gleaned from the patient. Option 3 is the correct answer because adherence with a medication administration schedule will influence the effectiveness of the medication.

MODIFY THE PLAN OF CARE

After it is determined that a plan of care is ineffective, the plan must be modified. The changes in the plan of care are based on new patient assessments, nursing diagnoses, goals, outcomes, and/or nursing strategies that are designed to address the specific needs of the patient. The modified plan must then be implemented and the whole evaluation process begins again. The process of evaluation is continuous.

SAMPLE ITEM 6–38

A newly admitted patient was provided with a regular diet consisting of three traditional meals a day. After a week it was identified that the patient was eating only approximately 50 percent of the meals and was losing weight. What should the nurse do?

(1) Assist the patient until meals are completed

(2) Schedule several between-meal supplements

(3) Change the plan of care to provide five small meals daily

(4) Secure an order to increase the number of calories provided

This item is designed to test your ability to identify that the nursing plan of care must be changed when care is ineffective. The new actions must be within the legal definition of nursing and address the specific needs of the patient.

Answers and Rationales for Sample Items in Chapter 6

ASSESSMENT

6-1 ① **An assessment must be made to determine if any intervention is necessary to stabilize an injured body part before moving a patient; moving an injured person can exacerbate an injury.**

② Moving an injured patient before assessment and stabilization can exacerbate an injury.

③ Moving an injured patient is unsafe because it can exacerbate an injury.

④ Reporting the incident should be done after the patient is safe; this does not address the need for an immediate assessment of the patient's condition.

6-2 ① This is unsafe because an overbed table is a movable object.

② **Nurses must always assess a patient before having the patient walk to ensure that the patient has the strength to ambulate safely.**

③ This is unsafe because it is concerned with implementing care before the patient is assessed.

④ The patient's strength must be assessed before the transfer to the wheelchair; not all patients using a wheelchair need a vest restraint to maintain safety.

6-3 ① 18 breaths per minute are within the expected range for an adult.

② 20 breaths per minute are within the expected range for an adult.

③ 16 breaths per minute are within the expected range for an adult.

④ **28 breaths per minute are outside the expected range for an adult; expected respirations should be between 14 and 20, effortless, and noiseless. This patient may be experiencing respiratory distress.**

6-4 ① A nurse may permit an alert and capable patient to insert a rectal thermometer; however, if the patient has physical or cognitive deficits, this may not be possible. When a patient self-inserts an electronic thermometer, the handle of the probe must be decontaminated after its use.

② When taking a rectal temperature, the patient can be safely positioned on either the right or left side.

③ The use of an electronic thermometer is not always practical. Electronic thermometers usually are not used in isolation because of the inconvenience related to the need to decontaminate equipment after use.

④ **Lubricating a rectal thermometer is always done to facilitate entry into the rectum; a lubricant reduces resistance when the thermometer is inserted past the anal sphincters.**

6-5 ① **To calculate ideal body weight, the nurse needs to know the patient's height, age, and extent of bone structure.**

② Daily intake reflects the amount of food the patient is ingesting; this information does not contribute to the calculation of ideal body weight.

③ Clothing size is determined by weight and inches reflecting circumference of the chest and waist; this information does not contribute to the calculation of ideal body weight.

④ Determining food preferences supports the patient's right to make choices about care; this information does not contribute to the calculation of ideal body weight.

6-6 ① The primary source is the patient, not the wife.

② A tertiary source provides information outside the patient's frame of reference.

③ The wife is not a subjective source. "Subjective" refers to a type of data; subjective data are collected when the patient shares feelings, perceptions, sensations, and thoughts.

④ **Family members are secondary sources. Secondary sources provide supplemental information about the patient.**

6-7 ① The nurse can examine between the patient's toes and visually verify the presence of sores. Because the sores can be visually verified this information is objective.

② The color of hair can be visually verified and, therefore, is considered objective information.

③ An altered gait can be visually verified and, therefore, is considered objective information.

④ **The experience of pain is subjective information because it can be verified only by the patient.**

6-8 (1) A letter is considered verbal communication; words are written.
(2) **Holding hands is nonverbal communication; a message is transmitted without using words.**
(3) Sounds may or may not communicate meaning; a sound that communicates a meaning is considered verbal communication.
(4) A telephone message is verbal communication; words generally are spoken in a telephone message.

6-9 (1) **The reading should be verified by retaking the blood pressure because the nurse may have made a mistake when originally taking the blood pressure.**
(2) Taking the other vital signs is done after the initial blood pressure is verified; once one vital sign is identified as outside the expected range, all the vital signs should be assessed.
(3) Notifying the nurse in charge may be done after the blood pressure is verified and all the vital signs are taken.
(4) Notifying the physician may eventually be necessary, but it is not the priority.

6-10 (1) Although a thready pulse may indicate a decrease in circulating blood volume and is a sign of dehydration, a straw-colored urine indicates that the patient probably is in fluid balance.
(2) Although decreased skin turgor is associated with dehydration, straw-colored urine is not.
(3) A thready pulse may indicate a decrease in circulating blood volume and is a sign of dehydration. However, a specific gravity of 1.015 is within the expected range of 1.010 to 1.030 and indicates that the patient is in fluid balance.
(4) **Skin turgor refers to normal skin fullness or the ability of the skin and underlying tissue to return to their regular position after being pinched and lifted. When there is decreased skin turgor because of dehydration, the skin remains pinched or "tented" for a longer period of time than well-hydrated skin after it is released. A urine specific gravity of 1.035 reflects concentrated urine, which indicates that the patient has a fluid volume deficit.**

ANALYSIS/NURSING DIAGNOSES

6-11 (1) Receptive aphasia is not associated with the data cluster presented in the stem. Receptive aphasia is an inability to understand either spoken or written language.
(2) **Difficulty swallowing can contribute to a risk for aspiration; it is associated with the data identified in the stem (paralysis of the right side, drooling, slurred speech), and together they present a cluster of information that is significant.**
(3) An inability to perform ADLs is not associated with the data cluster identified in the stem; this is associated with the inability of the patient to provide for self-care.
(4) Incontinence of stool is not associated with the data cluster identified in the stem; this is associated with hygiene needs and supports the fact that the patient is at risk for impaired skin integrity, not aspiration.

6-12 (1) **Patients who are immobilized are subject to increased pressure over bony prominences with a subsequent decrease in circulation to tissues.**
(2) A psychiatric diagnosis is unrelated to the development of pressure ulcers.
(3) Respiratory distress is unrelated to the development of pressure ulcers.
(4) A need for close supervision is unrelated to the development of pressure ulcers.

6-13 (1) Acting-out behaviors commonly reflect anger.
(2) Refusing to believe or accept a situation is reflective of denial.
(3) **Depression commonly is exhibited by patients with adaptations, such as avoiding contact with others, withdrawing, loss of appetite (anorexia), and difficulty falling asleep (insomnia).**
(4) Acceptance is related to the final step of grieving; a patient reconciles and accepts the situation and is at peace.

6-14 (1) The patient is not trying to be left alone. Avoiding others reflects this need.
(2) A patient who wants to be accepted usually will follow directions.

③ The patient is attempting to perform self-care to demonstrate the ability to be self-sufficient and independent.

④ Manipulation is associated with intrigue, scheming, and conniving. This patient's behavior is clear and direct.

6-15 ① Pain generally is not associated with hemorrhage.

② Jaundice is associated with a problem with the liver or biliary system.

③ **Tachycardia, an increased heart rate, is a compensatory mechanism to increase oxygen to all body cells and is associated with hemorrhage.**

④ Hyperthermia, increased body temperature, is unrelated to hemorrhage.

6-16 ① This statement is identifying a need, not a nursing diagnosis.

② This statement is an incorrectly worded nursing diagnosis; a stroke is not something a nurse can diagnose or treat.

③ This statement is a combination of an expected outcome and an intervention, not a nursing diagnosis.

④ **This statement is an appropriately worded nursing diagnosis that uses NANDA terminology; it contains a health problem appropriate for nursing interventions.**

PLANNING

6-17 ① This is correct wording for a goal, but it is unrealistic; it takes 3 to 5 days for a new colostomy to function.

② This is a long-term goal, not a short-term goal.

③ This is the problem statement, the first part of a nursing diagnosis.

④ **This is a short-term goal; it is patient centered, specific, and the word "remain" reflects the time frame.**

6-18 ① **This statement contains an expected outcome. The phrase "50 percent of every meal" is a specific (measurable) outcome. The goal associated with this expected outcome may be "The patient will gain 2 pounds a week."**

② This statement is the problem statement of a nursing diagnosis, not an expected outcome.

③ This statement is the nurse's goal, not an expected outcome.

④ This statement is a planned intervention, not an expected outcome.

6-19 ① Observing the dressing for drainage is important, but it is not the priority.

② **Providing for a patient's oxygenation is essential to maintain life and is always the priority.**

③ Checking for infiltration is important, but it is not the priority.

④ Monitoring vital signs is important, but it is not the priority.

6-20 ① **Washing the hands with soap and water mechanically removes microorganisms from the skin; handwashing is the most effective way to prevent cross-contamination.**

② Usually this is necessary only when a patient has a virulent microorganism.

③ Antibiotics usually are given not to prevent infection, but to treat it.

④ Although foot-operated linen hampers contain and limit the spread of microorganisms, they are not the most effective intervention to prevent cross-contamination.

6-21 ① **An occupied bed is made for a patient on complete bed rest; this patient is not permitted out of bed.**

② All the linens should be changed regularly and whenever necessary.

③ An occupied bed can be made without a mechanical lift just by turning the patient.

④ A patient on bed rest is not allowed out of bed for any reason unless directed by a physician's order.

6-22 ① An obese patient can be transferred out of bed while the linen is changed.

② A patient in a cast can be transferred out of bed while the linen is changed.

③ An immobile patient can be transferred out of bed while the linen is changed.

④ **Patients on bed rest must remain in bed when the linens are changed; this is called "making an occupied bed."**

6-23 ① **The nurse manager has an obligation to ensure that all patients' needs will be appropriately met; this is the only option that addresses this concept.**

② All patients must have their needs met.

③ Providing only essential care does not ensure that appropriate care will be provided; this action will increase anxiety and cause patients to doubt the quality of care being provided.

④ Once the nurse assumes a course of duty, the nurse is responsible for the care that is delivered.

6-24 ① Giving care as quickly as possible will increase the demand on the patient's cardiopulmonary system. This increases activity, which in turn increases oxygen needs; rushing may cause the patient to become upset.

② This does not address the patient's physical needs. The patient needs a full bath because of the diaphoresis.

③ **Providing rest periods conserves energy; this reduces the strain of activity by decreasing the demand for oxygen, which in turn decreases the rate and labor of respirations.**

④ The patient's dyspnea cannot be ignored. Continuing the bath will further jeopardize the patient's status.

6-25 ① When a patient is unresponsive to common nursing interventions for large pressure ulcers, there are other more appropriate resources available for consultation than a plastic surgeon.

② The physical therapist is a specialist in the area of assisting a patient to achieve or maintain physical mobility and is not an expert in providing nursing care.

③ The physician is responsible for the patient's medical care and is not an expert in providing nursing care.

④ **The clinical nurse specialist is educated and prepared to provide expert assistance when other members of the health team seek solutions to difficult clinical nursing problems.**

IMPLEMENTATION

6-26 ① There are other things the nurse must do first.

② Gathering equipment for this procedure is premature.

③ **Inserting an indwelling urinary catheter is a dependent nursing intervention and requires a physician's order that first must be verified by the nurse implementing the order.**

④ Washing the hands is not the first step in this procedure.

6-27 ① **Salt used to season meals contains sodium; sodium must be avoided when a patient is receiving a 2-gram sodium diet.**

② Sugar is avoided when a patient is receiving a reduced-calorie or diabetic diet, not a 2-gram sodium diet.

③ Fluids need to be avoided when the patient has fluid restrictions, not when receiving a 2-gram sodium diet; however, the patient must be alert to avoid fluids that are high in sodium such as diet sodas.

④ Margarine is to be avoided when a patient is receiving a low-fat diet, not a 2-gram sodium diet.

6-28 ① Positioning the head between the knees does not support or protect the vomiting patient.

② The high-Fowler's, not low-Fowler's, position may facilitate the exit of vomitus from the mouth.

③ Vomiting takes energy and can cause the patient to become weak during the transfer.

④ **Turning the patient on the side drains the mouth via gravity and reduces the risk of aspiration.**

6-29 ① Oral hygiene is sufficient every 8 hours and whenever necessary.

② Delaying meals is inappropriate; nausea may be a long-standing problem.

(3) **An emesis basin provides physical and emotional comfort; the emesis basin collects vomitus rather than soiling the bed linens and reduces the patient's concern regarding soiling.**

(4) This action provides false reassurance; the nurse cannot predict when nausea will subside.

6-30

(1) **Turning relieves pressure from body weight and permits circulation to return to the area; prolonged pressure can cause cell death from lack of oxygen and nutrients needed to sustain cellular metabolism.**

(2) Although skin condition should be assessed, it is not the primary reason for turning a patient every 2 hours.

(3) The nurse should ensure the skin is clean and dry, but this is not the primary reason for turning a patient every 2 hours.

(4) Although massage to bony prominences can be done, it is not the primary reason for turning a patient every 2 hours.

6-31

(1) Asking a patient his or her name is unsafe; the patient may be cognitively impaired.

(2) **Checking the identification band is the safest method to identify a patient; it is the most reliable because each patient on admission receives an identification bracelet with his or her name and an identification number.**

(3) Calling the patient's name and observing the response are unsafe interventions since the patient may be cognitively impaired.

(4) Checking the medication administration record will not verify the name of the person.

6-32

(1) **Using different parts of the washcloth with each stroke provides a clean surface for each stroke when washing; it avoids contaminating the meatus with soiled portions of the cloth.**

(2) Applying deodorant spray to the perineal area can be irritating to some patients, and can contribute to the risk of impaired skin integrity; also it does not remove bacteria.

(3) Talcum powder is contraindicated because its application may aerosolize toxins that may be inhaled contributing to lung disease.

(4) Using a circular motion to cleanse the labia is unsafe because it brings soiled matter into contact with the urinary meatus.

6-33

(1) A nurse can delegate tasks to other qualified nursing staff members as long as delegated tasks are supervised and their delivery evaluated.

(2) It is inappropriate to refuse to implement delegated tasks as long as the tasks are within the legal definition of LPN practice and the LPN can safely implement the task. The question is asking which of the options is accurate in terms of the responsibility of the RN, not the LPN.

(3) This is a true statement; however, the question is asking which of the options is accurate in terms of the responsibility of the RN, not the LPN.

(4) **This is an accurate statement; the delegating nurse is responsible for supervising and evaluating the delivery of delegated tasks.**

6-34

(1) Although a backrub with lotion should be implemented when a patient is turned and positioned, it is not the purpose of a turning and positioning form.

(2) **This indicates that turning and positioning were implemented as planned.**

(3) Although the patient should receive range-of-motion exercises, this is not the purpose of a turning and positioning form.

(4) A patient must actually be turned and positioned before the nurse signs the turning and positioning flow sheet; although a patient might be encouraged to turn, it does not mean that the patient was actually turned.

EVALUATION

6-35 ① A food intake diary for 3 days might be done later if initial reassessments are inadequate.

② It is unnecessary to wait until the end of the week; the patient's nutritional status can be assessed immediately by comparing a current weight with the patient's weight history.

③ It is not necessary to request a dietary assessment. The patient's nutritional status can be done easily and immediately by the nurse.

④ **Measuring a patient's weight and comparing the weight with a previous weight is a quick and easy way to determine a patient's nutritional status.**

6-36 ① Milk has more sodium than the nutrient in the correct option.

② **Fruit has the least amount of sodium compared to the other options.**

③ Celery has more sodium than the nutrient in the correct option.

④ Vegetables have more sodium than the nutrient in the correct options.

6-37 ① Arranging for the physician to order a different antibiotic is inappropriate before collecting additional data associated with the present plan of care; this may be necessary later.

② Obtaining another urine sample for a culture and sensitivity is inappropriate before collecting additional data about the present plan of care.

③ **Determining adherence to the medical regimen is the priority. Antibiotics must be taken routinely and consistently to maintain adequate blood levels of the drug.**

④ Making an appointment for the patient is inappropriate before collecting additional data associated with the present plan of care.

6-38 ① Patients must not be forced to eat all their meals; the portions may be too large for an anorectic patient to ingest.

② Adding between-meal supplements is a dependent intervention and requires a physician's order.

③ **Arranging for five small meals daily is an independent intervention and does not require a physician's order. Small, frequent feedings spread the meals throughout the day and provide a volume that is not as overwhelming as a full meal.**

④ The problem is not the number of calories provided on the tray but the amount of food the patient is able to ingest at any one time.

Test-Taking Techniques

Performing well on nursing questions requires both roots and wings. The previous chapters provided you with roots by giving you information about formulating a positive mental attitude, using critical thinking, employing time-management strategies, exploring a variety of study skills, and developing an understanding of the multiple-choice question and the nursing process. This chapter attempts to provide you with the wings necessary to "fly through" multiple-choice questions. Flying through multiple-choice questions has nothing to do with speed; it relates to being test wise and able to navigate through complex information with ease.

Tests in nursing involve complex information that has depth and breadth. In addition to having its own body of knowledge, nursing draws from a variety of disciplines, such as sociology, psychology, and anatomy and physiology. To perform well on a nursing examination, you must understand and integrate the subject matter. Nothing can replace effective study habits or knowledge about the subject being tested. However, being test wise can maximize the application of the information you possess. Being test wise entails specific techniques related to individual question analysis and general techniques related to conquering the challenge of an examination. One rationale for learning how to use these techniques is to provide you with skills that increase your command over the testing situation. If you are in control, you will maintain a positive attitude and increase your chances of selecting the correct answers. When you have knowledge and are test wise, you should fly through a test by gliding and soaring, rather than by flapping and fluttering.

Specific Test-Taking Techniques

A specific test-taking technique is a strategy that uses skill and forethought to analyze a test item before selecting an answer. A technique is not a gimmick but a method of examining a question with consideration and thoughtfulness to help you select the correct answer. When an item has four options, the chance of selecting the correct answer is one out of four, or 25 percent. When you eliminate one distractor, the chance of selecting the correct answer is one out of three, or 33.3 percent. If you are able to throw out two distractors, the chance of selecting the correct answer is one out of two, or 50 percent. Each time you successfully eliminate a distractor, you dramatically increase your chances of correctly answering the question.

Before you attempt to answer a question, break the question down into its components. First, read the stem. What is it actually asking? It may be helpful to paraphrase the stem to focus on its content. Then, try to answer the question being asked in your own words before looking at the options. Often, one of the options will be similar to your answer. Then examine the other options and try to identify the correct answer. If you know, understand, and can apply the information being tested, you can often identify the correct answer.

However, do not be tempted to select an option too quickly, without careful thought. An option may contain accurate information, but it may not be correct because it does not answer the question asked in the stem. Be careful. Each option deserves equal consideration.

Use test-taking techniques for every question. The use of test-taking techniques becomes more important when you are unsure of the answer, because each distractor that you are able to eliminate will increase your chances of selecting the correct answer. Most nursing students are able to reduce the number of plausible answers to two. However, contrary to popular belief, multiple-choice questions in nursing have only one correct answer. Use everything in your arsenal to conquer the multiple-choice question test: effective studying, a positive mental attitude, and, last but not least, test-taking techniques.

The correct answers for the sample items in this chapter and the rationales for all the options are at the end of the chapter.

IDENTIFY KEY WORDS IN THE STEM THAT INDICATE NEGATIVE POLARITY

Read the stem slowly and carefully. Look for key words such as **not, except, never, contraindicated, unacceptable, avoid, unrelated, violate,** and **least.** These words indicate negative polarity, and the question being asked is probably concerned with what is false. Some words that have negative polarity are not as obvious as others. A negatively worded stem asks you to identify an exception, detect an error, or recognize nursing interventions that are unacceptable or contraindicated. If you read a stem and all the options appear correct, reread the stem because you may have missed a key negative word. These words are sometimes brought to your attention by an underline (not), italics (*except*), boldface (**never**), or capitals (VIOLATE). Many nursing examinations avoid questions with negative polarity. However, examples of these items are included for your information.

SAMPLE ITEM 7–1

Which action violates medical asepsis when the nurse makes an occupied bed?

(1) Wearing gloves when changing the linen
(2) Returning unused linen to the linen closet
(3) Using the old top sheet for the new bottom sheet
(4) Tucking clean linen against the frame of the bed

The key term in this stem is *violates*. The stem is asking you to identify the option that does **not** follow correct medical aseptic technique. If you misread the stem and were looking for the answer that indicated correct medical aseptic technique, there would be more than one correct answer. When this happens, reread the stem for a word with negative polarity. In this item, you had to be particularly careful because the word *violate* is not emphasized for your attention.

SAMPLE ITEM 7–2

A patient is receiving a low-sodium diet. Before discharge, the nurse should teach the patient to *avoid*:

(1) Stewed fruit
(2) Luncheon meats
(3) Whole-grain cereal
(4) Green, leafy vegetables

The key word in this stem is *avoid*. The stem is asking you to select the food that a patient receiving a low-sodium diet should **not** eat. If you misread the question and were looking for foods that are permitted on a low-sodium diet, there would be more than one correct answer. When there appears to be more than one correct answer, reread the stem for a key negative word that you may have missed.

SAMPLE ITEM 7–3

When rubbing a patient's back, the nurse should NEVER:

(1) Knead the skin

(2) Wipe off excess lotion

(3) Use continuous strokes

(4) Apply pressure over the vertebrae

The key word in this stem is NEVER. The stem is asking you to identify which option is **not** an acceptable practice associated with a backrub. If you missed the word NEVER and were looking for what the nurse should do for a backrub, there would be more than one correct answer. This should alert you to the fact that you may have missed a key negative word.

IDENTIFY KEY WORDS IN THE STEM THAT SET A PRIORITY

Read the stem carefully while looking for key words such as **first, initially, best, priority, safest,** and **most.** These words modify what is being asked. This type of question requires you to put a value on each option and then place them in rank order. If the question asks what the nurse should do first, what the initial action by the nurse should be, or what the best response is, then rank the options in order of importance from 1 to 4 with the most desirable option as number 1 and the least desirable option as number 4. The correct answer is the option that you ranked number 1. If you are having difficulty ranking the options, eliminate the option that you believe is most wrong among all the options. Next, eliminate the option you believe is most wrong from among the remaining three options. At this point, you are down to two options, and your chance of selecting the correct answer is 50 percent. When key words such as "most important" are used, frequently all of the options may be appropriate nursing care for the situation. However, only one of the options is the most important. When all the options appear logical for the situation, reread the stem to identify a key word that asks you to place a priority on the options. These words occasionally are emphasized by an <u>underline</u>, *italics*, **boldface,** or CAPITALS.

SAMPLE ITEM 7–4

The nurse is assigned to care for a patient who is incontinent of urine and stool. What should the nurse apply to *best* protect this patient's skin?

(1) An incontinence pad

(2) A petroleum jelly

(3) Talcum powder

(4) Cornstarch

The key term in this stem is *best.* Each of these options is something a nurse might do for the incontinent patient. The stem is asking you to place a value on each option and decide which nursing intervention **best** protects the skin when compared to the other options. If you are having difficulty ranking these options, eliminate the option that is most wrong. Although an incontinence pad absorbs urine and is often used for incontinent patients, it holds excreta next to the skin and actually promotes skin breakdown. Eliminate option 1. Continue to eliminate options you believe are wrong, and then make your final selection of the correct answer.

SAMPLE ITEM 7–5

What should be the nurse's <u>first</u> action before administering an enema?

(1) Verify the physician's order.

(2) Collect the appropriate equipment.

(3) Arrange for the bathroom to be empty.

(4) Inform the patient about the procedure.

The key word in this stem is <u>first</u>. Each of these options includes a step that is part of the procedure for administering an enema. You must decide which option is the first step among the four options presented. Before you can teach a patient, collect equipment, or actually administer the enema, you need to know the type of enema ordered. The type of enema will influence the other steps of the procedure. If option 1 were different, such as "Use medical asepsis to dispose of contaminated articles," the correct answer among these four options would be option 4. You can choose the first step of a procedure only from among the options presented.

SAMPLE ITEM 7-6

A patient has significant short-term memory loss and does not remember the primary nurse from day to day. When the patient asks, "Who are you?" what is the most appropriate response?

(1) "You know me. I take care of you every day."

(2) "Don't worry. I'm the same nurse you had yesterday."

(3) Say nothing, because it probably will upset the patient.

(4) State your name and say, "I am the nurse caring for you."

The key words in this stem are *most appropriate*. Potential responses by the nurse are the options in this question. You are asked to select the **best** or **most suitable** response from among the four options presented. You may dislike all of the statements. You may even think of a response that you personally prefer to the offered options. You cannot rewrite the question. You must select your answer from the options presented in the item. The words "most appropriate" are not highlighted in this item, and therefore you must be diligent when reading the stem.

Answering a test question that asks you to establish a priority (which is "most important," "best," "initial," and "first") requires you to make a decision using clinical judgment. It requires you to use perceptual, inferential, and/or diagnostic judgment to arrive at the correct answer based on the data in the question and options. To do this, you must draw upon your knowledge of theory, concepts, principles, and nursing standards of practice. The student who has a strong foundation of knowledge and who is a critical thinker is best equipped to arrive at the correct answer. For additional information about making clinical decisions and types of clinical judgments, refer to Chapter 2, Critical Thinking, in the section titled Clinical Judgments.

A strategy you can draw on to help you answer priority questions is to refer to basic guiding theories that are part of the foundation of nursing. Maslow's Hierarchy of Needs, The Nursing Process, Kübler-Ross's Theory of Death and Dying, Man as a Unified Being, the theory that the patient is the center of the health team, teaching/learning theory, emotional support and communication theory, and the ABCs (airway, breathing, and circulation), to name a few, present clear parameters of practice that are the building blocks of the foundation of nursing practice. Keeping these theories in mind when answering test questions, you should recognize that:

- Physiologic needs generally need to be met first before higher-level needs.
- Disbelief and denial are generally a person's first response to news of a loss or anticipated loss.
- Meeting the needs of the patient come first over other tasks.
- Patient readiness to learn must be assessed first before designing a teaching program.
- A patient's emotional status must be assessed as part of the first step in the nursing process.
- Nurses need to use interviewing techniques to effectively communicate in a nonthreatening way with patients.
- The nurse must deliver care in a nonjudgmental manner.
- Maintaining a patient's airway is always a priority.
- The patient's safety is always a priority.
- A thorough assessment must be completed before other steps in the nursing process.

Choosing which theory or principle to draw on when answering a test question comes with practice. You first have to identify "what is happening" and "what should I do." You then have to identify which theory or principle applies best in the scenario presented in the question in light of the options offered. Practice the questions in Chapter 11 that ask you to set a priority and study the rationales for the right and wrong answers. Priority questions are identified by the statement, "Identify the word in the stem that sets a priority" that appears in the TEST-TAKING TIP after the question. This will help you build a body of knowledge associated with determining what the nurse should do first in different clinical situations presented in practice questions.

IDENTIFY CLUES IN THE STEM

Generally, the stem is short and contains only the information needed to make it clear and specific. Therefore, a word or phrase in the stem may provide a hint for choosing the correct answer. A clue is the intentional or unintentional use of a word or phrase that leads you to the correct answer. Most often a clue is a word or phrase that is important because of its relationship to another word or phrase in the stem (see Sample Item 7–7). Sometimes a word or phrase in the stem is significant because it is similar to or a paraphrase of a word or phrase in the correct answer (see Sample Item 7–8). Occasionally a word or phrase in the stem is identical to a word or phrase in the correct answer and is called a **clang association** (see Sample Item 7–9). Every word in the stem is important, but some words are more significant than others. The identification of important words and the analysis of the significance of these words in relation to the stem and the options require critical thinking.

SAMPLE ITEM 7–7

To meet a patient's basic physiologic needs according to Maslow's Hierarchy of Needs, what should the nurse do?

(1) Pull the curtain when the patient is on a bedpan.

(2) Maintain the patient in functional alignment.

(3) Respond to the call light immediately.

(4) Raise both side rails on the bed.

An important word in the stem is *physiologic*. It is an intentional use of a word to specifically limit consideration to one aspect of Maslow's theory.

SAMPLE ITEM 7–8

What should the nurse do to help meet a patient's self-esteem needs?

(1) Encourage the patient to perform self-care when able.

(2) Suggest that the family visit the patient more often.

(3) Anticipate needs before the patient requests help.

(4) Assist the patient with bathing.

An important word in the stem is *self-esteem*. The word "self-esteem" is similar to the word "self-care." Thoughtfully examine option 1. An option that incorporates words that are similar to words in the stem is often the correct answer. In addition, the word "self-esteem" in the stem is the intentional use of a word that focuses on one aspect of Maslow's theory. This question exemplifies the use of two clues in the stem when answering a question.

SAMPLE ITEM 7–9

What should the nurse do to meet a patient's basic physical needs?

(1) Pull the curtain when providing care

(2) Answer the call bell immediately

(3) Administer physical hygiene

(4) Obtain vital signs

An important word in the stem is *physical*. It is a clue that should provide a hint that option 3 is the correct answer. The use of the word "physical" in both the stem and the option is called a *clang association*. It is the repetitious use of a word. Examine option 3 because when a clang association occurs, it is often the correct answer.

IDENTIFY THE CENTRAL PERSON IN THE QUESTION

Test questions usually require the nurse to respond to the needs of a patient. When a stem is limited to just the patient and the nurse, the patient is almost always the central person in the question. However, some questions focus on the needs of others, such as a child, parent, spouse, or roommate. To select the correct option, you have to identify the central (significant) person in the stem. The significant person is the person who is to receive the care. Sometimes, in addition to the patient, a variety of people are included in the stem. The inclusion of others may set the stage for the question or test your ability to discriminate. These people also may distract you from who is actually the significant person in the stem. Therefore, to answer the question accurately, you must determine WHO is the central person in the question.

SAMPLE ITEM 7–10

A nurse will be going on vacation. To involve the patient in the excitement, what is the <u>best</u> thing the nurse should say?

    (1) "Do you want to hear about the plans for my vacation?"

    (2) "Tell me about some of your past vacations."

    (3) "I'll bring the brochures for you to see."

    (4) "What do you think about vacations?"

There are two people in this stem, the patient and the nurse. There are two clues in the stem. The first clue is "involve the patient." To involve the patient, the patient has to be active. Therefore, options 1 and 3 can be eliminated because they focus on the nurse, who is not the central person in the question. The second clue is the word <u>best</u>. The word <u>best</u> is asking you to set a priority. More than one option may include appropriate nursing care, but only one is the best action. Options 2 and 4 include appropriate nursing care. However, option 2 requires a more detailed response than option 4. Reminiscing involves more than just giving an opinion.

SAMPLE ITEM 7–11

A patient who has experienced the surgical removal of a breast (mastectomy) says to the nurse, "My husband can't look at my incision and hasn't suggested having sex since my surgery." What should be the initial action of the nurse?

    (1) Arrange to speak with the husband about his concerns.

    (2) Plan to teach the husband that the wife needs his support.

    (3) Explore the patient's feelings about her husband's behavior.

    (4) Make an appointment with Reach for Recovery for the patient.

There are three people in this stem: the patient, the husband, and the nurse. There are two clues in the stem. The first clue is the quoted statement by the patient about her husband's behavior. The second clue is the word *initial*. The word "initial" is asking you to set a priority. The situation may require one or more of these responses, but only one of them should be done first. The patient's statement reflects the patient's concern. Addressing the patient's concern should come first. The patient is the central person in this question, not the husband. Options 1 and 2 focus on the husband, who is not the central person in this question and can be eliminated. In option 4, the nurse is using a referral to sidestep the issues involved and avoid professional responsibility.

SAMPLE ITEM 7–12

A patient is friendly, has many visitors, and appears happy. However, when the patient's daughter visits, the patient cries and complains of pain. When the daughter becomes upset, the nurse should:

(1) Explore the situation with the daughter

(2) Encourage the patient to be more positive

(3) Continue to observe this situation from a distance

(4) Tell the daughter that the patient usually does not cry

There are many people in this situation: visitors, the patient, the daughter, and the nurse. The question asks the nurse to follow one course of action when the daughter becomes upset. The phrase "when the daughter becomes upset" shifts the focus of the question to the daughter. Options 1 and 4 focus on the daughter. By eliminating two options (options 2 and 3), you have increased your chances of getting this question correct to 50 percent.

IDENTIFY PATIENT-CENTERED OPTIONS

Nursing is a profession that is involved with providing both physical and emotional care to people. Therefore, the focus of the nurse's concern should be the patient. Items that test your ability to be patient centered tend to explore patient feelings, identify patient preferences, empower the patient, afford the patient choices, or in some other way put emphasis on the patient. Because the patient is the center of the health team, the patient usually is the priority.

SAMPLE ITEM 7–13

When assisting a patient who recently had an above-the-knee amputation to transfer into a chair, the patient starts to cry and says, "I am useless with only one leg." What is the nurse's best response?

(1) "You still have one good leg."

(2) "Losing a leg can be very difficult."

(3) "A prosthesis will make a big difference."

(4) "You'll feel better when you can use crutches."

Option 2 is patient centered. It focuses on the patient's feelings by using the interviewing technique of reflection. Option 1 denies the patient's feelings, and options 3 and 4 provide false reassurance. When a patient's feelings are ignored or minimized, the nurse is not being patient centered. To be patient centered, the nurse should concentrate on the patient's feelings or concerns.

SAMPLE ITEM 7–14

An oriented patient states, "I always forget the questions I want to ask when my doctor visits me." What is the nurse's best response?

(1) Remind the patient of the doctor's next visit

(2) Suggest that a family member question the doctor

(3) Give the patient materials to write down questions

(4) Offer to stay with the patient when the doctor visits

Option 3 is patient centered. It focuses on the patient's ability, fosters independence, and empowers the patient. Option 1 does not address the patient's concern, and options 2 and 4 promote dependence, which can lower self-esteem. Avoiding patient concerns and promoting dependence are actions that are not patient centered. To be patient centered, the nurse should encourage self-care.

SAMPLE ITEM 7–15

What should the nurse do first when combing a female patient's hair?

(1) Moisten the hair with tap water

(2) Apply a hair conditioner to the hair

(3) Begin at the roots and comb with long strokes

(4) Ask the patient how she prefers to wear her hair

Option 4 is patient centered. It allows choices and supports the person as an individual. Options 1, 2, and 3 do not take into consideration patient preferences. Option 3 also is wrong because combing should begin at the ends of the hair with combing progressively moving toward the roots as tangles are removed. A procedure that is begun before determining patient preferences or teaching the patient about the procedure is not patient centered. The Patient's Bill of Rights mandates that the patient has a right to considerate and respectful care and to receive information before the start of any procedure and/or treatment.

SAMPLE ITEM 7–16

A patient enjoys television programs about animals. After one of these programs, the patient sadly talks about a beloved cat who died. What should be the nurse's initial response?

(1) Tell the patient a story about a cat

(2) Ask the patient to share more about the cat

(3) Hang a picture of a cat in the patient's room

(4) Obtain a book about cats for the patient from the library

Option 2 is patient centered. It encourages the patient to communicate further. Options 1, 3, and 4 may eventually be done because they take into consideration the patient's interest in cats. However, they should not be the initial actions because they do not focus on the patient's feelings at this point in time. The nurse is being patient centered when encouraging additional communication and verbalization of feelings and concerns from the patient.

IDENTIFY SPECIFIC DETERMINERS IN OPTIONS

A specific determiner is a word or statement that conveys a thought or concept that has no exceptions. Words such as **just, always, never, all, every, none,** and **only** are absolute and easy to identify. They place limits on a statement that generally is considered correct. Statements that use all-inclusive terms frequently represent broad generalizations that usually are false. Frequently these options are incorrect and can be eliminated. However, some absolutes, such as "all patients should be treated with respect," are correct. Because there are few absolutes in this world, options that contain specific determiners should be examined carefully. Be discriminating.

SAMPLE ITEM 7–17

The nurse is giving a patient a bed bath. How can the nurse best improve the patient's circulation during the bath?

(1) Apply soap to the washcloth

(2) Keep the patient covered

(3) Use only hot water

(4) Use firm strokes

In option 3 the word *only* is a specific determiner. It allows for no exceptions. Hot water can burn the skin and also is contraindicated for patients with sensitive skin such as children, older adults, and people with dermatologic problems. Because option 3 allows for no exceptions, it can be eliminated as a viable option.

SAMPLE ITEM 7–18

When providing perineal care for patients, by what action can nurses most appropriately protect themselves from microorganisms?

    (1) Washing their hands before giving care

    (2) Wearing clean gloves during perineal care

    (3) Discarding the contaminated water in the toilet

    (4) Encouraging patients to provide all of their own care

In option 4 the word *all* is a specific determiner. It is a word that obviously includes everything. Expecting patients to provide all of their own care is unreasonable, unrealistic, and could be unsafe. Option 4 can be eliminated. This raises your chances of choosing the correct answer because you have to choose from among only three options rather than four.

SAMPLE ITEM 7–19

A patient complains that the elastic straps of the oxygen face mask feels too tight. The nurse should:

    (1) Explain that the mask must always stay firmly in place.

    (2) Replace the face mask with a nasal cannula.

    (3) Pad the straps with gauze.

    (4) Adjust the elastic straps.

In option 1 the word *always* is a specific determiner. It is an absolute term that places limits on a statement that might otherwise be true. This option can be eliminated. By deleting option 1, the chances of your selecting the correct answer become 33.3 rather than 25 percent.

IDENTIFY OPPOSITES IN OPTIONS

Sometimes an item contains two options that are the opposite of each other. They can be single words that reflect extremes on a continuum, or they can be statements that convey converse messages. When opposites appear in the options, they must be given serious consideration. One of them will be the correct answer, or they both can be eliminated from consideration. When one of the opposites is the correct answer, you are being asked to differentiate between two responses that incorporate extremes of a concept or principle. When options are opposites, more often than not, one of them is the correct answer. When the opposites are distractors, they are attempting to divert your attention from the correct answer. If you correctly evaluate opposite options, you can increase your chances of selecting the correct answer to 50 percent because you have reduced the plausible options to two.

SAMPLE ITEM 7–20

The nurse understands that the progress of growth and development in all older adults:

    (1) Slips backward

    (2) Moves forward

    (3) Becomes slower

    (4) Becomes stagnant

Options 1 and 2 are opposites. They need to be considered carefully in relation to each other and then in relation to the other options. These options are the reverse sides of a concept, movement in relation to growth and development. Options 3 and 4, although true for some individuals, are not true statements about *all* older adults as indicated in the stem. You now must select between options 1 and 2. Option 2 is the correct answer. By focusing on options 1 and 2 and then progressively examining and deleting options 3 and 4, you have systematically scrutinized this item.

SAMPLE ITEM 7–21

The physician orders anti-embolism stockings for a patient. When should the nurse apply the anti-embolism stockings?

(1) While the patient is still in bed

(2) Once the patient complains of leg pain

(3) When the patient's feet become edematous

(4) After the patient gets out of bed in the morning

Options 1 and 4 are opposites. Examine these options first. They are contrary to each other in relation to before or after an event, getting out of bed. Now assess options 2 and 3. These options expect the nurse to apply anti-embolism stockings after a problem exists. The purpose of these stockings is to foster venous return, thereby preventing edema and discomfort. Options 2 and 3 can be omitted from further consideration. The final selection is between options 1 and 4. You have increased your chances of correctly answering the question from 25 to 50 percent. Because edema occurs when the feet are dependent, anti-embolism stockings should not be applied after the patient gets out of bed. You have arrived at the correct answer, option 1, using a methodical approach.

SAMPLE ITEM 7–22

The physician orders a wrist restraint for a patient on bed rest. The nurse should tie the restraint to the:

(1) Side rails

(2) Footboard

(3) Bed frame

(4) Headboard

Options 2 and 4 are opposites. Consider these options first in relation to securing a restraint. These options are the opposite ends of a hospital bed. Neither option is more appropriate than the other. They are probably both distractors. Now examine options 1 and 3. Side rails are movable, and a restraint must be applied to something that is stationary. Now consider option 3. The bed frame is immovable. Options 1, 2, and 4 can be eliminated, and option 3 is the correct answer. In this question, the options that are opposites (2 and 4) are distractors and can be eliminated.

SAMPLE ITEM 7–23

In relation to extracellular body fluids, normal saline is:

(1) Hypertonic

(2) Hypotonic

(3) Isotonic

(4) Acidotic

Options 1 and 2 are opposites. Appraise these words in relation to each other and their relationship to body fluids and normal saline. They are extremes in the concentration of solutes. Because normal saline is equal to body fluids in the concentration of solutes, these options are probably distractors. Now examine options 3 and 4. Body fluids have a neutral pH (between 7.35 and 7.45). Acidosis, which is referred to in option 4, has a pH below 7.35. Option 4 can be deleted from consideration. In this question, the options that are opposites (1 and 2) are distractors and can be eliminated.

IDENTIFY EQUALLY PLAUSIBLE OR UNIQUE OPTIONS

Sometimes items contain two or more options that are similar. It is difficult to choose between two similar options because they are comparable. One option is no better or worse than the other option in relation to the statement presented in the stem. Usually equally plausible options are distractors and can be eliminated from consideration. You have now improved your chances of selecting the correct answer to 50 percent. If you find three equally plausible options when initially examining the options, the fourth option probably will be different from the others and appear unique. Children's activity books and a popular children's television program present a game based on this concept. Four pictures are presented, and the child is asked to pick out the one that is different. "Which one of these is not like the others? Which one of these is not the same?" For example, the picture contains three types of fruit and one vegetable, and the child is asked to identify which one is different. The correct answer to a test item can sometimes be identified by using this concept of similarities and differences.

SAMPLE ITEM 7–24

What should the nurse do to most effectively help meet a patient's basic safety and security needs?

(1) Serve adequate food

(2) Provide sufficient fluid

(3) Place the call bell near the patient

(4) Store the patient's valuables in the hospital safe

Options 1 and 2 are similar because they both provide nutrients. They are equally plausible when compared to each other and particularly when assessed in relation to the concepts of safety and security. These options are distractors and can be eliminated from consideration. By just having to choose between options 3 and 4, you have raised your chances of correctly answering the question to 50 percent.

SAMPLE ITEM 7–25

How can the nurse best promote circulation when providing a backrub?

(1) Place the patient in the prone position

(2) Use moisturizing cream

(3) Apply Keri lotion

(4) Knead the skin

Options 2 and 3 use substances when performing the backrub. Because no specifics about the patient's adaptations—such as extent of perspiration or dryness of skin—are provided, these two options are comparable. Because equally plausible options are usually distractors, you can delete these options. Now evaluate the remaining options. One of them is the correct answer.

SAMPLE ITEM 7–26

What is the main reason why passive range-of-motion (PROM) exercises are performed?

(1) Increase endurance

(2) Prevent loss of mobility

(3) Strengthen muscle tone

(4) Maximize muscle atrophy

Options 1, 3, and 4 all include words (increase, strengthen, and maximize) that address improvement of something (endurance, muscle tone, and atrophy). They are alike. Option 2 is different. It prevents something from happening, loss of mobility. Option 2 is unique when compared to the presentation of the other options, and it should be given careful consideration. Even if you do not know the definition of "atrophy" and do not recognize that the loss of muscle mass should not be maximized, you can still use the test-taking technique of identifying similar and unique options. "Which one of these is not like the others? Which one of these is not the same?"

Immediately before performing any patient procedure, the nurse should plan to:

(1) Shut the door

(2) Wash the hands

(3) Close the curtain

(4) Drape the patient

Options 1, 3, and 4 are similar in that they all somehow enclose the patient and provide for patient privacy. They are all plausible interventions when providing patient care. It is difficult to choose the most correct answer from among these three options. Option 2 is different. It relates to microbiologic safety rather than emotional safety. Because this option is unique when compared to the other options, it should be thoroughly examined in relation to the stem because it is likely to be the correct answer.

IDENTIFY THE GLOBAL OPTION

The global option is more comprehensive and general than the other options. Although unspoken, the global option may include under its mantle a specific concept identified in one or more of the other options. Identifying global options is similar to identifying unique options. The global option usually is a broad general statement, whereas the three distractors are specific. You must pick out the option that is different. "Which one of these is not like the others? Which one of these is not the same?"

SAMPLE ITEM 7–28

The most effective way for the nurse to prevent the spread of infection in a nursing home is by:

(1) Administering antibiotics to sick patients

(2) Limiting the spread of microorganisms

(3) Isolating residents who are sick

(4) Keeping all unit doors closed

Options 1, 3, and 4 are all incorrect as indicated in the rationales. However, if you did not know that they were incorrect and you just examined the four options, you should have noticed that options 1, 3, and 4 all identify specific actions while option 2 is broad and general and is different from the other options.

SAMPLE ITEM 7–29

When the nurse is repositioning a patient, what is the *most* important principle of body mechanics?

(1) Elevating the arms on pillows

(2) Maintaining functional alignment

(3) Preventing external rotation of the hips

(4) Placing a small pillow under the lumbar curvature

Options 1, 3, and 4 is something you might do to support a patient in a specific position. However, option 2 is comprehensive and broad and identifies something the nurse should do when positioning all patients regardless of the specific position.

IDENTIFY DUPLICATE FACTS AMONG THE OPTIONS

Sometimes items are designed so that each option contains two or more facts. Usually identical or similar facts appear in at least two of the four options. If you identify a fact as incorrect, you can eliminate all the options that contain this fact. By deleting distractors, you increase your chances of selecting the correct answer.

SAMPLE ITEM 7–30

A patient has a vest restraint. While making this patient's occupied bed, what must the nurse do to promote patient safety?

(1) Keep the vest restraint tied and lower both side rails

(2) Keep the vest restraint tied and lower one side rail

(3) Untie the vest restraint and lower both side rails

(4) Untie the vest restraint and lower one side rail

This item is testing two concepts: whether a vest restraint should be tied or untied when providing direct care, and whether one or both side rails should be lowered when providing direct care. If you only know the fact that the side rail should be lowered just on the side on which you are working, you can eliminate options 1 and 3. If you only know the fact that a vest restraint can be untied when the nurse is at the bedside providing direct care, you can eliminate options 1 and 2. In either case, you can eliminate two options as distractors, and you have raised your chances of selecting the correct answer from 25 to 50 percent.

SAMPLE ITEM 7–31

The physician orders a 2-gram sodium diet. Which group of nutrients are most appropriate for this diet?

(1) Fruit, vegetables, and bread

(2) Hot dogs, mustard, and pickles

(3) Hamburger, onions, and ketchup

(4) Luncheon meats, rolls, and vegetables

This item is testing your knowledge about the sodium content of foods. If you recognize that hot dogs and luncheon meats are both processed foods that are high in sodium, you can eliminate options 2 and 4. If you recognize that ketchup and mustard are both condiments that are high in sodium, you can delete options 2 and 3. By knowing either fact, you can reduce the final selection to between two options. The similarities between these options are less clear than if the parts were identical, but the technique of identifying duplicate facts in options can still be used.

SAMPLE ITEM 7–32

When monitoring a patient who is at risk for hemorrhage, the nurse should assess the patient for:

(1) Warm, dry skin; hypotension; bounding pulse

(2) Hypertension; bounding pulse; cold, clammy skin

(3) Weak, thready pulse; hypertension; warm, dry skin

(4) Hypotension; cold, clammy skin; weak, thready pulse

This item is testing your knowledge about patient adaptations associated with hemorrhage. Three patient adaptations are presented: the condition of the skin, the blood pressure, and the characteristic of the pulse. Even if you know only one of these facts about hemorrhage, you can reduce your final selection to between two options. If you know that hypotension is associated with hemorrhage, you can eliminate options 2 and 3. If you know that cold, clammy skin is related to hemorrhage, you can delete options 1 and 3. If you know that a weak, thready pulse is associated with hemorrhage, you can eliminate options 1 and 2. If you know only one or two of the facts presented, you can maximize your chance of correctly answering this type of item. Options that have two or three parts work to your advantage if you use the technique of identifying duplicate facts in options.

IDENTIFY OPTIONS THAT DENY PATIENT FEELINGS, CONCERNS, AND NEEDS

Because nurses are human and caring, and primarily want their patients to get well, they often assume the role of deliverer, champion, protector, or savior. However, by inappropriately adopting these roles, nurses often diminish patient concerns, provide false reassurance, and/or cut off further patient communication. To be a patient advocate, the nurse cannot always be a Pollyanna. Pollyanna, the heroine of stories by Eleanor Hodgman Porter, was a person of irrepressible optimism who found good in everything. Sometimes nurses must focus on the negative rather than the positive, acknowledge that everything may not have the desired outcome, and recognize patients' feelings as a priority. Options that imply everything will be all right deny patients' feelings, change the subject raised by the patient, encourage the patient to be cheerful, or transfer nursing responsibility to other members of the health team usually are distractors and can be eliminated from consideration.

SAMPLE ITEM 7–33

The day before surgery for a hysterectomy, a patient says to the nurse, "I am worried that I might die tomorrow." What is the nurse's most appropriate response?

(1) "It is really routine surgery."

(2) "You need to tell your doctor about this."

(3) "The thought of dying can be frightening."

(4) "Most people who have this surgery survive."

Options 1 and 4 minimize the patient's concerns because these messages imply that there is nothing to worry about; the surgery is routine and most patients survive. In option 2 the nurse avoids the opportunity to encourage further discussion of the patient's feelings and surrenders this responsibility to the physician. After collecting more information, the nurse should inform the physician of the patient's concern about death. Options 1, 2, and 4 deny the patient's feelings and can be eliminated because they are distractors. Option 3 is the correct answer because it encourages the patient to focus on the expressed feelings about death.

SAMPLE ITEM 7–34

After surgery, a patient complains of mild incisional pain while performing deep-breathing and coughing exercises. What is the nurse's best response?

(1) "Each day it will hurt less and less."

(2) "This is an expected response after surgery."

(3) "With a pillow, apply pressure against the incision."

(4) "I will get the pain medication the physician ordered."

Option 1 is a Pollyanna-like response that may provide false reassurance. The nurse does not know that the pain will get less and less for this patient. Option 1 can be deleted from consideration. Although option 2 is a true statement, it cuts off communication because it diminishes the patient's concern and does not explore a solution for minimizing the pain. Option 2 can be eliminated as a distractor. You now must choose between options 3 and 4. The stem indicates that the patient has pain when coughing; the pain is not continuous. Option 4 can be deleted because it is inappropriate to administer an analgesic at this time. Mild pain should subside after the activity is completed. The correct answer is option 3 because it recognizes the mild pain and offers an intervention to help relieve the temporary discomfort. Each time you eliminate an option that denies a patient's feelings, you raise your chances of selecting the correct answer.

SAMPLE ITEM 7–35

An older woman with a right-sided hemiplegia and tears in her eyes sadly states, "I used to brush my hair 100 strokes a day and now I have to rely on others to do it." What should be the initial response by the nurse?

(1) "It's hard not being able to do things for yourself."

(2) "With physical therapy you will be able to brush your own hair some day."

(3) "Let me brush your hair 100 strokes, and then I'll help you with breakfast."

(4) "That's true, but there are lots of other things you are capable of doing for yourself."

Option 2 is a Pollyanna-like response because it implies that everything will be all right eventually. Option 3 changes the subject and cuts off communication. Option 4 initially accepts the patient's statement but then attempts to refocus the patient on the positive. Options 2, 3, and 4 in one way or another deny the patient's feelings, concerns, and/or needs. The correct answer is option 1 because it is an open-ended statement that focuses on the patient's feelings.

USE MULTIPLE TEST-TAKING TECHNIQUES

You have just been introduced to a variety of test-taking techniques. As you practice applying each of these techniques to test items, you will become more skillful at being test wise. As you become better at applying test-taking techniques, you can further maximize success in choosing the correct option if you use more than one test-taking technique within an item.

SAMPLE ITEM 7–36

A patient's plan of care indicates that passive range-of-motion (PROM) exercises of the right leg are to be done every 4 hours while the patient is awake. What should the nurse do?

(1) Demonstrate how to perform PROM exercises

(2) Explain that all patients do PROM by themselves

(3) Move the patient's leg through PROM when indicated

(4) Take the patient to physical therapy for PROM exercises

Option 2 includes the specific determiner *all* and should be carefully evaluated. Some patients are able to perform PROM exercises themselves (e.g., a patient with hemiplegia can perform PROM on the affected arm and hand with the extremity that is unaffected), whereas some patients are unable to perform PROM (e.g., a patient with quadriplegia). Because some patients cannot perform PROM exercises, there are exceptions to the statement in option 2. This option can be deleted from consideration by using the technique Identify Specific Determiners in Options. Option 4 transfers the responsibility for care that the nurse is educated and licensed to provide. This option can be eliminated from consideration by using the technique Identify Options That Deny Patient Feelings, Concerns, and Needs. By using two test-taking techniques, you have eliminated options 2 and 4, reduced the number of options to two, and increased your chances of selecting the correct answer to 50 percent.

SAMPLE ITEM 7–37

Which patient adaptations are unexpected in response to the General Adaptation Syndrome (GAS)?

(1) Dilated pupils and bradycardia

(2) Mental alertness and tachycardia

(3) Increased blood glucose and tachycardia

(4) Decreased blood glucose and bradycardia

By carefully reading the stem, you should identify that the word *unexpected* is a significant word in this item. You have just used the test-taking technique Identify Key Words in the Stem That Indicate Negative Polarity. If you know that tachycardia is associated with the GAS, you can eliminate options 2 and 3. This reasoning uses the test-taking technique Identify Duplicate Facts Among the Options. If you recognize that options 3 and 4 are opposites, you should give these options particular consideration. By seriously considering these options, you are using the test-taking technique Identify Opposites in Options. A variety of test-taking techniques can be applied to analyze and answer this item.

SAMPLE ITEM 7–38

When the nurse administers a backrub to reduce the physical discomfort of a backache, what patient needs are being met?

(1) Safety

(2) Security

(3) Self-esteem

(4) Physiologic

By thoughtfully reading the stem, you should identify that the important words are *reduce the physical discomfort of a backache.* When reviewing the options, you should recognize that the word "physiologic" in option 4 is closely related to the word "physical" in the stem. Option 4 should be given serious consideration. This reasoning uses the test-taking technique Identify Clues in the Stem. Options 1 and 2 present the words "safety" and "security." They are comparable, and choosing between them is difficult. They are distractors. This reasoning uses the test-taking technique Identify Equally Plausible Options. Options 1, 2, and 3 all begin with the letter "S" while option 4 begins with the letter "P." Option 4 is different from the others and should be considered carefully because it may be the correct answer. You have just used the test-taking technique Identify the Option That Is Unique. The use of multiple test-taking techniques in considering an item can facilitate the deletion of distractors and the selection of the correct answer.

General Test-Taking Techniques

A general test-taking technique is a strategy that is used to conquer the challenge of an examination. To be in command of the situation, you must be able to manage your internal and external domains. The test taker who approaches a test with physical, mental, and emotional authority is in a position to regulate the testing situation, rather than to have the testing situation dominate.

FOLLOW YOUR REGULAR ROUTINE THE NIGHT BEFORE A TEST

Follow your usual routine the night before a test. This is not the time to make changes that may disrupt your balance. If you do not normally eat pepperoni pizza, exercise, or study until 2 AM, do not start now. Go to bed at your usual time. Avoid the temptation to have an all-night cram session. Studies have demonstrated that sleep deprivation decreases reaction times and cognitive skills. An adequate night's sleep is necessary to produce a rested mind and body that provide the physical and emotional energy required to maximize performance on an examination.

ARRIVE ON TIME FOR THE EXAMINATION

Plan your schedule so that you arrive at the testing site about 15 to 30 minutes early. Arrange extra time for unexpected events associated with traveling. There may be a traffic jam, a road may have a detour, the car may not start, the train may be late, the bus could break down, or you may have to park in the farthest lot from the testing site. If the location of the testing site or classroom is unfamiliar to you, it is wise to take a practice run at the same time of day of the scheduled test and locate the room. On the day of the examination, this should avoid getting lost or being late.

By arriving early, you have an opportunity to visit the rest room, survey the situation, and collect your thoughts. Because anxiety is associated with an autonomic nervous system response, you may have urgency, frequency, or increased intestinal peristalsis. Visit the rest room before the test to avoid using testing time to meet physical needs. The test may or may not be administered in the room in which the content is taught. Arriving early allows you to survey the situation and become more comfortable in the testing environment. Decide where you want to sit if seats are not assigned. Students have preferences such as sitting by a window, being in the back of the room, or surrounding themselves with friends. Selecting your own seat allows you to manipulate one aspect of your environment. In addition, this time before the test provides you with an opportunity to collect your thoughts. You may desire to review content on a flash card, perform relaxation exercises, or reinforce your positive mental attitude. However, avoid comparing notes with other students. They may have inaccurate information or be anxious. Remember, anxiety is contagious. If you are the type who is affected by the anxiety of other people, avoid these people until after the test.

BRING THE APPROPRIATE TOOLS

To perform a task, you need adequate tools. Pens, pencils, an eraser, and a watch are essential. A pen may be required to complete the identifying information on the answer sheet. A pencil usually is necessary to record your answers on the answer sheet if it is a computer answer form. Use number 2 pencils because they have soft lead that facilitates the computer scoring of the answer sheet. Bring at least two pens and two or more pencils. Backup equipment is advisable because ink can run out and points can break. Sharpen all your pencils and/or bring a small, self-contained pencil sharpener if you prefer to work with a sharp point on your pencil. Have at least one eraser. You may decide to change an answer or need to erase extraneous marks that you make on the question book or the answer sheet. A watch also is a necessary tool for taking every test. Some proctors will announce time frames as the test progresses and others will not. Bringing your own watch provides you with a sense of independence and control. Depending on your individual needs, other tools might include eyeglasses, a hearing aid, or a calculator. Assemble all your equipment the night before the test, and be sure to take them with you to the testing site.

UNDERSTAND ALL THE DIRECTIONS FOR THE TEST BEFORE STARTING

It is essential to understand the instructions before beginning the test. On some tests you are responsible for independently reading the instructions, whereas on others, the proctor verbally announces the instructions. However, more often than not you will have a written copy of the instructions while the proctor reads them aloud. In this instance, do not read ahead of the proctor. The proctor may elaborate on the written instructions, and you do not want to miss any of the additional directions. If you do not understand a particular part of the instructions, immediately request that the proctor explain them again. You must completely understand the instructions before beginning the examination.

MANAGE THE ALLOTTED TIME TO YOUR ADVANTAGE

All tests have a time limit. Some tests have severe time restrictions in which most test takers do not complete all the questions on the examination. These are known as "speed tests." Other tests have a generous time frame in which the majority of test takers have ample time to answer every question on the examination. These are known as "power tests." The purpose of tests in nursing is to identify how much information the test taker possesses about the nursing care of people. Most nursing examinations are power tests. Regardless of the type of test, you must use your time well.

To manage your time on an examination, you must determine how much time you have to answer each item, leaving some time for review at the end of the testing period. To figure out how much time you should allot for each item, divide the total time you have for the test by the number of items on the test. For example, if you have 90 minutes to take a test that has 50 items, divide 90 by 50. This allots 1 minute and 48 seconds for each item. If you actually allot 1½ minutes per item, you will leave 15 minutes for a final review. Be aware of the time as you progress through a test. If you determine that you have approximately 1½ minutes for each question, by the time you have completed 10 items, 15 minutes should have passed. Pace yourself so that you do not spend more than 1½ minutes on an item if possible. If you answer an item in less than 1½ minutes, you can use the extra time for another item that may take slightly longer than 1½ minutes or add this time to the end for review. The allocation of time for test completion depends on the complexity of the content, the difficulty of the reading level, and the number of options presented in the items. Timed multiple-choice nursing examinations generally allot 1 minute per item when there are four options.

Use all the time allocated for the examination. The test constructors calculated that the time parameters for the test were appropriate for a thoughtful review of the items. Read each item slowly and carefully including all four options. It may be necessary to read the question twice. If you process items too quickly, you may overlook important words, become careless, or arrive at impulsive conclusions. If you find that you are spending too much time, you may want to immediately eliminate obvious distractors and not belabor them. Then only work with the remaining viable options. In addition, you want to avoid getting bogged down on a difficult question because you can lose valuable time, become flustered, and lose focus and concentration when upset. Clearly indicate the question so that you can return to it later. Move on; this puts you back in control! Work at your own pace. Do not be influenced by the actions of other test takers. If other test takers complete the examination early, ignore them and do not become concerned. Just because they finish early does not indicate that they will score well on the test. They may be imprudent speed demons. A cautious, discriminating, and judicious approach is to your advantage. Be your own person and remember that time can be your friend rather than your enemy.

Time allocation varies for tests taken on a computer. See Chapter 9, Computer Applications in Education and Evaluation, for more information.

CONCENTRATE ON THE SIMPLE BEFORE THE COMPLEX

Answer the easy questions before the difficult questions. This uses the basic teaching/learning principle of moving from the simple to the complex. By doing this, you can maximize your use of time and maintain a positive mental attitude. Begin answering questions. When you are confronted with a difficult item, have already used your allotted time to answer it, and still do not know the answer, skip over this item and move on to the next one. Make a notation on scrap paper, next to the item in the question booklet, and/or next to the number of the skipped item on the answer sheet so that you can return to this item later in the test. Making a mark on the answer sheet should prevent you from making the error of recording the next answer in the previous item's location on the answer sheet. These and any other extraneous marks must be erased from the answer sheet before handing it in to the proctor. Extraneous marks confuse the computer, and you probably will lose credit because the mark will be scored as an incorrect answer. When you reach the end of the test, return to those items that you saved for the end. You should have time to spend on these items, and you may have accessed information from other items that can assist you in answering these questions. Concentrating on the simple before the complex permits you to answer the maximum number of items in the time allocated for the examination.

On computer-administered examinations this strategy may not be applicable. You may be required to enter an answer before the next item will appear on the screen.

AVOID READING INTO THE QUESTION

A multiple-choice question has two parts. The first part is known as the stem. The stem is the statement that asks a question. The second part contains the possible responses, which are called options. The stem of a question also has two parts. One part presents information about a clinical event, topic, concept, or theory. The other part asks you to respond in some way. The response part asks you to choose the best option that answers the question based on the information presented in the stem. The information presented in the stem needs to be separated in your mind from the response part of the stem. In some questions the information and response parts of the question are very clear. Other questions are presented in a manner that is less clear about which is the information part and which is the response part.

The following questions illustrate the difference between the information and the response parts of the stem. In each example, the information part of the stem is boldfaced and the response part is italicized.

While walking, a patient becomes weak and the patient's knees begin to buckle. *What should the nurse do?*

Which is an example of **a patient goal?**

Before administering medication for pain, *what should the nurse do first?*

Questions generally are designed to test common principles and concepts. Therefore it is important that you avoid overanalyzing the facts in the question. In an attempt to achieve this goal, consider the following suggestions.

When reading the stem:

- Underline the important words.
- Do not add information from your own mind.
- Do not make assumptions (read between the lines) about the information presented in the stem.

When reading the options:

- Read all the options before choosing the correct answer.
- Refer back only to the words that you underlined as being important in the stem.
- Do not add information to an option.
- Relate an option to just what is being asked in the response part of the stem.
- Focus on commonalities, principles, and concepts associated with your level of learning that is being tested.
- Do not focus only on your experiences, which may be too narrow for a point of reference.
- Recognize that an option can contain correct information but it may or may not have anything to do with the information and response parts of the stem.

When reading options, it is important that you read all four options before selecting the correct answer. This may sound like a ridiculous suggestion; however, we found that students often selected options 1, 2, or 3 over option 4. We tested this theory by placing the correct answer as option 1 and then placing it as option 4 on a different examination. When the correct answer was 4 instead of 1, fewer students selected the correct option. When we asked students who got the question wrong when the correct answer was option 4, the students admitted that they did not read all the options.

Most students find it helpful when they can separate the information part of the question from the response part of the question. By incorporating these suggestions, you should have a better ability to identify what information is in the scenario and what you are being asked to do. As a result, your chances of answering the question correctly, without reading into the question, should increase.

MAKE EDUCATED GUESSES

An educated guess is the selection of an option based on partial knowledge, without knowing for certain that it is the correct answer. When you have reduced the final selection to two options, usually it is to your advantage to reassess these options in the context of the knowledge you do possess and make an educated guess. Making a wild guess by flipping a coin or choosing your favorite number should depend on whether or not the test has a penalty for guessing.

Some examinations assign credit when you answer a question correctly and do not assign credit when you answer a question incorrectly. The directions for these examinations may state that only correct answers will receive credit, that you should answer every question, that you should not leave any blanks, or that there are no penalties for guessing. In these tests it is to your advantage to answer every question. First, select answers based on knowledge. If you are unsure of the correct answer, reduce the number of options and then make an educated guess. If you have absolutely no idea what the answer can be, then make a wild guess because you will not be penalized for a wrong answer.

Some tests assign credit when you answer a question correctly and subtract credit when you answer a question incorrectly. The instructions for these examinations may inform you not to guess, that credit will be subtracted for incorrect answers, or that there is a penalty for guessing. In these tests a statistical manipulation is performed to mathematically limit the advantage of guessing. When taking these tests, it is still to your advantage to make an educated guess if through knowledge you can reduce your final selection to two options. However, wild guessing is not to your advantage because your chance of selecting the correct answer is only 25%.

MAINTAIN A POSITIVE MENTAL ATTITUDE

It is important that you foster a positive mental attitude and a sense of relaxation. A little apprehension can be motivating, but too much can interfere with your attention, concentration, and problem-solving ability. Use the positive techniques you have practiced and that work for you to enhance relaxation and a positive mental attitude. For example, feel in control by skipping the difficult questions; enhance relaxation by employing diaphragmatic breathing for several deep breaths, rotating your shoulders, or flexing and extending your head; foster a positive mental attitude by telling yourself, "I am prepared to do this well!" or "I know I have studied hard and I will be successful!"

CHECK YOUR ANSWERS AND ANSWER SHEET

It is important to record your answers accurately, particularly when using a computer scoring sheet. Computer-scored tests usually use separate answer sheets in which each item has numbers or letters that represent the corresponding responses to each item in the test. You do not want to lose points because you placed your answer in the wrong bubble or in the wrong row. You need to verify the number of the question with the number on the score sheet at least two times when recording. You should conscientiously do this every time you record an answer.

At the end of the exam, again review your answer sheet for accuracy. Make sure that every mark is within the lines, heavy and full, and in the appropriate space. Erase any extraneous marks on the answer sheet. Additional pencil marks, inadequately erased answers, and marks outside the lines will confuse the computer and alter your score. Also, make sure that you have answered every question, especially on tests that do not penalize for guessing. An effective and thorough review should leave you with a feeling of control and a sense of closure at the end of the examination.

If you take an examination on a computer you may be able to select or change an answer before submitting your final choice. Double check your selected response before hitting the key that finalizes your answer.

Answers and Rationales for Sample Items in Chapter 7

7-1
① Used linens may be contaminated with body secretions; wearing gloves is part of Standard Precautions.
② **Linens cannot be returned to a linen storage area once they are removed because they are exposed to microorganisms in the hallways and/or patient rooms.**
③ Reusing a top sheet for the bottom sheet is an acceptable practice if the sheet is not wet or soiled.
④ Tucking clean linen against the frame of the bed is an acceptable practice; the entire bed is washed with a disinfectant between patients.

7-2
① Stewed fruit is low in sodium.
② **Luncheon meats generally are processed with large amounts of sodium.**
③ Whole-grain cereal is low in sodium.
④ Green, leafy vegetables are low in sodium.

7-3
① Kneading the skin increases circulation and should be part of a backrub unless contraindicated.
② Excess lotion can be an irritant to the skin and should be removed.
③ Using continuous, firm strokes is soothing and relieves muscle tension; this action is based on the gate-control theory of pain relief.
④ **Applying pressure over the vertebrae should be avoided because it can cause unnecessary pressure over bony prominences; backrub strokes should massage muscle groups, not vertebrae.**

7-4
① Although incontinence pads are often used for patients who are incontinent, they tend to hold urine and feces against the skin, promoting maceration and skin breakdown.
② **Ointments and jellies generally have an oil base that provides a barrier; also, they hold in moisture, which prevents drying and cracking of skin.**
③ Although talcum powder and cornstarch may be used by people in their homes, they are not used in health-care settings because, when airborne, they become respiratory irritants. In addition, when mixed with urine or perspiration, they result in a paste that irritates the skin and promotes the growth of microorganisms.
④ Same as #3.

7-5
① **The physician's order should be verified first. It is essential that the specific type of enema ordered be given; enemas have different solutions, volumes, and purposes.**
② This is not done first because each type of enema has different equipment requirements.
③ Arranging for an empty bathroom should be done after all the equipment and the patient are prepared and ready.
④ This is not done first because the nurse's explanation depends on the type of enema being administered.

7-6
① This statement is a demeaning response and does not answer the patient's question.
② This statement denies the patient's concern and does not answer the question.
③ Not responding may make the patient more upset; the patient has a right to know who is providing care.
④ **This statement answers the question, which meets the patient's right to know; also, it is a respectful response.**

7-7
① Pulling the curtain supports the patient's need for self-esteem; it provides privacy.
② **Maintaining functional alignment supports a basic physiologic need; this reduces physical strain and potential injury to joints, muscles, ligaments, and tendons and can prevent the formation of contractures.**
③ Responding to the call light immediately supports the patient's need for security and safety; patients need to know that help is available immediately when needed.
④ Raising both side rails on the bed supports the patient's need for safety and security; bed rails prevent a patient from falling out of bed.

7-8
1. **Self-care encourages a patient's independence, which increases self-esteem.**
2. Family member visits generally meet the patient's need for love and belonging, not self-esteem.
3. When a person is dependent on another, such dependency often lowers self-esteem.
4. Same as #3.

7-9
1. Pulling a curtain when providing care supports the patient's self-esteem needs.
2. Answering a call bell immediately meets the patient's safety needs.
3. **Administering physical hygiene meets a patient's basic physiologic need to be clean.**
4. Vital signs are not a physiologic need of the patient. They are an assessment done by the nurse to determine the patient's needs.

7-10
1. This response focuses on the nurse rather than the patient.
2. **This response directly involves the patient and invites the patient to relive a past vacation.**
3. Same as #1.
4. This question by the nurse asks for an opinion, which can be answered with a short response.

7-11
1. This might be done later. It is not the initial action.
2. Same as #1.
3. **The fact that the patient raised the issues about her husband indicates that she is concerned about his behavior. Her feelings need to be explored and her self-esteem supported.**
4. Same as #1.

7-12
1. **This intervention provides the daughter with an opportunity to explore her feelings with regard to her mother's behavior. All behavior has meaning and talking about the situation may provide insight. Eventually the situation should be explored with the patient and the daughter together.**
2. This approach denies the patient's feelings and ignores the daughter's feelings; both cut off communication.
3. The nurse has a responsibility to intervene.
4. This information could further upset the daughter and may precipitate feelings such as guilt or anger.

7-13
1. This statement denies the patient's feelings.
2. **This statement focuses on the patient's feelings by the use of reflection.**
3. This statement offers false reassurance.
4. Same as #3.

7-14
1. Reminding the patient of the physician's next visit does not address the patient's concern; the patient forgets the questions to be asked, not when the physician will visit.
2. This may foster feelings of dependence and could violate the patient's privacy if the questions to be asked are personal.
3. **Providing a paper and pen to write down questions promotes independence, self-esteem, and privacy.**
4. Same as #2.

7-15
1. This may be done after obtaining the patient's permission.
2. Same as #1.
3. Combing from the roots is unsafe; combing should begin at the ends and progressively move toward the roots as tangles are removed.
4. **Seeking preferences promotes individualized care by allowing personal choices.**

7-16
1. Although this may eventually be done, it is not the primary intervention.
2. **Asking the patient to share more encourages verbalization of feelings.**
3. Same as #1.
4. Same as #1.

7-17
1. Soap lowers the surface tension of water, which promotes cleaning.
2. Keeping the patient covered prevents chilling.

③ Hot water can damage delicate tissue and should be avoided; bath water should be between 110 and 115°F.

④ **Pressure and friction produce local heat, which dilates blood vessels, improving circulation.**

7-18 ① Handwashing before care protects the patient from the nurse.

② **Gloves are a barrier against body secretions and are used with Standard Precautions.**

③ The nurse is still exposed to body secretions if not wearing gloves when discarding contaminated water.

④ Expecting patients to provide all of their own care is unreasonable and inappropriate; some patients need assistance with meeting their needs.

7-19 ① Straps and a mask that are firm against the skin can cause tissue trauma.

② Changing the method of oxygen delivery requires a physician's order.

③ Padding the straps with gauze without adjusting the straps will make the mask tighter against the face.

④ **Loosening the elastic straps will reduce the pressure of the mask against the face; the elastic straps can be adjusted for comfort while keeping the edges of the mask gently against the skin.**

7-20 ① Aging is progressive and does not move backward.

② **Aging, from conception to death, advances and moves onward.**

③ Although this may be true for some older adults, it is not true for all.

④ Same as #3.

7-21 ① **Dependent edema is minimal while the feet are still elevated; anti-embolism stockings should be applied before the legs are moved to a dependent position.**

② The purpose of anti-embolism stockings is to promote venous return, not reduce pain.

③ This will cause tissue trauma because of the presence of fluid in the interstitial compartment; anti-embolism stockings are applied to prevent, not treat, edema.

④ Anti-embolism stockings should be applied before the feet are moved to a dependent position.

7-22 ① Side rails do not provide a stable base of support. Injury can occur if the rails are lowered before the straps are removed.

② Tying a restraint to the footboard requires an excessively long strap in which the patient's legs may get entangled.

③ **The bed frame is a stable base of support and is beyond the patient's reach.**

④ Tying a restraint to the headboard may result in an uncomfortable line of pull with the arm above the head.

7-23 ① A solution is hypertonic when the total electrolyte content is 375 mEq/L or greater.

② A solution is hypotonic when the total electrolyte content is less than 250 mEq/L.

③ **A solution is isotonic when the total electrolyte content is approximately 310 mEq/L; normal saline (sodium chloride) is isotonic.**

④ Acidotic refers to excessive levels of hydrogen ions in the blood affecting pH values.

7-24 ① Serving adequate food meets basic physiologic needs, not safety and security needs.

② Providing sufficient fluid meets basic physiologic needs, not safety and security needs.

③ **Being able to summon help when needed provides a sense of security and physical safety for the patient.**

④ Storing a patient's valuables in the hospital safe provides emotional safety.

7-25 ① Placing the patient in the prone position exposes the entire area to permit a thorough backrub; it does not promote circulation.

② Lotions or creams moisturize the skin and make it supple; they do not promote circulation.

③ Same as #2.

④ **Kneading causes friction and pressure against the skin that promotes localized heat, precipitates vessel dilation, and improves circulation.**

7-26

① Active range-of-motion (AROM), not passive range-of-motion (PROM), exercises can increase endurance.

② **PROM exercises prevent shortening of muscles, ligaments, and tendons, which causes joints to become fixed in one position, limiting mobility.**

③ Active, not passive, range-of-motion exercises can strengthen muscle tone.

④ Maximizing muscle atrophy would never be a patient goal. Atrophy is the loss of muscle mass because of lack of muscle contraction. Active range-of-motion exercises will minimize, not maximize, muscle atrophy.

7-27

① This action provides privacy and prevents drafts, but it may contaminate the nurse's hands.

② **Between patients and before and after providing care, the nurse must wash the hands to remove dirt and microorganisms; otherwise, equipment and the patient will be affected by cross-contamination. Medical asepsis is a priority.**

③ Same as #1.

④ Draping the patient provides for privacy and prevents chilling, but if the nurse's hands are not clean, they will contaminate the linen and patient.

7-28

① Antibiotics are administered to treat patients with infections, not all sick patients.

② **This is a broad statement that incorporates under its mantle many different actions that may be implemented to prevent the spread of microorganisms.**

③ This is not necessary; implementing Standard Precautions is sufficient.

④ Same as #3.

7-29

① This is not required for all positions.

② **Functional alignment refers to maintaining the body in an anatomic position that supports physical functioning, minimizes strain and stress on muscles, tendons, ligaments, and joints, and prevents contractures.**

③ Same as #1.

④ Same as #1.

7-30

① Both actions may injure the patient. The patient may fall out of bed on the side opposite the nurse, and moving a restrained patient exerts stress on the patient's musculoskeletal system.

② Although one side rail can be lowered, moving a restrained patient may injure the patient.

③ Although the vest restraint can be untied while the nurse is at the bedside, lowering the rail on the side opposite to which the nurse is working may result in the patient falling out of bed.

④ **Untying a restraint permits free movement, which limits stress on the patient's musculoskeletal system. Lowering one side rail allows the nurse to provide direct care. Keeping the side rail raised on the side opposite to which the nurse is working provides a barrier to prevent the patient from falling out of bed.**

7-31

① **These foods—fruit, vegetables, and bread—contain the least amount of sodium compared to the foods listed in the other options.**

② Hot dogs, mustard, and pickles all contain a high level of sodium and should be avoided.

③ Ketchup is high in sodium and should be avoided.

④ Luncheon meats are processed foods that contain a high level of sodium and should be avoided.

7-32

① With hemorrhage, the patient's skin will be cold and clammy, not warm and dry, and the pulse will be weak and thready, not bounding.

② Because of the reduced blood volume associated with hemorrhage, the patient's blood pressure will decrease, not increase, and the pulse will be weak and thready, not bounding.

③ With hemorrhage, the patient's blood pressure will decrease, not increase, and the skin will be cold and clammy, not warm and dry.

④ **Because of the decreased blood volume associated with hemorrhage, the blood pressure will be reduced and the pulse will be weak and thready; because of the autonomic nervous system response and the constriction of peripheral blood vessels, the patient's skin will be cold and clammy.**

7-33

① This statement denies the patient's feelings about death and cuts off further communication.

② This statement abdicates the responsibility of the nurse (to explore the patient's feelings) to the physician; it cuts off communication and does not meet the patient's immediate need to discuss fears of death; eventually the physician should be notified of the patient's feelings.

③ **This statement uses reflective technique because it focuses on the underlying feeling expressed in the patient's statement.**

④ Same as #1.

7-34

① Although this is true for most patients, it may not be true for this patient. This is a Pollyanna-like response that may provide false reassurance.

② Although this is a true statement, it cuts off communication and does not present an intervention to help limit the patient's present discomfort.

③ **This response recognizes the mild pain and offers the patient an intervention to help limit the temporary discomfort.**

④ This response is inappropriate at this time. If more than mild pain is expected, analgesics should be administered before pain-inducing activities.

7-35

① **This response identifies the patient's concern and offers an opportunity to further discuss the topic.**

② This is a Pollyanna-like response that provides false reassurance; the patient may never be able to brush her own hair.

③ This response offers a solution before allowing the patient to discuss concerns, thereby cutting off communication.

④ After the patient's present feelings are explored, then pointing out the patient's abilities is appropriate.

7-36

① PROM exercises of a leg cannot be performed independently; this is appropriate for AROM exercises.

② Some patients are not capable of performing PROM exercises, depending on the strength of the unaffected extremity and their physical, mental, and/or emotional status.

③ **PROM exercises are interventions within the role of the nurse and meet the patient's need to prevent contractures.**

④ Taking the patient to physical therapy transfers the nurse's responsibility to other members of the health team.

7-37

① Tachycardia, not bradycardia, is associated with the General Adaptation Syndrome (GAS); dilated pupils are expected.

② Both these adaptations are expected autonomic nervous system responses that occur during the alarm stage of the GAS.

③ Same as #2.

④ **During the alarm stage of the GAS, both the blood glucose level and heart rate of the patient increase, not decrease.**

7-38

① Safety and security needs, the second level of needs according to Maslow, are met when the patient is protected from harm.

② Same as #1.

③ Self-esteem needs, a third level need, are met when the patient is treated with dignity and respect.

④ **Being free from pain or discomfort is a basic physiologic need; a backrub improves local circulation, reduces muscle tension, and limits pain.**

Testing Formats Other Than Multiple-Choice Questions

Teachers make many decisions that influence students. Some are instructional decisions. What teaching strategies should be used to teach certain content? Some decisions are curricular decisions. What information should be included in a unit of instruction? The decisions teachers make that produce the most anxiety for most students are the measurement and evaluation decisions. What does the student know? What can the student do? To make these decisions, teachers use tests to appraise progress toward curricular goals, assess mastery of a skill, and evaluate knowledge of what was taught in a course. Three factors are involved in making measurement and evaluation decisions.

- **What knowledge or ability is to be measured?**
  Generally, that which is most important or relevant is measured. Examples include the expected range of vital signs in an adult, the principles of patient teaching, legal and ethical implications of health-care delivery, and patient safety. You usually can identify what is most significant by the emphasis placed on the material. Content in a textbook that is highlighted, boldfaced, capitalized, or repeated several times usually is important. Information that appears in the textbook and is incorporated into the teacher's classroom instruction also is significant. Concepts that are introduced in the classroom setting and then applied in a classroom laboratory or clinical setting are critical concepts. You often can predict the content that will be on a test and therefore use your study time more efficiently.

- **How can the identified knowledge or ability be measured?**
  A set of operations must be devised to isolate and display the knowledge or ability that is to be measured. Examples include multiple-choice questions, true-false questions, completion items, matching columns, extended essay questions, and the performance of a procedure. To feel in control when taking tests, you should be familiar with the various testing formats. Dealing with a particular test format is a skill, and to develop a skill you must practice. Student workbooks that accompany required textbooks, practice questions at the end of chapters, and books devoted to testing usually contain practice questions. Practice answering these questions. Experience promotes learning and practice makes perfect!

- **How can the results of the devised operations be measured or expressed in quantitative terms?**
  In other words, the unit of measure that indicates a passing grade or an acceptable performance must be identified by the instructor. Examples of acceptable results include a grade within 10 percent of the average grade in the class, a grade of 80 percent, or the correct performance of previously identified steps (critical elements) of a procedure. When taking tests, you should be aware of the criteria for scoring the test. You should ask the following questions: What is the passing grade? How many points are allocated to each question? Can partial credit be received for an answer? Is there a

penalty for guessing? What are the critical steps that must be performed for each skill to pass the test? Answers to these and other questions can help you make decisions such as how much time to devote to certain questions or whether or not to guess at an answer.

In previous chapters, the multiple-choice question was discussed in detail. In this chapter, testing formats other than multiple-choice questions are presented. Test questions can be classified as structured-response questions, restricted-response questions, extended essay questions, or performance appraisals.

A **structured-response question** requires you to select the correct answer from among available alternatives. Multiple-choice, multiple-response, true-false, and matching items are examples of structured-response questions.

A **restricted-response question** requires you to write a short answer. The response is expected to be a word, phrase, sentence, or product of a mathematical calculation. Short-answer, completion, and fill-in-the blank items are examples of restricted-response questions.

An **extended essay question** requires you to generate the answer, via a free-response format, in reply to a question or problem that is presented.

A **performance appraisal** presents a structured situation and requires you to demonstrate part or all of a skill.

The answers and rationales for all the sample items in this chapter are at the end of the chapter.

Structured-Response Questions

A structured-response item is one that asks a question and requires you to select an answer from among the options presented. These items include multiple-choice, multiple-response, true-false, and matching questions. These formats usually are efficient, dependable, and objective. Because multiple-choice questions are discussed in Chapter 5, only multiple-response, true-false, and matching questions are presented here.

MULTIPLE-RESPONSE QUESTIONS

A multiple-response question is a variation of a regular multiple-choice question. A regular multiple-choice question asks a question and then provides three or four potential answers. The test taker must select the one correct answer from among the presented potential answers. (For additional information, see Chapter 5.) A multiple-response question is similar in that it presents a question and potential answers. However, it varies in that it requires the test taker to identify several correct answers from among numerous potential answers.

SAMPLE ITEM 8-1

When assessing a Stage III pressure ulcer, the nurse identifies the extent of tissue damage. Select all that apply.

(1) _____ Undermining of neighboring tissue

(2) _____ Limited to partial-thickness loss

(3) _____ Damage to subcutaneous tissue

(4) _____ Extension through the fascia

(5) _____ Damage to muscle

SAMPLE ITEM 8-2

What actions must be implemented to meet the criteria of Transmission-Based Precautions to reduce the spread of infection when the nurse is caring for a patient with primary pulmonary tuberculosis? Indicate all the actions that apply.

(1) _____ Donning a gown when entering the room

(2)	_____	Putting on gloves when delivering a food tray
(3)	_____	Placing a mask on the patient during transport
(4)	_____	Admitting the patient to a private room that has negative air pressure
(5)	_____	Wearing a respiratory device when entering the room (N95 respirator)
(6)	_____	Keeping the door to the room closed except when entering or leaving

TRUE-FALSE QUESTIONS

A true-false question also is known as an **alternate-response item.** A question is presented and only two options are given from which to select an answer. This item frequently is used to test knowledge of facts because the response must be absolutely true or false. It can be a demanding format because no frame of reference is provided. The question usually is constructed out of context, and the truth or falsity of the statement can be difficult to evaluate. However, true-false questions can work to your benefit because you have a 50 percent chance of getting the answer right. If you do not know the answer and there is no penalty for guessing, make an educated guess. Never leave a blank answer if there is no penalty for guessing. Follow the instructions for selecting the correct answer; for example, you may be told to circle your answer or instructed to place an X on a line next to your answer.

SAMPLE ITEM 8–3

When providing a bed bath, the nurse understands that soap helps in cleaning because it lowers the surface tension of water.
True _____   False _____

SAMPLE ITEM 8–4

When transferring a patient from the bed to a wheelchair, the nurse should assume a broad stance.
True _____   False _____

SAMPLE ITEM 8–5

The nurse should teach a patient experiencing insomnia that exercising just before going to bed promotes sleep.
True _____   False _____

SAMPLE ITEM 8–6

When obtaining a patient's vital signs the nurse is aware that pulse pressure is the difference between the apical and radial pulse rates.
True _____   False _____

Variations of true-false items have been developed to simplify and clarify what is being asked. These questions may also obtain more information about what you know and limit guessing. **Highlighting a word or phrase in the question** (by CAPITALIZING it or by using **bold type**, *italics*, or underlining) is a simple variation that helps to reduce ambiguity and increase precision. You can also use this technique when answering true-false questions in which certain words are not highlighted. Underline key words, as well as words that modify key words, to focus your attention on the most important part of the statement.

SAMPLE ITEM 8-7

Palpation is the examination of the body using the sense of **touch.**
True _____   False _____

SAMPLE ITEM 8-8

The process in which solid, particulate matter in a fluid moves from an area of higher concentration to an area of lower concentration is known as <u>osmosis</u>.
True _____   False _____

Grouping short true-false items under a common question, another variation of the true-false question, attempts to arrange affiliated information together. It is an effective approach to assess knowledge about related categories, classifications, or characteristics. Each statement that is being evaluated must be considered in relation to the original question. This variation reduces the amount of reading and provides a greater frame of reference for evaluating each statement. This type of question increases specificity and clarity.

SAMPLE ITEM 8-9

Indicate if the following choices are true or false in relation to the introductory statement.
Surgical asepsis is maintained when the nurse:
  (1) Removes the drape from a sterile package by touching the outer 1 inch with ungloved hands.
    True _____   False _____
  (2) Dons the first sterile glove by touching just the inside of the glove.
    True _____   False _____
  (3) Holds the hands below the elbows during a surgical hand scrub.
    True _____   False _____
  (4) Holds a sterile object below waist level.
    True _____   False _____

SAMPLE ITEM 8-10

Signify whether or not each procedure employs the principle of positive pressure.
  (1) Mechanical ventilation
    True _____   False _____
  (2) Continuous bladder irrigation
    True _____   False _____
  (3) Chest tubes (chest drainage system)
    True _____   False _____
  (4) Instillation of fluid into a nasogastric tube with a piston syringe
    True _____   False _____

Requiring the test taker to correct false statements is another variation of the true-false question. With this type of question, you are instructed to rewrite the question whenever you determine that the statement is false. This approach guarantees that you understand the information underlying a false statement. It also decreases guessing because you will receive credit only if able to revise the question to make it a correct statement. This variation is sometimes combined with the true-false variation that highlights a word or phrase in the original question.

SAMPLE ITEM 8–11

Mark your answer with an X in the space provided. If you identify the statement as false, revise the statement so that it is accurate.
The expected range of the heart rate for an adult is 75 to 120 beats per minute.
   True _____   False _____   Correction _____

SAMPLE ITEM 8–12

Indicate if the statement is true or false. Correct the underlined words if the statement is false.
According to Erikson's developmental theory, the central task of <u>young adulthood</u> is identity versus role confusion.
   True _____   False _____   Correction _____

True-false items can be asked in relation to specific stimulus material included with the question. This variation of the true-false question provides a frame of reference for the specific questions being asked within the item. Examples of stimulus material include a graph, map, chart, table, or picture. Memorization of information generally is not sufficient for answering these types of questions because they test more than the recall or regurgitation of facts. These questions test comprehension, interpretation, application, and reasoning, which are higher levels of cognitive ability.

SAMPLE ITEM 8–13

The vital signs sheet on page 122 reflects an adult patient's 7-day hospitalization. Determine if each statement is true or false in relation to the information plotted on the vital signs sheet.

   (1) On June 7 at 10 PM, the patient's temperature was 101.2°F.
      True _____   False _____
   (2) During the last 3 days of the patient's hospitalization, the patient's temperature reflected a normal circadian rhythm.
      True _____   False _____
   (3) During the first 4 days of the patient's hospitalization, the patient's blood pressure was consistent with a developing fluid volume deficit.
      True _____   False _____
   (4) During hospitalization, the patient's pulse rate ranged from 76 to 110 beats per minute.
      True _____   False _____
   (5) The patient's baseline pulse rate on admission to the hospital was within expected limits.
      True _____   False _____
   (6) When the patient's temperature increased during the acute phase of the illness, the patient's respirations decreased.
      True _____   False _____

SAMPLE ITEM 8–14

A patient's daily intake and output (I&O) record for the 7 AM to 3 PM shift is illustrated on page 123. Identify whether the following statements correctly or incorrectly reflect the information presented in the I&O record.

   (1) If the intravenous solution infused at an equal volume per hour, the hourly rate was 75 mL per hour.
      True _____   False _____

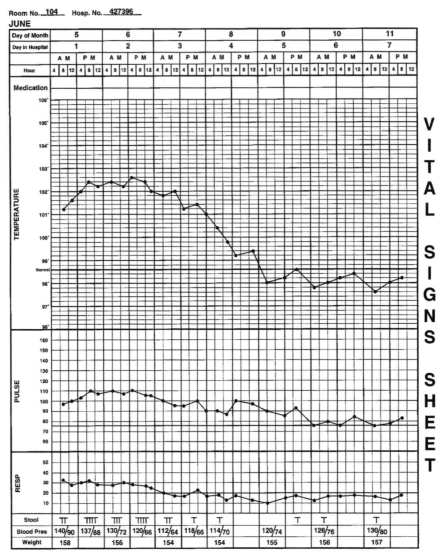

Room No. __104__ Hosp. No. __427396__

JUNE

Day of Month	5		6		7		8		9		10		11	
Day in Hospital	1		2		3		4		5		6		7	
	A M	P M	A M	P M	A M	P M	A M	P M	A M	P M	A M	P M	A M	P M
Hour	4 8 12	4 8 12	4 8 12	4 8 12	4 8 12	4 8 12	4 8 12	4 8 12	4 8 12	4 8 12	4 8 12	4 8 12	4 8 12	4 8 12

Stool	TT		TTTT		TTT		TTTT		TT		T		T				T		T				T		
Blood Pres	140/90		137/88		130/72		120/66		112/64		118/66		114/70				120/74				126/76				130/80		
Weight	158				156				154				154				155				156				157		

(2) If the patient had 4 oz of orange juice with breakfast at 8:30 AM, the patient also drank another 10 oz of fluid with breakfast.
True _____   False _____

(3) The patient's intake and output was equal at the completion of the 7 to 3 shift.
True _____   False _____

(4) The additive to the patient's intravenous solution was 20 mg of vitamin K.
True _____   False _____

MATCHING QUESTIONS

A matching question begins by establishing a frame of reference for the question. It explains the topic of the question and the basis on which matches should be made. The item then divides into a double-column format. It presents a statement in Column I and then requires you to select a corresponding, related, or companion statement from among a list of possible options in Column II. Usually the question assesses information about related categories, classifications, or characteristics. Sometimes the items in the two columns are equal in number, and

DAILY INTAKE AND OUTPUT RECORD

DATE   JUNE 5

	INTAKE							OUTPUT			
	I.V. FLUIDS			Medication and Dosage	*ABS.	∓LIB	ORAL	URINE	EMESIS	N.G. TUBE	HEMOVAC
Time	Bottle	Amount	Solution								
8	1	1000	NS	20 mEq KCl				650			
8:30							360				
10:00							120				
11:30							240	150			
12:00									160		
1:40									90		60
2:15					↓			250			
3:00					525	475					45
7-3 TOTAL		8-HR TOTAL			525	475	720	1050	250		105
3-11 TOTAL		8-HR TOTAL									
11-7 TOTAL		8-HR TOTAL									
24 HOUR TOTAL											

INTAKE GRAND TOTAL [   ]   OUTPUT GRAND TOTAL [   ]

*ABS. = amount absorbed   ∓LIB = Left in bag

sometimes Column I will have fewer statements than Column II. When the columns are equal in length, the format can work either for you or against you. If the columns have seven items each and you know six of the answers, you will automatically get the last answer correct, whether or not you understand the content. On the other hand, if you make an incorrect choice, you will automatically get two answers wrong. These problems are minimized if the response column (Column II) has more options than the question column (Column I).

You must first read the directions for the matching questions carefully because they specify the basis for the matching. In addition, they will tell you where to place the correct answer and the number of times an option can be selected. Next, match items that you are absolutely certain are correct matches. This eliminates the options that you have correctly matched, leaving a reduced list on which to focus. Now consider the remaining options, moving from the simple to the complex as determined by your frame of reference.

The matching question is a relatively superficial testing format that lends itself to factual information that usually is memorized. Therefore, another strategy is to cover Column II and for each item in Column I attempt to recall the memorized information without being cued by the content in Column II. Hopefully, the information you memorized will appear as an option in Column II. By doing this, you may become less confused or distracted by the list of options. If you do not know the answer and there is no penalty for guessing, make an educated guess.

SAMPLE ITEM 8–15

Column I contains terminology used to describe types of breathing exhibited by patients. Match each term to its correct description in Column II. Place the number you select from Column II on the line at the left of the term in Column I. Use each number only once.

Column I	Column II
_____ a. Bradypnea	1. Respirations that are increased in depth and rate
_____ b. Apnea	2. Difficulty breathing
_____ c. Hyperpnea	3. Respiratory rate less than 10 breaths per minute
_____ d. Tachypnea	4. Absence of breathing
_____ e. Eupnea	5. Respiratory rate greater than 20 breaths per minute
_____ f. Dyspnea	6. Normal breathing
	7. Shallow breathing interrupted by irregular periods of apnea

SAMPLE ITEM 8–16

Column I lists types of exercises. Match a type of exercise with its most therapeutic value or outcome. Indicate, in the space provided, the number from Column I that matches the letter in Column II. Options from Column I can be used more than once.

Column I—Exercises

1. Passive range of motion
2. Aerobic
3. Isometric
4. Kegel

Column II—Outcomes

a. Promote urinary continence (_____)
b. Improve strength of pelvic floor muscles (_____)
c. Promote pulmonary functioning (_____)
d. Improve cardiovascular conditioning (_____)
e. Increase muscle mass, tone, and strength of an extremity in a cast (_____)
f. Maintain joint mobility (_____)

Restricted-Response Questions

Restricted-response questions are also known as **free-response questions.** Completion and short-answer questions are examples of restricted-response questions. These questions pose a simple question and expect you to furnish the answer. The response can be a word, phrase, sentence, or product of a mathematical calculation. Because these types of questions usually have an uncomplicated, direct format, they are most effective for assessing the understanding of simple concepts, the definition of terms, the knowledge of facts, or the ability to solve mathematical problems.

COMPLETION QUESTIONS

A completion question generally is a short statement with one or more blanks. You are required to furnish the word, words, or phrase that accurately completes the sentence. In a completion question, the key word or words are the ones that are omitted. This forces you to focus on the important information reflected in the question rather than trivia. This type of question does not permit flexibility or creativity in your response. The question anticipates a particular word or phrase that will produce an accurate statement.

SAMPLE ITEM 8–17

Flexion and fixation of a joint is called a _____.

SAMPLE ITEM 8–18

Postural drainage uses gravity to drain secretions from the _____.

SAMPLE ITEM 8–19

The expected respiratory rate for an adult is _____ to _____ breaths per minute.

The inclusion of two possible answers to fill in the blank is a simple variation of a completion question. This format resembles an alternate-response question because you are asked a question and two choices are presented from which to pick an answer. This type of question gives you an advantage because the words presented are clues. These words nudge your memory and the recall of information necessary to answer the question. When faced with a question that has only two possible options, the chance of selecting the correct answer is 50 percent.

SAMPLE ITEM 8–20

When describing "radiating pain," the nurse is referring to its (intensity/location).

SAMPLE ITEM 8–21

The feeling that a person needs to void immediately is called (frequency/urgency).

SHORT-ANSWER QUESTIONS

A short-answer question is a free-response item because it asks a question and expects you to compose an answer. It provides some flexibility and creativity because the response does not have to complete a sentence or fill in a blank. You usually can use anywhere from one word to several sentences to answer the question. A short-answer question that needs only a word or a phrase to answer the question is similar to a completion question, but the original question is a complete sentence rather than an incomplete sentence. A short-answer question that requires several sentences to answer the question goes beyond the standards or criteria of a completion question, but it still focuses on the knowledge of facts, terminology, simple concepts, or the ability to perform mathematical computations. The more relevant information you include in the response, the better you can demonstrate comprehension of the information being tested. Short-answer questions do not lend themselves to test-taking strategies. However, write as much as the format permits in the hope that what you include answers the question and contains the specific information expected by the teacher.

Short-answer and completion questions can be used interchangeably to address the same content. For example, compare Sample Items 8–17 through 8–19 with Sample Items 8–22 through 8–24, respectively.

SAMPLE ITEM 8–22

What is the definition of the word *contracture?*

SAMPLE ITEM 8–23

What is the purpose of postural drainage?

SAMPLE ITEM 8–24

What is the normal range of respirations per minute in an adult?

SAMPLE ITEM 8–25

The physician orders an intravenous solution of 1000 mL of D5W to be administered at 100 mL per hour. The drop factor of the intravenous administration set is 15 drops per mL. How many drops per minute should the patient receive?

126 ## Extended Essay Questions

An extended essay is a free-response question because the answer is drafted by you in reply to a question. It requires higher cognitive skills than just recall and comprehension. Essay questions expect you to select, arrange, organize, integrate, synthesize, compare, or contrast information. You must be able to use language constructively, be creative when solving problems, and use critical thinking to manipulate complicated information. The extended essay is most suitable for evaluating mastery of complex material.

When writing responses to extended essay questions, it is wise to follow a three-part format when possible. First, begin with an introduction. The **introduction** should, in a general way, indicate what will be discussed. It introduces the topic and serves as a preface or prologue for what will follow. Next, present the central part or body of the answer. The **central part** of the answer should explore all the information that is being presented to answer the question. Organize this part of the answer by writing a topical outline. This blueprint promotes an orderly flow of information, prevents departure from your script, and ensures that significant material is included. Finally, complete the answer with a summary. The **summary** should recap what was discussed and come to several conclusions. It serves as a finale and brings closure to your answer.

Generally, instructors examine your writing from the viewpoint of **writing for evaluation.** Instructors measure your knowledge by evaluating an end product such as a written assignment or essay question on an examination. To answer an essay question, you must be able to put your thoughts on paper in a logical manner using correct spelling, grammar, and punctuation. There is no easy way to develop effective writing skills without practice. Most learning institutions today have writing centers that provide specialized faculty to assist you with writing activities. To maximize your success in formulating written assignments, you must view writing from the perspectives of **learning to write** and **writing to learn.**

LEARNING TO WRITE

When learning to write, you are not looking at an end product that will be evaluated by the instructor, but rather focusing on the process of writing. Writing requires a basic understanding of the English language. For example, you need to have an adequate vocabulary, understand the rules of grammar and punctuation, and be able to spell. When learning to write, you also must focus on the organizational and analytical skills that help you to assess, advise, teach, argue a point of view, and challenge new and old theories. Critical thinking is an essential skill needed to process the information that is to be written. Techniques that can be used to promote learning to write include brainstorming, setting priorities, and editing and revising previously written material.

Brainstorming is a method of exploring a topic by spontaneously listing thoughts or ideas. Making lists of words or phrases that relate to a topic allows you to explore a topic and your perspectives on the topic. For example, when students were asked to make a list of everything and anything relevant to patient progress notes, interesting insights developed. Some students were content oriented, in that they listed everything a health-care provider should include in progress notes, such as vital signs, specific care provided, and patients' responses to care. Other students were process oriented, in that they stated that notes should be specific, legible, and comprehensive. Brainstorming not only helps you to learn to write but also to explore topics through writing. If you take the time to examine what you have written, it also may tell you a lot about yourself.

Setting priorities is an analytical skill that requires you to compare and contrast information and identify that which is most important or significant. Use a systematic method or theoretical base to make priority setting easier. Maslow's Hierarchy of Needs is an excellent framework because it also helps to organize information. Data can be clustered in each of the five levels or categories of needs. These needs are ranked according to how critical they are to survival. The physiologic needs are the most basic and carry the highest priority; safety and security, love and belonging, self-esteem, and self-actualization follow. You can practice setting priorities each day just by ranking your activities for the day in order of importance.

Analyzing, editing, and revising previously written material are other ways to learn to write. Consider writing directly on a computer. On a computer, it is easy to move around words, phrases, and sentences as you edit and revise your writing. Seeing your words in print helps to separate you from your own handwriting, making it easier to examine the content of your writing. When you have the luxury of time, it is always to your advantage to write an assignment one day and then several days later review this first draft. Your analytical skills may improve; you may acquire new information since you first wrote the material; or your perspective may be different or clearer. Also, you probably will be more open to constructive criticism when it comes from within. Analyzing, editing, and revising your own written work are excellent ways to improve your writing abilities.

The hardest thing to overcome when engaging in learning-to-write activities is the feeling that, because you may not have completed a project, you have not learned. Remember, learning takes place in the learner and is a lifelong process.

WRITING TO LEARN

When writing to learn, you are focusing on what you will eventually understand or remember, not on the process of writing. You learn content by the very act of writing because at least two cognitive domains are being integrated: cognitive (thinking) and psychomotor (writing). You learn the course content you are writing about and discover what you know, what you need to know, and what you think about certain topics. When you are writing to learn, you are writing for yourself, and what you learn is the end product. Techniques that can be used to promote writing to learn include writing lists, writing journals, posing and answering questions, and note taking.

Writing a list can be a simple or complex task. A simple list would be repetitiously writing a phrase or fact in an effort to reinforce learning. This requires a low-level thinking process that involves the recall of information. For example, writing common equivalents in the apothecaries' and metric systems (15 to 16 grains = 1 gram). A complex list might require the writer to discriminate between the commonalities and differences of content material. This requires higher levels of the thinking process and includes comprehension, application, and analysis. For example, making a list of nursing interventions that use the concept of gravity (IV infusion, urinary catheter, elevation of an extremity to promote venous return). To compile this list, you must comprehend a concept and be able to identify the commonalities among the applications of this concept.

Writing a journal focuses on the use of words, the expression of ideas and feelings, and the documentation of activities; no consideration should be given to format, grammar, or punctuation. For 5 to 10 minutes each day, write a diary. It will improve your thinking and learning as well as document where you have been, where you are, and where you are going.

Posing and answering questions can lead to a better understanding of the content you are learning as well as improve your critical-thinking skills. Many textbooks have a companion study guide or workbook. Answering questions from these books and questions that you make up for yourself are excellent ways to reinforce the understanding of information. Putting your thoughts into concrete words and using the psychomotor skill of writing helps you to learn.

Note taking can be a simple or complex task. A simple note-taking strategy is the rewriting of class notes. When you rewrite notes, you revise information so that it is more organized and clear. A complex note-taking strategy is to add relevant information from the textbook to your class notes. You can even add to your notes your own thoughts and reactions.

SAMPLE ITEM 8–26

Compare and contrast critical thinking and problem solving and include at least three characteristics of each.

Performance Appraisal

Nursing care is an art and a science. Nurses must not only comprehend information but be able to perform skills safely. Therefore, testing the ability to identify and implement steps in a procedure accurately is essential in evaluating the achievement of skills. Skills can be tested in a variety of ways. Questions that require you to identify a step in a procedure are asked in the typical multiple-choice format. For example: "What should the nurse do first when preparing to give a bed bath to a patient?" This question requires you to select one correct answer out of four presented options. See Chapter 5 for additional information about multiple-choice questions. Questions that require you to select related steps in a procedure are presented in the multiple-response format. For example, "Identify all the actions that should be implemented when maintaining Airborne Transmission-Based Precautions." This question requires you to select more than one response to answer the question. See Multiple-Response Questions in this chapter for more information.

Questions that ask you to demonstrate knowledge about a skill in relation to a realistic image such as a graphic, table, chart, or picture expect you to respond in some way. For example, "Identify the area on the picture where the nurse should place a stethoscope to best auscultate the apical heart rate." This question requires you to implement just one step of a procedure in relation to a visual cue. See The Performance of Part of a Procedure via a Realistic Image in subsequent paragraphs for additional information.

The ability to demonstrate a procedure safely can also be evaluated when you actually implement the skill on a mannequin or person. This testing situation presents a skill that must be performed and you are required to meet all the critical elements when completing the skill. See The Performance of a Procedure in subsequent paragraphs for additional information on these types of questions.

Because multiple-choice questions and multiple-response questions are discussed elsewhere in this book, only the performance of part of a procedure via a realistic image and the performance of a procedure will be presented next.

THE PERFORMANCE OF PART OF A PROCEDURE VIA A REALISTIC IMAGE

It is impossible to physically demonstrate an entire psychomotor skill on paper-and-pencil or computer-administered examinations. Therefore, alternate items have been developed to test the knowledge of one or more parts of a procedure via realistic images such as graphs, charts, tables, or pictures. These questions require the test taker to apply knowledge using visual cues. The test taker may be required to identify an anatomic landmark as part of a procedure, recognize the significance of information on a chart, insert or find data on a graph, or identify safe or unsafe practice in a picture. The following sample items are examples of questions that test the performance of part of a procedure via a realistic image.

SAMPLE ITEM 8-27

Place a dot over the area where the nurse must place the fingers to take a radial pulse.

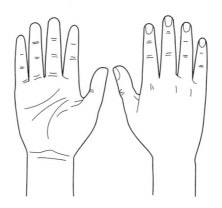

What was the patient's temperature on June 10th at 4 AM?
Answer: _____

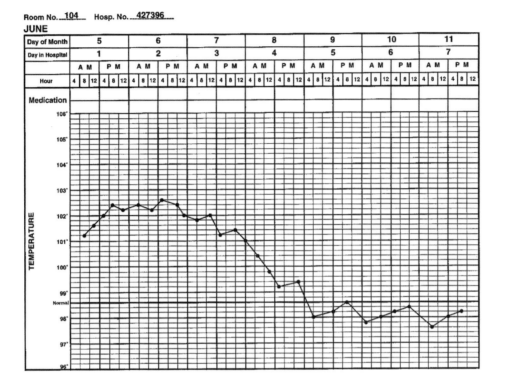

THE PERFORMANCE OF A PROCEDURE

A performance appraisal evaluates the ability to complete an entire procedure. Psychomotor skills, the motor effects of mental processes, are most effectively assessed by performance appraisals. Obtaining a blood pressure, changing a sterile dressing, administering a tube feeding, and performing tracheal suctioning are examples of psychomotor skills. When evaluating these skills, the criteria for passing should be identified before you attempt the procedure. For example, the criteria in obtaining a blood pressure reading might be that you must obtain accurate systolic and diastolic readings. In another testing situation, the criteria for passing might be previously identified steps of the procedure such as washes hands, checks functioning of equipment, places cuff evenly around the upper arm, places stethoscope over brachial artery, inflates cuff 20 mm Hg above palpated systolic reading, deflates cuff at 2 to 3 mm Hg per second, obtains accurate systolic reading, and obtains accurate diastolic reading.

A **critical element** is any step that must be performed accurately to receive a passing score. Critical elements are very specific criteria. Other criteria may be more general. For example, when obtaining a temperature reading, you must maintain medical asepsis, provide for physical safety, and ensure privacy. These are less specific because there are numerous ways to meet each of these criteria. For example, physical safety can be provided by holding the thermometer while it is in place or taking a tympanic temperature when the patient is confused.

Performance appraisals should be objective and the criteria for an acceptable performance identified. Clinical techniques and skills textbooks are helpful when practicing procedures and preparing for performance appraisals. A clinical skills checklist of step-by-step elements can be used by another student to assess your performance of a psychomotor skill in a laboratory setting. This is a nonthreatening way to practice, and it supports reciprocal study relationships. Also, it provides an opportunity to simulate a testing situation and helps with desensitization, which may give you a feeling of control.

Alternate Question Formats Reflective of NCLEX

Before April 2003, all of the questions on NCLEX examinations were presented in the typical multiple-choice format. This type of question requires you to select one correct answer out of four presented options. In April 2003, The National Council of State Boards of Nursing (NCSBN) incorporated item formats other than the typical multiple-choice question. These items are called alternate-item formats. **Alternate-item formats** use the benefits of computer technology to assess knowledge via questions that require you to identify multiple answers, perform a calculation, prioritize information, or respond to a question in relation to a graphic image, picture, table, or chart/exhibit. The NCSBN believes that test takers can demonstrate their entry-level nursing competence in ways that are different from the typical multiple-choice format and that some nursing content will be more readily and authentically evaluated. The NCSBN predicts that a candidate who takes a minimum length exam, which is the majority of candidates, may be administered just one question with an alternate item format.

Alternate-item formats include fill-in-the-blank items; hot spot items; multiple-choice items using a chart or graphic image; drag and drop/ordered response items; multiple response items; and chart/exhibit items. The following sample questions are examples of these types of alternate-item formats.

FILL-IN-THE-BLANK ITEMS

A fill-in-the-blank item asks a question that requires you to perform a calculation and type in your answer. Only numbers and decimal points can be entered. If the test is taken on a computer usually you can access a calculator on the computer to assist you with your computation.

SAMPLE ITEM 8–29

> The physician orders 1500 mL to be administered every 24 hours. At what hourly rate should the nurse set the infusion pump?
> Answer: _____ mL/hr

SAMPLE ITEM 8–30

> The physician orders 500 mg of an antibiotic to be administered IVPB every 6 hours.
> 1 gram of the medication is supplied in a vial that states: "add 2.5 mL of sterile water to yield 3 mL of solution." How much solution should the nurse administer?
> Answer: _____ mL

HOT SPOT ITEMS

A hot spot item asks a question in relation to a presented illustration. When taken on the computer, you need to place the cursor on the area you want to select and left click on the mouse.

SAMPLE ITEM 8–31

> A patient is on complete bed rest in the semi-Fowler's position because of excessive fluid volume and difficulty breathing. Put an X over the area of the body that is at the greatest risk for dependent edema.

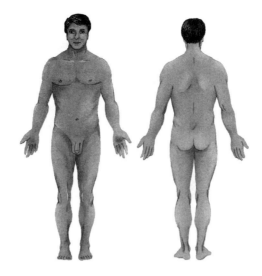

SAMPLE ITEM 8–32

The nurse must administer an intramuscular injection. Place an X over the area where the nurse should insert the needle of the syringe when utilizing the *vastus lateralis* muscle.

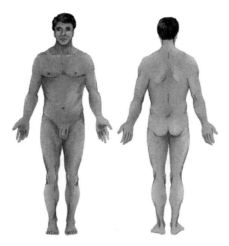

MULTIPLE-CHOICE ITEMS USING A CHART, TABLE, OR GRAPHIC IMAGE

This type of multiple-choice item presents a question with four options as potential answers. A chart, table or graphic image is presented along with the question. You must analyze the image and select the correct answer from the presented options.

SAMPLE ITEM 8–33

Identify which colostomy site along the large intestines would produce stool that is formed but soft. Select site a, b, c, or d.

(1) a

(2) b

(3) c

(4) d

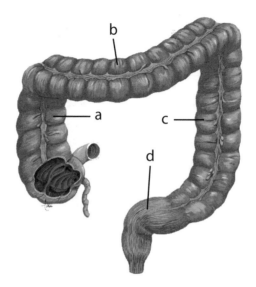

SAMPLE ITEM 8-34

Referring to the Intake and Output flow sheet for a patient admitted at 8:00 AM, what was the patient's total fluid intake for the 7 hours between 8:00 AM and 3:00 PM?

(1) 527 mL

(2) 720 mL

(3) 1245 mL

(4) 1405 mL

DAILY INTAKE AND OUTPUT RECORD

DATE JUNE 5

	INTAKE							OUTPUT			
	I.V. FLUIDS						ORAL	URINE	EMESIS	N.G TUBE	HEMOVAC
Time	Bottle	Amount	Solution	Medication and Dosage	*ABS.	∓LIB					
8	1	1000	NS	20 mEq KCl				650			
8:30							360				
10:00							120				
11:30							240	150			
12:00									160		
1:40									90		60
2:15								250			
3:00					525	475					45
7-3 TOTAL		8-HR TOTAL			525	475	720	1050	250		105
3-11 TOTAL		8-HR TOTAL									
11-7 TOTAL		8-HR TOTAL									
24 HOUR TOTAL											

INTAKE GRAND TOTAL [   ]   OUTPUT GRAND TOTAL [   ]

*ABS. = amount absorbed   ∓LIB = Left in bag

DRAG AND DROP/ORDERED RESPONSE ITEMS

A drag and drop item presents a situation followed by a list of statements. You are asked to place them in order of priority. For example, it may be steps in a procedure or actions that need to be placed in order of importance. When taken on a computer each option must be highlighted and dragged with your mouse and then dropped in a designated area in rank order. When included on a written test you may be asked to write the numbers of the options in the rank order you identify.

SAMPLE ITEM 8–35

The nurse discovers a fire in the dayroom where a patient is watching television. Rank the following actions from 1 to 4 in the order in which they should be performed in accordance with the RACE acronym associated with fire safety.

(1) Pull the fire alarm

(2) Shut the doors on the unit

(3) Take the patient out of the dayroom

(4) Move patients out of rooms adjacent to the dayroom

Answer: _____.

SAMPLE ITEM 8–36

A person who was in a motor vehicle collision is brought to the emergency department via an ambulance. When the patient arrives in the emergency department, the nurse identifies that the patient is unresponsive and initiates the assessment for CPR. List the following assessments in order of priority.

(1) Level of consciousness

(2) Patency of airway

(3) Breathing pattern

(4) Urinary output

(5) Heart rate

Answer: _____

MULTIPLE RESPONSE ITEMS

A multiple response item requires you to identify one or more correct options from among a list of presented options.

SAMPLE ITEM 8–37

The nurse assesses a patient and concludes that the patient has a fluid volume deficit. Which assessments supports this conclusion? Select all that apply.

(1) _____ Tenting of skin

(2) _____ Decreased pulse

(3) _____ Sudden weight loss

(4) _____ Increased blood pressure

(5) _____ Longitudinal furrows in the tongue

SAMPLE ITEM 8–38

The nurse manager of a medical/surgical unit is making the assignments for the day for the nursing members of the health team. Select those activities that can be assigned to a nursing assistant.

(1) _____ Changing the linen of a patient in traction.

(2) _____ Teaching a patient who is receiving an opioid how to prevent constipation.

(3) _____ Massaging the back of a patient who is on complete bed rest.

(4) _____ Transferring a patient from the bed to a chair by using a mechanical lift.

(5) _____ Reinforcing a postoperative dressing that is saturated with a bloody discharge.

(6) _____ Obtaining the vital signs of a patient who is returning from the postanesthesia care unit.

CHART/EXHIBIT ITEMS

A chart/exhibit item presents a situation and asks a question. It provides information that can be accessed via a variety of tabs. Each tab must be reviewed to collect information within the tab. When taken on a computer you must click on one tab to collect the information within the tab before moving onto the next tab. When included on a written test you probably will be able to view the information within all the tabs at the same time. You must identify significant information within each tab and integrate the information from among the tabs. From this analysis you can make inferences, deductions, and/or conclusions that eliminate options and support the correct answer.

SAMPLE ITEM 8–39

A 90-year-old man is admitted to the hospital with a diagnosis of change in mental status. A family member states that the patient has not eaten much for the last week and seemed very confused this morning. After the nurse completes a physical assessment and reviews the patient's medical record, the most likely inference is, "The patient:

(1) Is dehydrated."

(2) Has hypervolemia."

(3) Has a urinary tract infection."

(4) Is experiencing hyperglycemia."

CHART/EXHIBIT

Laboratory Results: Sodium 155 mEq/L
WBC 8000 µL
Hct 60%
FBS 114 mg/dL

Vital Signs: 2:00 PM 100°F, P 88, R 24

Nursing Progress Note: Patient is oriented to place and person but is easily distracted, is unable to follow directions, voided a small amount of clear amber urine, tongue has furrows and there is tenting of the skin.

A patient comes to the emergency department with concerns about extreme fatigue and prolonged episodes of menstruation. The practitioner performs a battery of tests. When reviewing the patient's record, the nurse identifies that the patient's oxygen problem is related to impaired:

(1) Osmosis

(2) Diffusion

(3) Transport

(4) Ventilation

CHART/EXHIBIT

Laboratory Tests: RBC 2.9×10^6
WBC 7000 mm³
Hgb 8.5 g/dL
Hct 34%

Radiologic Reports: Chest x-ray: normal findings; all bones aligned and symmetrical; normal positioned soft tissues, mediastinum, lungs, pleura, heart, and aortic arc.

Vital Signs Sheet: Temperature: 98.8°F (oral temperature)
Pulse: 92 and regular
Respirations: 24 per minute, regular rhythm, and unlabored

Summary

To promote success when challenged by an examination with a variety of testing formats, it is wise to be familiar with the various formats. Structured-response, restricted-response, extended-essay, and performance-appraisal formats are commonly used in schools of nursing in addition to the alternate-item formats found on NCLEX such as fill-in-the-blank items, multiple-response items, hot spot items, multiple-choice items using a chart, table or graphic image; drag and drop/ordered response items; and chart/exhibit items. These questions have some commonalities, but each is unique. Understanding the commonalities and differences in these formats and using a variety of test-taking techniques facilitates a feeling of control, which contributes to a positive mental attitude.

TEST SUCCESS: TEST-TAKING TECHNIQUES

Answers and Rationales for Sample Items in Chapter 8

8-1 **Answer: 1 and 3.** A stage III pressure ulcer involves a full-thickness skin loss (through the dermis and epidermis) extending to the subcutaneous tissue, but not through underlying fascia of muscle. It does not involve underlying bone or supportive structures. It presents as a deep crater that may or may not undermine adjacent tissue.

8-2 **Answer: 3, 4, 5, and 6.** To protect others from the infected patient, providers of care must wear masks when entering the room and the patient must wear a mask when being transported outside the room. The door should be kept closed except when entering or exiting the room. A negative airflow room prevents room air from flowing through the door to the nursing unit and expels the room air to the outside environment. A gown and gloves are not necessary when entering the room of a patient who is on Airborne Transmission-Based Precautions unless there is a likelihood of splashing of blood, body fluids, body secretions, or excretions. Standard Precautions are followed when caring for any patient.

8-3 TRUE—Soap lowers the surface tension of water. Surface tension is the tendency of a liquid to minimize the area of its surface by contracting. Lowering the surface tension increases the ability of water to wet another surface.

8-4 TRUE—A broad stance widens the nurse's base of support, which promotes stability.

8-5 FALSE—Exercise is a stimulating activity that should be avoided before bedtime. Adequate exercise during the day promotes sleep later in the day.

8-6 FALSE—Pulse pressure is the difference between the systolic and diastolic blood pressures. Pulse deficit is the difference between the apical and radial pulse rates.

8-7 TRUE—Palpation is a technique in which the examiner applies the fingers or hands to the body to assess the texture, size, consistency, and location of body parts.

8-8 FALSE—The process in which solid, particulate matter in a fluid moves from an area of higher concentration to an area of lower concentration is known as *diffusion*. The process in which a pure solvent, such as water, moves through a semipermeable membrane from an area that has a lower solute concentration to one that has a higher solute concentration is known as *osmosis*.

8-9 ① TRUE—The outer border of a drape is considered contaminated. After sterile gloves are donned, the nurse can touch only inside this border to maintain sterility of the field.
② TRUE—Because the hands are not sterile, the nurse avoids contaminating the sterile glove by touching only the inside of the glove. The second sterile glove is donned by touching just the outside of the glove with the hand that is already covered by the first sterile glove.
③ FALSE—During a surgical hand scrub, the hands are held above the elbows; this allows water to flow downward by gravity without contaminating the nurse's hands. Handwashing associated with medical asepsis requires the hands to be held below the elbows.
④ FALSE—Sterile objects held below the waist are not within the nurse's direct visual field and inadvertently may become contaminated.

8-10 ① TRUE—Mechanical ventilation uses positive pressure to push air and/or oxygen into the lungs during the inspiratory phase of the respiratory cycle. Positive pressure is pressure greater than that of the atmosphere.
② FALSE—A continuous bladder irrigation uses the principle of gravity to instill fluid into the bladder as well as to promote the flow of fluid out of the bladder through the triple-lumen indwelling urinary catheter. Gravity is the force that draws all masses in the earth's sphere toward the center of the earth.
③ FALSE—Chest tubes (chest drainage system) exert negative pressure to remove air and fluids from the pleural space. Negative pressure is pressure less than that of the atmosphere, and it is the opposite of positive pressure.
④ TRUE—Positive pressure is exerted when the plunger of a piston syringe is pushed toward its cone tip.

8-11　　**FALSE**—This statement can be revised in two different ways. The expected range of the heart rate for an adult is *60 to 100* beats per minute, or the expected range of the heart rate for a *6-year-old child* is 70 to 110 beats per minute. Either of these revisions results in a correct statement.

8-12　　**FALSE**—To revise this question as directed, the words *young adulthood* must be changed to *adolescence.* You would not receive credit for this question if you changed *identity versus role confusion* to *intimacy versus isolation.* Although this statement is accurate, the instructions for revising the statement have not been followed.

8-13　　① **FALSE**—The patient's temperature was 101.4°F. Each line above 101 is 2/10 of a degree.
　　　　② **TRUE**—Body temperature varies throughout the day with the lowest temperature in the early morning and the highest temperature between 8 PM and midnight. A circadian rhythm (diurnal variation) is a pattern based on a 24-hour cycle.
　　　　③ **TRUE**—With fluid volume deficit, the volume in the intravascular compartment decreases (hypovolemia), resulting in a decreased blood pressure (hypotension).
　　　　④ **TRUE**—This patient's pulse rate per minute ranged from 76 (on June 10th and 11th) to 110 (on June 5th and 6th).
　　　　⑤ **TRUE**—A pulse rate of 96 is within the expected range of 60 to 100 beats per minute.
　　　　⑥ **FALSE**—During the acute phase of the illness, the patient's temperature, pulse, and respirations were all elevated.

8-14　　① **TRUE**—The intravenous solution was hung at 8 AM and infused 525 mL over the next 7 hours. The total volume (525) divided by the number of hours (7) equals 75 mL per hour.
　　　　② **FALSE**—If each ounce is equal to 30 mL, 4 ounces is equal to 120 mL. If you subtract 120 from the total volume of fluid taken at 8:30 AM (360), the amount of additional fluid consumed was 240 mL. If you divide 240 mL by 30 mL, it equals 8 ounces, not 10.
　　　　③ **FALSE**—The intake was 525 + 720 = 1245 mL. The output was 1050 + 250 + 105 = 1405 mL. The output exceeded the intake by 160 mL.
　　　　④ **FALSE**—The additive to the patient's intravenous solution was 20 mEq of potassium chloride (KCl).

8-15　　**a. 3.**　*Bradypnea* is abnormally slow breathing (less than 10 breaths per minute) with a regular rhythm.
　　　　b. 4.　*Apnea* is the temporary cessation of breathing.
　　　　c. 1.　*Hyperpnea* is deep, rapid, labored respirations, usually associated with strenuous exercise.
　　　　d. 5.　*Tachypnea* is abnormally rapid breathing (more than 20 breaths per minute) with a regular rhythm.
　　　　e. 6.　*Eupnea* is breathing that is expected in rate (12 to 20 breaths per minute) and depth (tidal volume of approximately 500 mL).
　　　　f. 2.　*Dyspnea* is difficulty breathing characterized by an increased effort and use of accessory muscles.

　　　　"Shallow breathing interrupted by irregular periods of apnea" (option 7) was an extra option included in Column II that did not have a matching term in Column I.

8-16　　**a. 4.**　Kegel exercises consist of repetitive contractions of the muscles of the pelvic floor. These muscles facilitate voluntary control of urination.
　　　　b. 4.　Kegel exercises, which are performed by voluntarily starting and stopping the urinary stream, tone the perineal muscles of the pelvic floor.
　　　　c. 2.　Aerobic exercises involve activity that demands that oxygen be taken into the body at a rate greater than the amount the body usually requires, promoting respiratory functioning.
　　　　d. 2.　Aerobic exercises involve sustained muscle movements that increase blood flow, heart rate, and metabolic demand for oxygen over time, promoting cardiovascular functioning.
　　　　e. 3.　Isometric exercises cause a change in muscle tension but no change in muscle length; no muscle or joint movement occurs.
　　　　f. 1.　Passive range-of-motion exercises occur when another person moves each of the patient's joints through their full range of movement, maximally stretching all muscle groups within each plane over each joint.

8-17 *Contracture* is the only acceptable answer to this question. Contractures are permanent flexion deformities of joints caused by disuse, atrophy, and shortening of muscles.

8-18 *Respiratory passages* or *lung* would both be acceptable answers to this question. With postural drainage, the patient is placed in various positions to promote the movement of secretions from smaller to larger pulmonary airways, where they can be removed by coughing or suctioning.

8-19 The correct answer for this question is *12 to 20.*

8-20 The correct answer is *location.* Radiating pain is a description that relates to where the pain is experienced in the body. It includes the initial site of the pain and its extension to other parts of the body. Intensity refers to the perceived severity of the pain; intensity can be measured on a scale of 0 (no pain) to 10 (severe pain).

8-21 The correct answer is *urgency.* Urgency is the feeling that the person must void whether or not there is much urine in the bladder. It is precipitated by psychologic stress and/or irritation of the vesical trigone and/or urethra. Frequency is the increased incidence of voiding.

8-22 Acceptable answers include: permanent flexion and fixation of a joint; an abnormal shortening of a muscle that results in limited range of motion of a joint and eventually ankylosis. Compare this item with sample item 8–17.

8-23 Acceptable answers include: mobilize respiratory secretions; loosen pulmonary secretions to facilitate their expectoration; promote a clear airway by draining respiratory secretions toward the oral cavity. Compare this item with sample item 8–18.

8-24 Acceptable answers may include just stating the numbers 12 to 20. A more complex answer might state: The expected (normal) number of breaths per minute for an adult ranges from 12 to 20 with an average of 16. The expected (normal) respiratory rate in relation to the heart rate usually is 1 respiration to every 4 heartbeats. The respiratory rate usually increases with exercise and decreases with rest or sleep. Compare this item with sample item 8–19.

8-25 Answer: 25 drops per minute. To arrive at the correct answer, you have to perform the following calculation:

$$\frac{\text{Volume to be infused} \times \text{drop factor}}{\text{Number of hours} \times 60 \text{ minutes}}$$

$$\frac{100 \times 15}{1 \times 60}$$

$$1500 \div 60 = 25 \text{ drops per minute}$$

8-26 To answer this question, use the three-part format.

INTRODUCTION: The introduction functions as a preface, preamble, or prologue for what information will follow.

Although there are many detailed definitions of the practice of nursing, in the simplest terms nursing consists of helping people meet needs. To do this, nurses must employ cognitive skills such as critical thinking and problem solving. The commonalities and differences of critical thinking and problem solving will be discussed.

CENTRAL PART: The central part of the answer presents and explores the information necessary to answer the question. Make a topical outline of the facts to be included, and then write a narrative that incorporates and elaborates on the information in the outline.

Definition of critical thinking
   Reasoning
   Goal directed
   Reaching conclusions from a new perspective

Definition of problem solving
   Identifies a problem
   Suggests solutions
   Implements interventions to resolve problems

Commonalities of critical thinking and problem solving
   Strong knowledge base
   Attitude of inquiry and intellectual humility
   Systematic process
   Identifies priorities

Differences of critical thinking
   Uses problem-solving techniques
   Proactive
   Focuses more on the positive
   Open-ended and focuses on continuous improvement

Differences of problem solving
   Reactive
   Focuses more on the negative
   Starts with a problem and ends with a solution

SUMMARY: The summary should briefly recap or review the general theme of the discussion and come to one or more conclusions. It serves to close the response to the essay question.

The nurse of today and especially of the future must be able to integrate critical thinking and problem solving to maximize human potential. The nurse must use critical thinking to effectively resolve problems, and the nurse must use problem-solving techniques to think critically. Although they have a common foundation, each mode of thinking is unique. Nurses should blend them into a repertoire of cognitive strategies.

8-27 The radial artery is located on the inner aspect of the forearm along the side of the radius bone on the thumb side of the wrist.

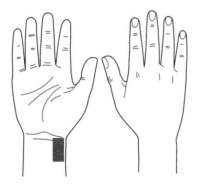

8-28 **Answer: 97.8°F.** Find the box in the top left that indicates "Day of Month." Read toward the right across the row until you see the box with the 10 (indicating the 10th day of the month). Look two rows down below the box with the 10 until you see the box with AM. Now look below the AM box for the box with the 4. Guide your eye down the column until you find a dot on a line. From the dot on the line guide your eye left across the row until you reach the numbers running along the left edge of the graph. Move down the column of numbers until you see the nearest dark line below the row with the dot that indicates a full degree of temperature. In this example, it is 97. The dot in the 4 AM column is 4 light-colored lines above the 97 line. Each of the light-colored lines indicates 2/10 of a degree of temperature. Therefore, the dot in the 4 AM column indicates a temperature of 97.8°F.

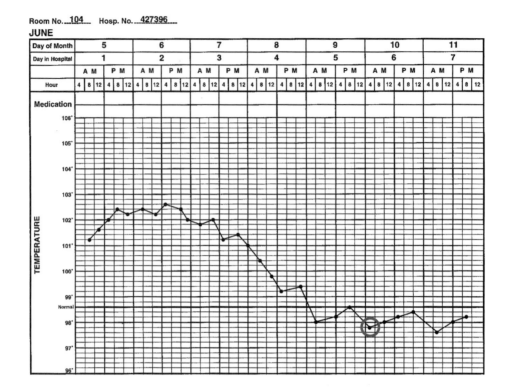

Room No. __104__   Hosp. No. __427396__

Alternate-Format Items Reflective of NCLEX

FILL-IN-THE-BLANK ITEMS

8-29 **Answer: 63 mL/hour.** 1500 ÷ 24 = 62.5 mL. When a portion of an mL is 0.5 or greater, round up to the next full number.

8-30 **Answer: 1.5 mL.**

1 gram is equal to 1000 mg. Solve the problem using ratio and proportion.

$$\frac{\text{Desired}}{\text{Have}} \quad \frac{500 \text{ mg}}{1000 \text{ mg}} = \frac{\text{x mL}}{3 \text{ mL}}$$

$$1000 \text{ x} = 1500$$

$$\frac{1000 \text{ x}}{1000} = \frac{1500}{1000}$$

$$\text{x} = 1.5 \text{ mL}$$

HOT SPOT ITEMS

8-31 The sacral area (shaded) is at greatest risk for dependent edema for this patient. Fluid volume excess increases capillary pressures causing fluid to move from the intravascular compartment into interstitial tissue. Because fluid flows by gravity, edema is observed in dependent tissues. A patient who has difficulty breathing is generally positioned in a semi- or high-Fowler's position. In the Fowler's position the sacrum is the most dependent area and is therefore at greatest risk for interstitial edema.

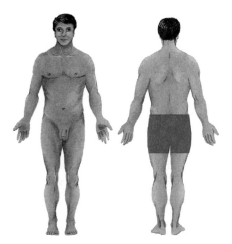

8-32   The *vastus lateralis* site (shaded) is located on the middle third and anterior lateral aspect of the thigh, one handbreadth above the knee (from the lateral femoral condyle) and one handbreadth below the greater trochanter.

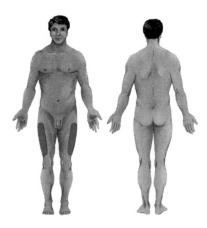

MULTIPLE-CHOICE ITEMS USING A CHART, TABLE, OR GRAPHIC IMAGE

8-33   ① a—This site is the ascending colon, which contains the most liquid stool because it is at the beginning of the large intestine, where little fluid has yet to be reabsorbed.
② b—The stool in the transverse colon is pasty.
③ c— Stool in the descending colon is formed but soft. As stool moves through the large intestines, fluid is reabsorbed and stool becomes more dry and formed.
④ d—Stool in the sigmoid colon is formed and firm.

8-34   ① 525 mL is the total amount of fluid absorbed via the intravenous infusion.
② 720 mL is the total amount of oral fluid intake.
③ 1245 mL: To arrive at the total intake for the 7 hours between 8 AM and 3 PM, the nurse has to add the 525 mL of IV fluid absorbed (indicated in the box at the bottom of the "Abs" column in the row labeled "7-3 total" and the 720 mL of oral intake (indicated in the box at the bottom of the "ORAL" column in the row labeled "7-3 total." 525 mL of IV fluids plus 720 mL of oral intake equals 1245 mL of total fluid intake for the 7 hours between 8 AM and 3 PM.
④ 1405 mL is the total amount of urine, emesis, and Hemovac output.

DAILY INTAKE AND OUTPUT RECORD

DATE   JUNE 5

	INTAKE						OUTPUT				
	I.V. FLUIDS						ORAL	URINE	EMESIS	N.G. TUBE	HEMOVAC
Time	Bottle	Amount	Solution	Medication and Dosage	* ABS.	∓ LIB					
8	1	1000	NS	20 mEq KCl				650			
8:30							360				
10:00							120				
11:30							240	150			
12:00									160		
1:40									90		60
2:15					↓			250			
3:00					525	475					45
7-3 TOTAL		8-HR TOTAL			525	475	720	1050	250		105
3-11 TOTAL		8-HR TOTAL									
11-7 TOTAL		8-HR TOTAL									
24 HOUR TOTAL											

INTAKE GRAND TOTAL [ ]   OUTPUT GRAND TOTAL [ ]

* ABS. = amount absorbed   ∓ LIB = left in bag

DRAG AND DROP/ORDERED RESPONSE ITEMS

8-35 Answer: 3, 1, 2, 4

③ Take the patient out of the dayroom—**R**emove: The priority is to remove the patient, who is in the immediate vicinity of the fire and is at risk for injury.

① Pull the fire alarm—**A**ctivate: Once the patient is protected from harm, the fire alarm can be activated.

② Shut the doors on the unit—**C**ontain: After the patient is protected from harm and the alarm is sounded, measures can be implemented to contain the fire by actions such as closing doors.

④ Move patients out of rooms adjacent to the dayroom—**E**vacuate: This is necessary only after the previous three steps are implemented and if it is determined that patients are at risk.

8-36 Answer: 1, 2, 3, 5, 4

① Level of consciousness. The initial step in CPR is to determine if the patient is unresponsive.

② Patency of airway. The airway must be unobstructed to ensure that inhalation and exhalation can occur.

③ Breathing pattern. Feeling and hearing air movement ensures gas exchange in and out of the lung; oxygen deprivation for 4 minutes or longer can cause brain damage.

⑤ Heart rate. Assessing the heart rate ensures cardiac output. This can be assessed via an apical or carotid pulse.

④ Urinary output. In an emergency situation this is the least important assessment. However, a urinary output of less than 30–50 mL per hour may indicate inadequate cardiovascular or kidney function.

MULTIPLE RESPONSE ITEMS

8-37 ① _X_ Tenting of skin occurs because of the decrease in interstitial and intracellular fluid.
② ____ The pulse increases to compensate for hypovolemia.
③ _X_ One liter of fluid weighs 2.2 pounds. The patient will lose weight as fluid is excreted.
④ ____ The blood pressure decreases because of the decreased intravascular fluid volume.
⑤ _X_ Interstitial and intracellular fluid shifts to the intravascular compartment to maintain cardiovascular function. As a result, the tongue becomes furrowed and dry.

8-38 ① _X_ Assisting patients with the activities of daily living, which includes maintaining clean linen for a patient in traction, is within the scope of practice of a nursing assistant.
② ____ Patient teaching is an independent role of a nurse, not a nursing assistant. This teaching requires the knowledge of anatomy, physiology, pharmacology, teaching/learning principles, and rationales for appropriate nursing interventions.
③ _X_ This is part of a bath, an activity of daily living, which is within the scope of practice of a nursing assistant.
④ _X_ Assisting patients with the activities of daily living, which includes transferring patients from the bed to a chair, is within the scope of practice of a nursing assistant.
⑤ ____ Caring for surgical dressings, which requires the use of sterile technique, is not within the scope of practice of a nursing assistant.
⑥ ____ Although nursing assistants can take the routine vital signs of patients who are physiologically stable, immediate postoperative patients and patients who are physiologically unstable should have their vital signs assessed by a nurse.

CHART/EXHIBIT ITEMS

8-39

CHART/EXHIBIT

Laboratory Results: Sodium 155 mEq/L
WBC 8000 μL
Hct 60%
FBS 110 mg/dL

Vital Signs: 2:00 PM 100°F, P 88, R 24

Nursing Progress Note: Patient is oriented to place and person but is easily distracted, is unable to follow directions, voided a small amount of clear amber urine, tongue has furrows, and there is tenting of the skin.

ANSWER & RATIONALES: 1. The physical assessment and laboratory results indicate that the patient is dehydrated. Oliguria, furrows of the tongue, tenting of the skin, and elevated vital signs are all signs of dehydration. The serum sodium level that is higher than the expected range of 135–145 mEq/L and the Hct that is higher than the expected range of 40%–54% indicate hemoconcentration associated with dehydration.
2. With hypervolemia, the patient's Hct would be low indicating hemodilution.
3. With a urinary tract infection there would not be just an elevation in the temperature; the WBCs also would be elevated and the urine would be cloudy.
4. The physical assessment data do not support the inference that the patient has hyperglycemia. The FBS is within the expected limits of 70–120 mg/dL in the older adult and there is an absence of polyuria, polyphagia, polydipsia, fatigue, weakness, and vision changes.

CHART/EXHIBIT

Laboratory Tests: RBC 2.9×10^6
WBC 7000 mm³
Hgb 8.5 g/dL
Hct 34%

Radiologic Reports: Chest x-ray: normal findings; all bones aligned and symmetrical; normal positioned soft tissues, mediastinum, lungs, pleura, heart, and aortic arc.

Vital Signs Sheet: Temperature: 98.8°F (oral temperature) Pulse: 92 and regular
Respirations: 24 per minute, regular rhythm, and unlabored

ANSWER AND RATIONALES: 1. Osmosis is related to fluid balance not respiratory status. Osmosis is the movement of water through a semipermeable membrane from an area of lower concentration of constituents to an area of higher concentration of constituents. This is unrelated to this patient situation.

2. The patient's respiratory status—an unlabored respiratory rate of 24 with a regular rhythm—does not reflect a problem with diffusion. The slight increase in respiratory rate is a compensatory response to the decreased number of RBCs that carry oxygen to all body cells. The chest x-ray rules out primary lung disease indicating that problems with diffusion do not exist.

3. **The patient has a problem with oxygen transport because of an inadequate number of red blood cells; the hemoglobin component of red blood cells carries oxygen to body cells. When comparing the patient's laboratory results to the expected values below, the results indicate that the patient's RBC, Hgb, and Hct are all low reflecting a reduced ability to transport oxygen on the hemoglobin molecule of the RBCs. The expected range for women:**
   RBC: 3.6 to 5.0×10^6
   WBC: 5000 to 7000 mm³
   Hgb: 12.0 to 16.0 g/dL
   Hct: 36% to 48%

4. Although the elevated pulse and respirations may indicate a problem with ventilation, the fact that the respirations are unlabored and the chest x-ray results are within expected limits, problems with these functions are not supported.

Computer Applications in Education and Evaluation

We are members of an informational society in which information is created, stored, retrieved, manipulated, and communicated. Exploding knowledge and technology, the emerging health-care reform initiatives, and the intensified and diversified role of the nurse all add to the complexity of functioning within this informational society. To process information efficiently, effectively, and economically, computers are essential. They have become a reality in every aspect of our world and are used in private homes, educational settings, industry, and health-care facilities. To prepare for a career in nursing, you must have the basic skills to use computers in a comfortable manner and be a willing learner to keep pace with rapidly advancing computer technology. Although computers are used in the practice of nursing, this chapter will focus on the use of computers only in relation to education and evaluation.

Computing across the curriculum is not new in the educational setting. Educators immediately identified the potential of interactive participation to facilitate learning. Programmed-instruction textbooks were the predecessors of computer programs. These textbooks present information within blocked narrative material. Each grouping of material is called a frame. Each frame requires a response from the learner before moving on to the next narrative frame. These textbooks require active involvement by the learner. Computers make this programmed approach more interactive by increasing the potential, richness, and variety of frame styles, which improve the effectiveness of the lesson. Computers also use graphics, color, and sound to facilitate learning in a way that programmed instruction textbooks are unable to do because of the limitations of the written format.

Students generally enjoy using the computer to facilitate learning because the programs hold their attention, provide immediate feedback, and never become impatient. Also, they are accessible, challenging, and fun. Computer-based instruction is not designed to replace the more traditional forms of teaching in most settings but to augment them. Computers allow you to review difficult material at your own rate, increase critical thinking, experience simulated clinical situations, and assess your knowledge. The greatest advantage of computer-based instruction is that you become an active participant, not just a passive spectator.

To be an active participant, you should have a simple understanding of a few essential keyboard keys. Most programs are "user friendly" and include on-screen instructions or help menus. Generally, students do not have difficulty manipulating the keyboard or mouse (handheld device to move an on-screen directional arrow). However, some students have "computer anxiety." Only exposure to computers in a secure and positive learning environment can lessen computer anxiety and promote computer literacy.

The following are examples of how computers can be used in education and evaluation. The computer can enhance student learning by accessing professional resources, managing information, teaching, simulating clinical situations, and evaluating knowledge.

The Computer as a Resource Tool

The computer is a resource tool that can be used to obtain information for academic assignments. A computerized literature search that uses national databases or networks can provide rapid access to current literature in nursing and its related fields. A modem (a device that allows transmission of data between computers over a telephone or cable line) connects you to the information retrieval system, and specific protocols may be required to gain entry to a database. These searches usually can be conducted in most libraries with the assistance of the research librarian. However, cost may be a factor because lines must be maintained to transmit and receive information. Most systems also have online connect charges for accessing the database as well as for the length of time the database is being used, and a fee may be charged for online or off-line printing. Online printing provides an immediate hard copy of the desired information, whereas off-line printing provides a hard copy that is sent by mail at a later date. Sometimes the fees incurred are beyond the financial means of the average student. Literature searches on the computer save time and energy. Therefore, you must decide whether these activities are cost effective for you by measuring the time saved against the money spent.

The Computer as an Information Manager

The computer has revolutionized the way in which information is managed, not only outside the home but inside the home. Many people now compose written material immediately on the computer. This is possible because you no longer need to have strong keyboard skills or expend extensive time and energy to learn how to use software programs. Today, user-friendly software programs have on-screen commands and effective help menus. Touch, a stylus, or a mouse also help facilitate computer use. The personal computer can be used for word processing, setting up spreadsheets, data processing, graphing data, and so on. You can now manipulate data, words, and images to complete your academic assignments with ease.

The Computer as an Instructor

Computer-assisted instruction (CAI) is an excellent addition to the repertoire of strategies available to educators and nursing students to facilitate the learning process. In CAI, information is communicated from the computer to the learner without direct interaction with the teacher. These instructional delivery systems can present principles and theory, enhance comprehension, promote creative problem solving, and provide immediate feedback to enrich independent learning.

Some computer programs display information in a textual format that has limited interaction between you and the computer. These programs really function as an automated textbook. Other tutorial approaches present new information in small steps or frames, then require you to make responses to demonstrate your comprehension of the material just delivered. Such programs function as an automated, programmed-instruction textbook. These types of programs generally use a linear format that proceeds from the beginning of the program to the end of the program without deviation. They present information in a straight line, with one beginning and one end, and every student is exposed to the same information. Although valuable, these programs do not recognize the learner as an individual with specific needs, interests, and abilities.

With the advent of CD-ROM (Compact Disk–Read-Only Memory) technology and sophisticated software programs, the computer learning experience has become more individualized. Programs that use a branching format allow you to select a path that focuses on information relevant to your ability and interest. When programs meet individualized needs, learning is more effective, use of time is more efficient, and student motivation increases.

The Computer as a Tool for Distance Education

Computers and the technology that affects their use are revolutionizing the existing parameters about what is a teaching/learning environment. The age of the Internet has enabled a shift from the typical classroom setting to distance learning/education via the Internet/Worldwide Web.

Distance education has created communities of learning that maximize communication between and among students and faculty. Many colleges and universities offer distance education courses in response to the needs of students who have part-time or full-time jobs, family responsibilities, study-time constraints, or who are geographically isolated. Originally, distance education involved print materials, instruction via audio or video cassettes, and communication via telephone, voice mail, and faxing. Today, technological advances including fixed computer media (e.g., CD-ROM), room-based video conferencing (e.g., interactive television), desktop video conferencing, the Worldwide Web (e.g., Internet-based programming), etc., provide multimedia methods of instruction that many students find more challenging and interesting than the traditional text-based materials. These new methods of delivery promote learning in the cognitive (thinking), affective (feeling), and psychomotor (skills) learning domains inherent in nursing practice, which is an intellectually challenging and social, behavioral, and practice-oriented profession.

Distance education has both advantages and disadvantages and requires a special type of learner.

Advantages of distance education include:

- Accessibility to education for those who are geographically isolated
- Opportunities for learning within a flexible time frame
- An individualized pace of learning
- Active participation
- Self-motivation
- Development of computer literacy

Disadvantages of distance education include:

- Lack of face-to-face communication
- A sense of isolation
- Difficulty with course content in the affective (feelings) and psychomotor (skills) learning domains
- Adjustment to innovative teaching/evaluation strategies
- Pressure to master the technology

Characteristics of students who participate successfully in distance education are:

- Risk takers
- Assertive
- Self-directed
- Responsible

Distance education, particularly in nursing education, is still in its infancy. Important questions exist regarding student financial aid, confidentiality, source of finances for infrastructure, availability of qualified nursing faculty, transferability of credit, delivery of academic support services, and valid and reliable methods of evaluation. These concerns have legal and ethical implications that must be addressed for distance education to be a viable alternative for students who want to become nurses. The computer as a tool for distance education has unlimited potential and has already revolutionized higher education. Only the future will tell if computers in relation to distance education will increase the number of graduate nurses and help reverse the nursing shortage.

The Computer as a Simulator

The role of the nursing educator is to assist you to move beyond the mere memorization of facts to the application of information in clinical situations. To do this, you must use critical thinking to integrate information into a meaningful frame of reference. Computer simulations are designed to enhance your ability to use critical thinking and safely make sound judgments in a fabricated situation. These simulation programs provide a supportive environment because they usually produce less anxiety and are obviously safe for the "patient." Although computer simulation has long been used in aeronautics and flight training, it is in its infancy in simulating experiences within the health-care professions.

Nursing simulations may present a patient database that requires you to input, sort, and retrieve data. Simulations may focus on the application of information processing skills, which assist you to select sources of data that are most appropriate, classify data, cluster and sequence data, and even evaluate data. Simulations may focus on components of critical thinking. A program addressing critical thinking may require you to identify relationships, recognize commonalities and differences, and use deductive and inductive reasoning to support inferences. Simulations may also be designed to improve decision making by requiring you to identify the nature of the problem, choose a course of action from multiple options, establish priorities, and evaluate the outcome of the final decision. In addition, simulations can present clinical situations that are difficult to present in a classroom setting or events that you may not have had the opportunity to experience in the clinical setting. Curricula cannot guarantee that every student will have an opportunity to experience each and every situation that may be important to learning. However, computer simulation may help to fill this void.

The disadvantage of simulation programs in nursing is that they cannot include all the unpredictable variables that occur in real-life situations. However, interactive videodisc instruction (IVD, IVI), a sophisticated form of computer-assisted instruction, uses the newest computer technology to enrich the clinical situations presented and encourage the highest degree of interaction between you and the computer. Studies have demonstrated that there is a highly significant degree of student satisfaction with interactive videodisc instruction and that a positive mental attitude is significant to the learning process because of its influence on student motivation, learning rate, and retention and application of information.

The Computer as an Evaluator

Evaluation (test-taking) programs are designed to measure your knowledge, skills, and abilities in relation to the practice of nursing. They can be self-administered or administered by a person in authority. Programs devised to be self-administered generally contain both a learning mode and a self-evaluation mode.

In the learning mode, you are presented with a question and are asked to select the correct answer. After you select an option, the program provides immediate feedback regarding the correctness of the choice. Rationales for the correct and wrong answers may be provided, depending on how the program is designed. The learning mode that provides rationales for all the choices has the potential to promote new learning or reinforce previous learning. These types of programs are a form of CAI.

The evaluation mode enables you to conduct an assessment of your test-taking abilities regarding a specific body of knowledge addressed in the program. The evaluation mode also allows you to experience a testing situation. Some programs provide rationales for all the options at the completion of the program. Other, more detailed programs may allow you to design self tests according to specific parameters (e.g., number of questions, clinical content, steps in the nursing process, difficulty level of the questions). Also, it may supply an individualized analysis of your performance after you take a test. This analysis may include information such as the questions you got wrong and why, the content areas that you need to study further, your performance in relation to other nursing students, or predictions for passing future examinations. Self-administered evaluation programs are particularly successful because they focus on competency and provide immediate feedback.

An evaluation program conducted by a person in authority may be administered to assess your ability to pass a course of study or to demonstrate your competency for certification or licensure. These programs use computer technology and replace paper-and-pencil tests. Some programs may use a format in which you and every other test taker are confronted by the exact same questions. Other programs may use **computerized-adaptive testing** (CAT), a unique format in which your examination is assembled interactively as you answer each question. In a typical CAT format, all the questions in the test bank have a calculated level of difficulty. You are presented with a question. If you answer the question correctly, you are presented with a slightly more difficult question. If you answer the question incorrectly, you are presented with a slightly easier question. This process is repeated for each question until a pass-or-fail decision is made. Passing is determined by your demonstration of knowledge, skills, and abilities in relation to a standard of acceptable performance. The advantages of the CAT format are that it individualizes each test, provides for self-paced testing, reduces the amount of time needed to complete the test, and produces greater measurement precision. The disadvantages of the CAT format are that you cannot review the entire test before starting, difficult questions cannot be skipped and returned to at a later time, and you cannot go back and change an answer once it is selected and entered.

In 1994 the NCLEX-RN and the NCLEX-PN, the licensure examinations for registered nurses and practical nurses, respectively, changed from standard paper-and-pencil tests to examinations using computerized-adaptive testing. Although no previous computer experience is necessary to take a test using CAT, it is always better to be familiar with the particular testing format used. There are many commercial products available that use the CAT format. Practice can only improve your performance on future CAT examinations.

Summary

Computers are causing major changes in the traditional ways things are done in health-care education and evaluation. In our informational society, some certainties exist: we are on information overload; the manipulation of information has become more sophisticated than ever before; and computers will be used more extensively in education, evaluation, and practice in the future. You must become computer literate and be willing to learn about new computer technology as it emerges. The most important implication of computer applications in learning, evaluation, and practice is that you can use the computer to increase the efficiency of your work and study, thereby leaving more time to interact with instructors, peers, and clients.

10

Analyze Your Test Performance

Students work hard at studying course content and learning and using test-taking strategies. However, they seldom progress to the important step of analyzing their test performance to determine their knowledge and information-processing strengths and needs. When reviewing a wrong answer, usually you are able to identify when you did not know the theory or principles being tested. However, without a performance analysis, you may not identify the trends in the gaps in your knowledge because you are lacking the "big picture." In addition, errors often occur because of inept information processing rather than because of lack of knowledge. When reviewing an exam, you might say, "What a silly mistake. I knew that content." This suggests that you probably made an information-processing error. Unless you identify your knowledge gaps and information-processing errors and take corrective action, you probably will continue to make the same mistakes over and over.

Students frequently do not review their test performance because they believe it is time-consuming or they do it in a haphazard, rather than a systematic, manner. A methodical analysis of your test performance is well worth the time and effort. It does take time because you have to stop and think critically about each item you answered incorrectly. However, you must spend time to save time. When you focus your study, you will study "better," not longer or harder. Also, the results of an analysis of your test performance should identify your information-processing errors. When you are aware of these errors, you can correct them, which should improve your test-taking abilities and ultimately your test grades.

You may find it threatening to analyze your test performance because it requires you to admit that you may be doing something wrong or that you are unprepared in some manner. You need to *get a grip!* Get over this kind of negative thinking! Finding fault is not the focus of a performance review. We all make mistakes. If we were perfect, we would not be human. The important point is that you must learn from your mistakes. If you are having difficulty with controlling negative thoughts, review Chapter 1, Empowerment. Your goal is to improve your test performance. Identifying your knowledge deficits and information-processing errors should provide a focus for corrective action. This places you in a position of control, which is essential if you are to be successful.

How to Use the Test-Analysis Tools

Two tools are presented in this chapter to analyze questions that you answer incorrectly. The first tool, **Identify Information-Processing Errors,** focuses on the "process" of test taking. It should disclose processing errors in relation to the stem of a question, the options in a question, and personal performance trends. It includes an area for comments for you to make notes about your reactions or questions you may want to explore with your instructor. The second tool, **Identify Knowledge Deficits,** focuses on the "content" aspect of a test. It may identify clusters of errors in specific knowledge categories. You can individualize these tools by further subdividing the areas under Processing Errors or Knowledge Categories. For example, if you find that on the Identify Information-Processing Errors tool you frequently got questions wrong because you read into the question, you might subdivide this area into "Added information from my own mind" and/or "Made assumptions." If you find that on the Identify Knowledge Deficits tool many of the questions you got wrong were in the area of perioperative nursing, you might subdivide this area into "Preoperative," "Intraoperative," and "Postoperative."

Complete each tool in the same way:

- Start by placing the number of the first question you got wrong in the first box on the left in the top row.
- Second, identify the Processing Error or Knowledge Category listed in the first column that relates to the question you answered incorrectly.
- Third, find the box where the column and row intersect and place an X in the box. Check all the boxes that apply for each question. Follow this process for every question you got wrong.
- Fourth, tally the total number of Xs for each row in the last column on the right. Students often will notice a clustering of errors in one area or another. With this information, you are able to develop a corrective action plan to address your individual needs.

IDENTIFY INFORMATION-PROCESSING ERRORS

PROCESSING ERRORS	QUESTION NUMBER														TOTAL
STEM															
Missed key word(s) indicating negative polarity															
Missed key word(s) setting a priority															
Missed important word(s) that were clues															
Misinterpreted information presented															
Missed the central point/theme															
Missed the central person															
Read into the question															
Missed the step in the nursing process (NP)															
Incompletely analyzed the stem; read it too quickly															
Did not understand what the question was asking															
Did not know or could not remember the content associated with the question															
OPTIONS															
Answered quickly without reading all the options															
Failed to respond to negative polarity in stem															
Misidentified the priority															
Misinterpreted information															
Read into option															
Did not know or could not remember the content															
Knew content but inaccurately applied concepts and principles															
Knew the right answer but recorded it inaccurately															

IDENTIFY INFORMATION-PROCESSING ERRORS

PERSONAL PERFORMANCE TRENDS	COMMENTS
1. I finished the exam with time to review YES { }　　　NO { }	
2. I was able to focus with little distraction YES { }　　　NO { }	
3. I felt calm and in control YES { }　　　NO { }	
4. When I changed answers, I got the questions right YES { }　　　NO { }	
5. Identify error clusters: 　First third of exam　　　　{ } 　Middle third of exam　　　{ } 　Last third of exam　　　　{ } 　No clusters identified　　　{ }	

IDENTIFY KNOWLEDGE DEFICITS

KNOWLEDGE CATEGORY	QUESTION NUMBER
Legal/ethical issues	
Health-care delivery systems	
Basic human needs	
Growth and development	
Communication	
Emotional needs	
Physical assessment	
Physical safety	
Mobility	
Hygiene	
Comfort	
Rest and sleep	
Nutrition	
Fluid balance	
Urinary elimination	
Bowel elimination	
Oxygen	
Microbiologic safety	
Administration of medications	
Pharmacology	
Perioperative	
Community setting	
Pathophysiology	
Anatomy and physiology	
Computations	
NURSING PROCESS	
Assessment	
Analysis and diagnosis	
Goal setting	
Planning intervention	
Implementation	
Evaluation	

Corrective Action Plan

The test analysis tools, Identify Information-Processing Errors and Identify Knowledge Deficits, were designed to ultimately affect the way you study and process information when answering test questions. After you complete the Identify Knowledge Deficits tool, you should devise study sessions that focus on the clustered areas of gaps in knowledge. For example, if you have 10 Xs in the row related to "Communication," you should study your class notes and required textbook readings that relate to communication theory, especially the specific content or principles being tested in the questions that you got wrong. Now review the practice questions in Chapter 11 that relate to communication content and evaluate your attainment of new information. With this approach, you can use your time wisely by focusing on what you still need to know and not waste time on what you already know.

After you complete the Identify Information-Processing Errors tool, you should use the **Corrective Action Guide for Information-Processing Errors.** The guide has three columns:

- The first column lists Processing Errors, which are identical to the Processing Errors in column 1 of the Identify Information-Processing Errors tool.
- Column 2 refers you to the chapters and sections in this textbook that address information related to the Processing Errors listed in column 1.
- Column 3 indicates the pages where you can find the information listed in column 2.

This guide directs you to information that you can review to correct your information-processing problems. For example, if you have multiple Xs in the row related to "Missed key word(s) setting a priority," you should review the information about Identify Key Words in the Stem That Set a Priority that is included in Chapter 7, Test-Taking Techniques. Now answer the practice questions in Chapter 11 and evaluate if you are better able to correctly identify key words in the stem that set a priority. With this approach, you can improve your information-processing abilities.

The Corrective Action Guide for Information-Processing Errors has a section titled Personal Performance Trends. **Personal Performance Trends** include issues such as:

- Time management (I finished the exam with time to review)
- Concentration (I was able to focus with little distraction)
- Empowerment (I felt calm and in control)
- Decisiveness/indecisiveness (When I changed answers, I got the questions right)
- Error clusters (Identify error clusters in first, middle, or last third of exam or no cluster errors)

If you answered No to any of the questions in the Personal Performance Trends section of the guide, refer to the appropriate area under Corrective Action to Address Problem Personal Performance Trends later in this chapter.

The Corrective Action Guide also has a "Comments" section for you to document your reactions to the exam or questions you may have about the exam that you can review with your instructor.

CORRECTIVE ACTION GUIDE FOR INFORMATION-PROCESSING ERRORS		
PROCESSING ERRORS	**REVIEW THE FOLLOWING SECTIONS IN THIS TEXTBOOK**	**PAGE NUMBER**
STEM		
Missed key word(s) indicating negative polarity	**Chapter 7,** Test-Taking Techniques (Identify Key Words in the Stem That Indicate Negative Polarity)	92
Missed key word(s) setting a priority	**Chapter 7,** Test-Taking Techniques (Identify Key Words in the Stem That Set a Priority)	93
Missed important word(s) that were clues	**Chapter 7,** Test-Taking Techniques (Identify Clues in the Stem)	95
Misinterpreted information presented	**Chapter 2,** Critical Thinking (Practice Critical Thinking and Apply Critical Thinking to Multiple-Choice Questions)	12 14

CORRECTIVE ACTION GUIDE FOR INFORMATION-PROCESSING ERRORS

PROCESSING ERRORS	REVIEW THE FOLLOWING SECTIONS IN THIS TEXTBOOK	PAGE NUMBER
Missed the central point/theme	**Chapter 2,** Critical Thinking (Practice Critical Thinking and Apply Critical Thinking to Multiple-Choice Questions)	12 14
Missed the central person	**Chapter 7,** Test-Taking Techniques (Identify the Central Person in the Question)	96
Read into the question	**Chapter 7,** Test-Taking Techniques (Avoid Reading into the Question)	108
	Chapter 2, Critical Thinking (Apply Critical Thinking to Multiple-Choice Questions)	14
Missed the step in the nursing process (NP)	**Chapter 6,** The Nursing Process (Focus on the Step That You Misidentify in the Identify Knowledge Deficits Tool)	63-89
Incompletely analyzed the stem	**Chapter 7,** Test-Taking Techniques (Avoid Reading into the Question and Identify Clues in the Stem)	108 95
	Chapter 2, Critical Thinking (Apply Critical Thinking to Multiple-Choice Questions)	14
Did not understand what the question was asking	**Chapter 7,** Test-Taking Techniques (Identify Clues in the Stem and Avoid Reading Into the Question)	95 108
	Chapter 2, Critical Thinking (Practice Critical Thinking and Apply Critical Thinking to Multiple-Choice Questions)	12 14
	Chapter 11, Practice Questions with Answers and Rationales (Study Answers and Rationales of Practice Questions)	159–294
Did not know or could not remember the content associated with the question	**Chapter 4,** Study Techniques (Specific Study Techniques Related to Cognitive Levels of Nursing Questions)	31
	Chapter 11, Practice Questions with Answers and Rationales (Study Answers and Rationales of Practice Questions)	159–294
OPTIONS Answered quickly without reading all the options	**Chapter 7,** Test-Taking Techniques (Avoid Reading into the Question)	108
Failed to respond to negative polarity in the stem	**Chapter 7,** Test-Taking Techniques (Identify Key Words in the Stem That Indicate Negative Polarity)	92
Misidentified the priority	**Chapter 7,** Test-Taking Techniques (Identify Key Words in the Stem That Set a Priority)	93
	Chapter 11, Practice Questions With Answers and Rationales (Study Answers and Rationales for Questions That Ask You to Set a Priority Indicated in the TEST-TAKING TIP)	159–294
Misinterpreted information	**Chapter 2,** Critical Thinking (Practice Critical Thinking and Apply Critical Thinking to Multiple-Choice Questions)	12 14
Read into options	**Chapter 7,** Test-Taking Techniques (Avoid Reading into the Question)	108
	Chapter 2, Critical Thinking (Apply Critical Thinking to Multiple-Choice Questions)	14
Did not know or could not remember the content	**Chapter 4,** Study Techniques (Specific Study Techniques Related to Cognitive Levels of Nursing Questions)	37
	Chapter 2, Critical Thinking (Apply Critical Thinking to Multiple-Choice Questions)	14
	Chapter 11, Practice Questions with Answers and Rationales (Study Answers and Rationales for Practice Questions)	159–294
Knew content but inaccurately applied concepts and principles	**Chapter 2,** Critical Thinking (Apply Critical Thinking to Multiple-Choice Questions)	14
	Chapter 11, Practice Questions with Answers and Rationales (Study Answers and Rationales for Practice Questions)	159–294

(Continued)

CORRECTIVE ACTION GUIDE FOR INFORMATION-PROCESSING ERRORS—*cont'd*

PERSONAL PERFORMANCE TRENDS	COMMENTS
1. I finished the exam with time to review YES { } NO { }	
2. I was able to focus with little distraction YES { } NO { }	
3. I felt calm and in control YES { } NO { }	
4. When I changed answers, I got the questions right YES { } NO { }	
5. Identify error clusters: First third of exam { } Middle third of exam { } Last third of exam { } No clusters identified { }	

Corrective Action to Address Personal Performance Trends

1. I finished the exam with time to review

If your answer was YES, you have managed your time well. If your answer was NO, you are not managing your time effectively and you need to identify why you are taking too long to proceed through the test. You need to answer the following questions:

- Am I taking too much time to answer each question?
- Am I getting bogged down and spending too much time on a few difficult questions that prevent me from finishing or reviewing the test?
- (Other) Identify your own questions.

Corrective Action—Review:

- Chapter 7, Test-Taking Techniques: Manage the Allotted Time to Your Advantage, page 107.
- Chapter 7, Test-Taking Techniques: Concentrate on the Simple Before the Complex, page 108.

2. I was able to focus with little distraction

If your answer was YES, you have sufficient concentration and the ability to block out distractions. If your answer was NO, you need to answer the following questions:

- Am I fatigued before and/or during the test?
- Do minor distractions in the environment cause me to lose focus?
- Was I physically uncomfortable during the test?
- (Other) Identify your own questions.

Corrective Action—Review:

- Chapter 1, Empowerment: Establish Control Before and During the Test, page 6.

3. I felt calm and in control

If your answer was YES, you have anxiety under control and are able to focus on the test rather than having to cope with anxious responses. If your answer was NO, you need to answer the following questions:

- Do I experience uncomfortable, fearful responses during exams?
- Do I experience internal mental stressors (negative self-talk) that block my confidence?
- Do I get flustered when confronted with a question that I am unable to answer?
- (Other) Identify your own questions.

Corrective Action—Review:

- Chapter 1, Empowerment: Develop a Positive Mental Attitude, page 1–7.
- Chapter 7, Test-Taking Techniques: Maintain a Positive Mental Attitude, page 110.

ANALYZE YOUR TEST PERFORMANCE

4. When I changed answers, I got the questions right

If you answered YES to this question, you are able to change answers based on careful thought and sound rationales. If you answered NO to this question, you need to ask yourself the following questions:

- What causes me to change my answers?
- Why do I bring an eraser to an exam when I know I always change correct answers to wrong answers?
- (Other) Identify your own questions.

Corrective Action—Analyze whether changing answers works to your advantage. The length of time allocated for most exams usually includes enough time for a short review at the end. If you have paced yourself appropriately, you should have 10 to 15 minutes for review. During your review, reassess your answers, particularly for those items for which you made an educated guess. Subsequent questions may contain content that is helpful in answering a previous question. You may access information you did not remember originally, or you may be less anxious at the end of the test and able to assess the question with more objectivity. Be aware of your success in changing answers on previous tests. Every time you review a test, evaluate your accuracy in changing answers. Keep score of how many answers you changed from wrong to right and how many you changed from right to wrong. If the number of items you changed from wrong to right is greater than the number of items you changed from right to wrong, it probably is to your advantage to change answers you ultimately believe you answered incorrectly. On the other hand, if you changed more answers from right to wrong, you should avoid changing your answers unless you are positive that your second choice is the correct choice. As the end of an exam approaches, people tend to experience more anxiety, which interferes with perception and the processing of information. This is the main reason why people change answers to the wrong answers at the end of a test. If you tend to change answers to the wrong answer, leave your eraser home!

5. Identify error clusters

If you identify a group of errors at the beginning, middle, or end of the exam, you need to analyze what is happening. You need to ask yourself the following questions:

- Am I too anxious?
- Do I get tired?
- Do I get flustered when confronted with a difficult question?
- Do I lose my ability to concentrate?
- (Other) Identify your own questions.

The purpose of identifying error clusters is to determine if fatigue or anxiety is affecting your performance. If your errors occur in the beginning of an exam, you may want to use anxiety reduction techniques just before the exam begins as well as control the testing environment to feel more in control and therefore less anxious. If you find that errors occur in clusters after every 20 or 30 questions, you may need to close your eyes, roll your shoulders, or take several deep breaths in an effort to reduce tension. We counseled a graduate nurse who did not pass the National Council Licensure Examination for Registered Nurses (NCLEX-RN) after two attempts. When assessing her performance on a practice exam, we identified the fact that every 30 minutes she made four or five errors in a row. We counseled her to take a break every 25 minutes until she completed the exam. On the third attempt, she passed the NCLEX-RN. A break every 25 minutes was the key change in her approach to the NCLEX-RN. In the classroom setting, this may be impossible; therefore, you should engage in a relaxation technique that works for you for 2 or 3 minutes. You can use positive self-talk by saying, "I can do this," or "I studied hard for this exam." In addition, you can visualize a person who supports you emotionally standing beside you and giving you encouragement. If you find that the majority of your errors occur during the last part of the exam, you may need to practice increasing your test-taking stamina by practicing test-taking for longer periods of time. Using the techniques identified previously during a test will be time well spent if you avoid unnecessary errors. Remember, relaxation techniques must be practiced to be effective and should be practiced in a simulated testing situation before a real testing situation. Recognize that if you implement relaxation techniques during a test, you need to adjust the time you allot for each question and your review.

Corrective Action—Review the following sections in Chapter 1, Empowerment:

- Establish Control Before and During the Test, page 6.
- Use Controlled Breathing (Diaphragmatic Breathing), page 2.

- Perform Muscle Relaxation, page 4.
- Use Imagery, page 5.
- Desensitize Yourself to the Fear Response, page 3.
- Challenge Negative Thoughts, page 2.

Summary

You should use these test-analysis tools to assess your test performance after taking a practice exam. Then you should use these tools when reviewing every exam you take in class. Do not be shy in asking your instructor for help with your analysis. Nursing instructors who are student centered will help you with this analysis during class or office hours because instructors have a vested interest in your success. Analysis of your test performance is essential if you are to identify your own individual learning needs. After your learning needs are identified using the presented tools, the Corrective Action Guide should direct you to information that can improve your abilities. Engaging in activities that analyze your test performance is time well spent!

Practice Questions with Answers and Rationales

Chapter 11 contains 400 questions divided into 14 categories of basic nursing practice. Each category contains between 25 and 35 test items. These items provide an opportunity for you to apply the test-taking techniques that were presented in Chapter 7. A test-taking technique is a strategy that uses skill and forethought to analyze a test item before selecting an answer. Every test item should be examined to determine if any of the test-taking techniques apply. When it is appropriate to use a test-taking technique, a **Test-Taking Tip** follows the item. Some items do not have a Test-Taking Tip because test-taking techniques do not pertain to every item.

The Test-Taking Tip cues you to one or more of the 12 different strategies that can assist you in arriving at the correct answer. These strategies were discussed in Chapter 7 under Specific Test-Taking Techniques. Use the Test-Taking Tip to examine the question with consideration and thoughtfulness. The rationales for items are given at the end of each category and address the following:

- Application of the Test-Taking Tip
- Identification of the correct answer
- Rationale for why the correct answer is correct
- Rationale for why each distractor is incorrect

The World of the Patient and Nurse

• • •

This section includes factors that influence the role of the nurse and the delivery of health care. Questions address ethics, legal aspects of nursing practice, the nursing process, the responsibilities associated with the management of nursing practice, meeting the spiritual needs of patients, patients' rights, the difference between dependent and independent roles of the nurse, supervision of the practice of subordinate staff members, the standards of nursing practice, and agencies that provide structure for the delivery of health care.

Questions

Please fill in the circle to mark your answer choice.

1   A patient tells the nurse, "My new bathrobe is missing." The nurse's MOST appropriate response is to:
   (1) Determine if the patient is angry
   (2) Initiate a search for the patient's bathrobe
   (3) Provide an isolation gown that can be used as a robe
   (4) State that it must have gone down with the soiled linen
   TEST-TAKING TIP ○ Identify the key word in the stem that sets a priority.

2   When comparing and contrasting examples of dependent, independent, and interdependent functions of the nurse, the nurse identifies which activity as a dependent function of the nurse?
   (1) Documenting perioperative nursing care
   (2) Changing a sterile dressing that is soiled
   (3) Assisting with selection of choices on the menu
   (4) Administering oxygen for acute shortness of breath
   TEST-TAKING TIP ○ Identify the clue in the stem.

3   The nurse must understand the scientific rationale for the actions that constitute a procedure. The most important reason why this is necessary is that the nurse should be able to:
   (1) Implement the procedure safely
   (2) Document the nursing care given
   (3) Explain the required nursing care
   (4) Formulate the nursing plan of care
   TEST-TAKING TIP ○ Identify the key word in the stem that sets a priority. Identify the unique option.

4   The nurse observes a patient going into another patient's room without permission, which upsets the other patient. When responding to the wandering patient's behavior, the nurse should initially:
   (1) Help the patient to the correct room
   (2) Place the patient in restraints temporarily
   (3) Determine the motivation for the patient's behavior
   (4) Share the observation about the patient with the health team
   TEST-TAKING TIP ○ Identify the key word in the stem that sets a priority. Identify the patient-centered options.

5   A voluntary agency is classified as such because it is:
   (1) Supported by volunteers and contributors
   (2) A health maintenance organization
   (3) Privately owned and operated
   (4) A nonprofit organization
   TEST-TAKING TIP ○ Identify the clue in the stem.

6   A primary nurse, responsible for a group of patients, is delegating responsibilities to the other members of the nursing team. Which task should the nurse include when formulating an assignment for the nursing assistant?
   (1) Monitoring patients' tube feedings
   (2) Ambulating patients outside their rooms
   (3) Regulating patients' intravenous solutions
   (4) Assisting patients with taking medications
   TEST-TAKING TIP ○ Identify the option that is unique.

7   The nurse in charge directs a nurse to do something that is outside the legal role of the nurse. The nurse to whom the task has been delegated should:
   (1) Notify the supervisor immediately
   (2) Inform the union representative

③ Decline to do the assigned task
④ Complete the delegated task

TEST-TAKING TIP ○ Identify opposites in options. Identify the option that is unique.

8 Which action by the nurse violates patient confidentiality and privacy?
① Interviewing a patient in the presence of others
② Writing patient statements in the progress notes
③ Sharing data about a patient at the change of shift report
④ Presenting the patient's problems at a team conference

TEST-TAKING TIP ○ Identify the key word in the stem that indicates negative polarity.

9 A patient dies three days after having extensive abdominal surgery. The nurse should begin post-mortem care:
① Only after the attending physician has been notified
② Once the nursing supervisor has been informed
③ After significant others have left
④ As soon as death is pronounced

TEST-TAKING TIP ○ Identify the option with a specific determiner.

10 A patient is angry about not being able to perform the activities of daily living (ADLs) without help. To best reduce the patient's anger, the nurse should:
① Disregard angry behavior
② Offer choices about care
③ Set firm limits on angry behavior
④ Encourage recognition of limitations

TEST-TAKING TIP ○ Identify the key word in the stem that sets a priority. Identify opposites in options.

11 Nurses must respect the rights of hospitalized patients and inform them of the Patient Bill of Rights. The nurse understands that a "right" of patients in a hospital is:
① Being able to smoke in their rooms
② Requesting meals at the times they prefer
③ Refusing treatment ordered by their physicians
④ Demanding that they be moved to private rooms

TEST-TAKING TIP ○ Identify the unique option.

12 A step in the nursing process involves facilitating the setting of goals with patients. An example of a goal is, "The patient will:
① Be assisted with meals."
② Be at risk for weight loss."
③ Need small, frequent feedings."
④ Maintain a weight of 140 pounds."

TEST-TAKING TIP ○ Identify the unique option.

13 The first task to be completed by the nurse when arriving on the unit for work is to:
① Count controlled drugs with the nurse going off shift
② Prioritize care to be completed during the shift
③ Make rounds to check the safety of patients
④ Receive a report on the status of patients

TEST-TAKING TIP ○ Identify the key word in the stem that sets a priority. Identify the clue in the stem.

14 The nurse breaks a patient's dentures because of carelessness. What specific legal term applies to this action?
① Battery
② Assault
③ Negligence
④ Malpractice

162

15 A patient is often argumentative and demanding. When planning care, the nurse's **best** intervention is to:
1. Bring another nurse as a witness
2. Involve the patient in decision making
3. Accept the behavior as probably a lifelong pattern
4. Explain that the staff would appreciate the patient's cooperation

TEST-TAKING TIP ○ Identify the key word in the stem that sets a priority. Identify opposites in options. Identify the patient-centered option.

16 Nurses are aware that the American Nurses' Association (ANA) Standards of Nursing Practice are:
1. Legal statutes that guide nursing practice
2. Progressive actions for a nursing procedure
3. Requirements for registered nurse licensure
4. Policy statements defining the obligations of nurses

17 A patient with dementia needs assistance with hygiene, grooming, eating, and toileting. When discharged from the hospital, the agency that best meets this patient's needs is:
1. A nursing home
2. A psychiatric institution
3. An adult daycare program
4. An outpatient care facility

TEST-TAKING TIP ○ Identify the key word in the stem that sets a priority.

18 The nurse observes a multivehicle collision where several people are seriously injured. When a nurse stops at the scene of this accident, the nurse is:
1. Given legal immunity by the Good Samaritan Law
2. Held responsible for the care provided at the scene
3. Meeting the legal trust that accompanies a nursing license
4. Immune from prosecution because a contract does not exist

TEST-TAKING TIP ○ Identify opposites in options. Identify equally plausible options.

19 A nurse says to a patient, "You should get a second opinion because your physician is not the best." The nurse could be sued for:
1. Libel
2. Assault
3. Slander
4. Negligence

20 A nurse obtains an informed consent from a patient who is to have an invasive procedure. The nurse's signature on the informed consent form indicates that the:
1. Surgeon described the procedure and its potential risks
2. Patient knows and understands expected outcomes
3. Patient actually signed the consent form
4. Surgeon is protected from being sued

TEST-TAKING TIP ○ Identify equally plausible options.

21 The nurse observes another nurse treating a patient in an abusive manner. The nurse's **initial** action should be to:
1. Tell the nurse in charge and write a report
2. Become a role model for the other nurse
3. Talk with the nurse about the incident
4. Reassure and calm the patient

TEST-TAKING TIP ○ Identify the key word in the stem that sets a priority. Identify the central person in the question.

22 The purpose of the National Council Licensure Examination for Registered Nurses (NCLEX-RN®) is to:
① Verify graduation
② Control nursing education
③ Accredit schools of nursing
④ Identify minimal safe practice
TEST-TAKING TIP ⊙ Identify equally plausible options.

23 When obtaining a health history, the nurse identifies that a patient has gained 10 pounds in the past week. When the nurse communicates this information to the physician, the nurse is performing which step in the nursing process?
① Planning
② Analysis
③ Evaluation
④ Assessment

24 The nurse assigns a Nursing Assistant to a patient who transfers to a chair with a mechanical lift. It has been a long time since the Nursing Assistant has used the lift. To ensure the safety of the patient, the nurse should:
① Assign the patient to another Nursing Assistant
② Explain to the Nursing Assistant how to use the lift
③ Ask the Nursing Assistant to demonstrate how to use the lift
④ Request that another Nursing Assistant assist with the transfer
TEST-TAKING TIP ⊙ Identify the equally plausible options.

25 The nurse is formulating a Nursing Assistant assignment. Which activity should the nurse delegate to the Nursing Assistant?
① Ensuring that patients swallow their medication
② Reporting unusual gross symptoms to the nurse
③ Orienting a new employee to the unit
④ Teaching patients personal hygiene

26 The nurse is planning to delegate patient care to a Nursing Assistant. Which is an appropriate activity for a Nursing Assistant?
① Evaluating vital signs
② Monitoring tube feeding
③ Providing patients with physical hygiene
④ Assisting postoperative patients with their first ambulation

27 A male patient has dementia. He is verbally and physically abusive and paranoid. When providing care the nurse should always:
① Compliment him on how nice he looks
② Administer care as quickly as possible
③ Tell him what he wants to hear
④ Explain what care is to be done
TEST-TAKING TIP ⊙ Identify equally plausible options.

28 A patient says, "I don't like anyone to go into my closet or drawers." When returning hygiene equipment, the nurse should:
① Store the equipment on the bedside stand
② Allow the patient to put the equipment away
③ Explain the safety hazard of not putting equipment away
④ Provide reassurance that personal things will not be taken
TEST-TAKING TIP ⊙ Identify the patient-centered option.

29 As an agency, Alcoholics Anonymous (AA) is classified under which category?

① Proprietary

② Voluntary

③ Official

④ Private

30 Ethics is concerned specifically with: Check all that apply.

① _____ Preventing a crime

② _____ Protecting civil law

③ _____ Making value judgments

④ _____ Identifying negligent acts

⑤ _____ Determining right or wrong

The World of the Patient and Nurse
Answers and Rationales

1 **TEST-TAKING TIP** ○ The word MOST in the stem sets a priority.
   ① Determining if the patient is angry does not address the problem of the missing bathrobe.
   ② **Patients have a right to expect that efforts will be implemented to ensure security for their belongings.**
   ③ Although this may be done, it does not address the problem of the missing bathrobe.
   ④ Explaining what may have happened does not address the feeling of loss.

2 **TEST-TAKING TIP** ○ The word "dependent" is a clue in the stem.
   ① Documenting nursing care is an independent function of the nurse and does not require a physician's order.
   ② **Dependent activities of the nurse are those activities that require a physician's order; changing a sterile dressing requires a physician's order.**
   ③ Selecting among choices of foods offered within a diet is an interdependent function; however, the type of diet is a dependent function.
   ④ In an emergency, the nurse may administer oxygen to a patient experiencing acute shortness of breath until a physician's order can be obtained.

3 **TEST-TAKING TIP** ○ The word *most* in the stem sets a priority. Option 1 is unique because it is the only option that does not use the words "nursing care."
   ① **The safety of the patient always takes priority; the nurse must perform only those skills that are understood and have been practiced.**
   ② Knowledge of the scientific rationale for care given is not necessary for the act of documentation.
   ③ Although it is important to explain all care to the patient, it is not the priority.
   ④ Although nurses need to understand scientific rationales to appropriately plan care, it is not the priority.

4 **TEST-TAKING TIP** ○ The word "initially" in the stem sets a priority. Options 1 and 2 are patient centered and focus on the patient who is the victim. However, Option 1 is correct because initially the patient who is upset must be protected.
   ① **Patients have a right to privacy and security for themselves and their belongings; helping the patient to the correct room protects the other patient.**
   ② Restraining patients for any reason other than their own physical safety or the safety of others is illegal.
   ③ This is not the priority. The nurse can explore the motivation for the behavior later.
   ④ Sharing the observation with the health team does not address the immediate need. After the behavior is addressed, it can be communicated.

5 **TEST-TAKING TIP** ○ The word "voluntary" in the stem is a clue.
   ① Although volunteers serve as helpers and contributors provide financial support to voluntary agencies, these are not the reason for the classification; voluntary agencies are nonprofit organizations.
   ② A health maintenance organization (HMO) is a form of health-care delivery and does not reflect how the organization is funded. An HMO can be voluntary (nonprofit) or proprietary (for profit) and, with emerging health-care reform, some may be official agencies (supported by government funds).
   ③ A privately owned and operated agency is a proprietary agency.
   ④ **Voluntary agencies may not make a profit; any money made must be applied to operating expenses and provision of services.**

6 **TEST-TAKING TIP** ○ Options 1, 3, and 4 all are associated with the intake of a substance. Option 2 is not like the others because it deals with an activity of daily living (ADL).
   ① Monitoring patients' tube feedings is the legal responsibility of the nurse, not the nursing assistant.
   ② **Nursing assistants are responsible for meeting patients' basic ADLs under the supervision of the nurse.**
   ③ Regulating patients' intravenous solutions is the legal responsibility of the nurse, not the nursing assistant.
   ④ Assisting patients with taking medication is the legal responsibility of the nurse, not the nursing assistant.

7 **TEST-TAKING TIP** ○ Options 3 and 4 are opposites. Option 3 is unique because of the extra words (to do) between the verb and the rest of the sentence.
   ① The nurse should notify the supervisor only if the nurse in charge continues to insist that the task be performed.
   ② Eventually the union representative may be notified if the nurse is threatened with repercussions for not following the order. Not all agencies are unionized.
   ③ **Performing a task that is outside the legal definition of the nurse is illegal; a nurse has the responsibility to refuse to follow an order that is illegal.**
   ④ Nurses should perform only those tasks that they are licensed to perform.

8 TEST-TAKING TIP ○ The word "violates" in the stem indicates negative polarity.

① **Interviewing a patient in the presence of others violates confidentiality; others may overhear information that should be kept confidential.**

② Documenting statements in the patient's chart is an acceptable practice.

③ Sharing information at change of shift report notifies nursing team members of the patient's changing status and is an appropriate practice.

④ A team conference enables professionals to share important information about patients and is an acceptable practice.

9 TEST-TAKING TIP ○ Option 1 contains the word "only," which is a specific determiner.

① Postmortem care should not begin until after death is pronounced and the family has an opportunity to make a last visit.

② Postmortem care at this time is premature.

③ **This allows the family members time to make a last visit before the body is prepared for transfer to a mortuary.**

④ This does not recognize the right of the family to see the deceased one last time before postmortem care.

10 TEST-TAKING TIP ○ The word "best" in the stem sets a priority. Options 1 and 3 are opposites and are distractors.

① All behavior has meaning and requires recognition.

② **Making decisions places the patient in control and supports feelings of independence.**

③ Setting firm limits only makes the patient more angry because it is a controlling intervention.

④ Pointing out limitations only intensifies the patient's feelings of dependence.

11 TEST-TAKING TIP ○ Option 3 is unique because it has a negative connotation; it relates to an action of refusal. Options 1, 2, and 4 are statements from the positive perspective and are therefore alike.

① Patients are not permitted to smoke in their rooms. The Joint Commission on Accreditation of Healthcare Organizations, the agency responsible for accrediting hospitals, requires that accredited facilities be "smoke free." However, some facilities still provide limited, designated smoking areas.

② Meals are generally scheduled during regular meal times. It is impractical to serve meals any time a patient prefers; however, if a special need arises, the nurse generally should attempt to individualize care.

③ **The patient has a right to refuse care against medical advice; the physician needs to explain to the patient the risks involved in lack of treatment.**

④ A private room is generally a privilege, not a right, that is provided at extra expense; it is not automatically provided on demand. However, a patient requiring isolation may be transferred to a private room at no additional expense to the patient.

12 TEST-TAKING TIP ○ Option 4 is unique because it is the only option with a number.

① This is an intervention, not a goal.

② This is an inference about the patient's status, not a goal.

③ This statement identifies a need or an intervention in response to an identified problem, not a goal.

④ **This is a goal statement that is specific and measurable and contains a time frame; "maintain" implies continuously.**

13 TEST-TAKING TIP ○ The word "first" is the key word in the stem that sets a priority. The word "arriving" in the stem establishes a time frame and is therefore an important clue.

① Controlled drugs can be counted at any time during the change of shift.

② Before the nurse can prioritize care, the nurse must first know about each patient's status.

③ Rounds are implemented after report. The nurse first needs to know the status of the patients; a report provides baseline data about patients that are needed before additional assessments can be planned. Some institutions have walking rounds in which report and assessment of patients are conducted simultaneously.

④ **Before care can be planned and implemented, the nurse needs to know the condition and immediate needs of patients.**

14 ① *Battery* is the purposeful, angry, or negligent touching of a patient without consent.

② *Assault* is an act intended to provoke fear in a patient.

③ ***Negligence*** **occurs when the nurse's actions do not meet appropriate standards and result in injury to another; negligence can occur with acts of omission or commission.**

④ *Malpractice* is misconduct performed in professional practice that results in harm to another.

15 TEST-TAKING TIP ○ The word **best** in the stem sets a priority. Options 3 and 4 are opposites and are distractors. Option 2 is patient centered.

① This is a defensive response. All behavior has meaning; the nurse should initially identify the reason for the behavior.

② **The patient is the center of the health team and has a right to be involved in the decision making concerning care; this individualizes care and promotes self-esteem, which often prevents argumentative and demanding behavior.**

③ This is an assumption; many people cope with anxiety by this behavior. This behavior may be an attempt to gain control in a situation in which the individual feels out of control and should be addressed.

④ This is judgmental and takes away the patient's coping mechanism.

16 ① Legal statutes are laws created by elected legislative bodies; they are not nursing standards.

② Step-by-step actions in a procedure or protocol are the critical elements for completing an intervention.

③ Requirements for licensure and the ANA Standards of Nursing Practice are unrelated. Most state licensing acts require a specified level of education and the passing of a special examination.

④ **The ANA has general resolutions that recommend the responsibilities and obligations of nurses; these standards help determine if a nurse has acted as any prudent, reasonable nurse would given similar education, experiential background, and environment.**

17 **TEST-TAKING TIP** ◉ The word "best" in the stem sets a priority.

① **This patient needs long-term nursing care as well as 24-hour supervision.**

② A psychiatric institution is inappropriate for this patient. Patients with dementia need supportive care for the rest of their lives. Psychiatric settings today generally provide acute care services for mentally ill patients.

③ Many daycare programs function five days a week from 8 AM until 6 PM to assist working family members. There are no data given that indicate the support of a family to meet the patient's needs or the ability of the patient to provide self-care when not at the daycare center.

④ Outpatient care facilities usually provide acute care services, not long-term nursing care or 24-hour supervision.

18 **TEST-TAKING TIP** ◉ Options 2 and 4 are opposites. Options 1 and 4 are equally plausible.

① The Good Samaritan Law does not provide legal immunity; the nurse can still be held accountable for gross departure from acceptable standards of practice or willful wrongdoing.

② **Nurses are responsible for their own actions, and the care provided must be what any reasonably prudent nurse would do under similar circumstances.**

③ Assistance at the scene of an accident is an ethical, not a legal, duty.

④ A contract does not have to exist for a nurse to commit negligence.

19 ① *Libel* is defamation of character via print, writing, or pictures, not spoken words.

② *Assault* is an attempt or threat to touch another person unjustifiably.

③ ***Slander* is defamation of character by spoken words.**

④ *Negligence* is the failure to do something a reasonably prudent nurse would do under similar circumstances or the commission of an act that a reasonably prudent nurse would not do under similar circumstances.

20 **TEST-TAKING TIP** ◉ Options 1 and 2 are equally plausible.

① The nurse's signature does not document that the physician described the procedure and its risks; the patient's signature documents that the procedure and its risks are understood.

② The nurse's signature does not document that the patient was properly informed about expected outcomes.

③ **The nurse only witnesses the patient's signature and examines the document for the correct date.**

④ The nurse's signature on an informed consent form does not protect the surgeon from being sued. Reasonably prudent practice protects the surgeon from being sued.

21 **TEST-TAKING TIP** ◉ The word **initial** in the stem is the key word that sets a priority. The patient is the central person in the question.

① Telling the nurse in charge about the behavior should be done later; another action is the priority.

② Becoming a role model would be done later; another action is the priority.

③ This may be done later but it is not the priority at this time.

④ **The patient is the priority at this point in time; after the patient is protected and safe, the actions of the abusive nurse must be addressed.**

22 **TEST-TAKING TIP** ◉ Options 2 and 3 are equally plausible.

① A degree or diploma, not NCLEX-RN®, verifies that the student has met the criteria for graduation from the granting institution.

② Controlling nursing education is not the purpose of NCLEX-RN®.

③ State boards of nursing, the National League for Nursing Accrediting Commission, and the American Association of Colleges of Nursing accredit schools of nursing.

④ **The NCLEX-RN® examination is designed to identify whether a candidate has met a minimum level of performance to safely practice as a licensed registered nurse.**

23 ① Planning is involved with setting goals, establishing priorities, identifying expected outcomes, identifying interventions designed to achieve goals and outcomes, ensuring that the patient's health-care needs are met appropriately, modifying the plan as necessary, and collaborating with other health team members to ensure that care is coordinated. Planning does not include the communication of data collected during assessment.

(2) Analysis is involved with the interpretation of data, collection of additional data, and identification and communication of nursing diagnoses. Analysis does not include the communication of data collected during the assessment phase of the nursing process.

(3) Evaluation is involved with identifying a patient's response to care, comparing a patient's actual responses with the expected outcomes, analyzing factors that affected the actual outcomes for the purpose of drawing conclusions about the success or failure of specific nursing activities, and modifying the plan of care when necessary; evaluation does not include the communication of data collected during the assessment phase.

(4) **Communicating important assessment data to other health team members is a component of the assessment phase of the nursing process.**

24 **TEST-TAKING TIP** ○ Options 1 and 4 are equally plausible.

(1) This does not address the Nursing Assistant's need to know how to move a patient safely with a mechanical lift.

(2) This teaching method does not take into consideration the need for the Nursing Assistant to practice the psychomotor skills associated with this task. Explaining is not sufficient.

(3) **Demonstration is the safest way to assess whether the Nursing Assistant has the knowledge and skill to safely transfer a patient using a mechanical lift.**

(4) Another Nursing Assistant should not be held accountable for the care assigned another staff member. The nurse is directly responsible for ensuring that delegated care is safely delivered to patients.

25 (1) It is illegal for the Nursing Assistant to administer drugs, even if under the supervision of the nurse.

(2) **The Nursing Assistant is trained to identify major abnormal signs and symptoms and to notify the nurse when they are outside the expected range or are changed from the patient's baseline; the nurse then completes a professional assessment of the patient's condition.**

(3) A Nursing Assistant should not be responsible for the supervision of other employees.

(4) The Nursing Assistant is not prepared for this responsibility. Teaching requires a strong scientific knowledge base and an ability to use scientific teaching/learning principles when planning and implementing an educational plan.

26 (1) Evaluating vital signs requires professional nursing judgment. The nurse is educationally prepared to determine the significance of vital sign measurements, not the Nursing Assistant.

(2) It is not legal for a Nursing Assistant to monitor tube feedings; this action is within the legal practice of nursing.

(3) **Nursing Assistants are trained to provide basic hygiene measures under the direction of a nurse.**

(4) Nurses should ambulate postoperative patients for the first time; nurses have the knowledge to analyze a patient's response to ambulating postoperatively; the Nursing Assistant can ambulate patients with simple, noncomplex needs.

27 **TEST-TAKING TIP** ○ Options 1 and 3 are equally plausible because neither option is better than the other.

(1) This may not be true; trust is based on honesty.

(2) This does not address the patient's needs. Rushing may increase the patient's anxiety.

(3) Telling a patient what he wants to hear is patronizing; when patients feel they are being humored, trust deteriorates.

(4) **This supports every patient's right to know what care is being given and why.**

28 **TEST-TAKING TIP** ○ Option 2 gives the patient control and therefore is the most patient-centered option.

(1) This does not support the patient's need to be in control of the immediate environment; equipment should be stored appropriately to protect it from pathogens in the environment.

(2) **This supports the patient's right to control personal space.**

(3) Logic generally does not reduce a patient's concern; the patient needs to feel in control, and this action does not support this need.

(4) This still results in a violation of the patient's personal space.

29 (1) Proprietary agencies are privately owned and operated to make a profit.

(2) **AA is a voluntary organization. Voluntary agencies are not for profit and rely on professional and lay volunteers, in addition to a paid staff.**

(3) Official health agencies are supported by local, state, and/or national taxes.

(4) Same as #1.

30 (1) _____ Criminal law is concerned with crimes.

(2) _____ Civil law is concerned with wrongs committed by one person against another.

(3) _X_ **Ethics is concerned with value judgments and behavior that is acceptable or unacceptable.**

(4) _____ Negligence is concerned with a careless act of commission or omission that results in injury to another.

(5) _X_ **Ethics is concerned with value judgments such as behaviors that are considered acceptable or unacceptable.**

Common Theories Related to Meeting Patients' Basic Human Needs

• • •

This section includes questions related to the work of theorists such as Kübler-Ross, Maslow, Selye, and Erikson. It also includes questions related to principles of teaching, growth and development, stress and adaptation, and the definition of health.

Questions

Please fill in the circle to mark your answer choice.

1   Of the human needs identified by Maslow's Hierarchy of Needs, the nurse understands that the most basic are:
   ① Physiologic needs
   ② Belonging needs
   ③ Security needs
   ④ Safety needs
   TEST-TAKING TIP ◉ Identify the key word in the stem that sets a priority. Identify the equally plausible options.

2   The nurse provides preoperative teaching for a patient scheduled for surgery. To ensure that the patient understands the content of the teaching session, the nurse should:
   ① Use simple vocabulary
   ② Ask the patient what was learned
   ③ Speak distinctly when giving directions
   ④ Speak slowly when talking with the patient
   TEST-TAKING TIP ◉ Identify the option that is unique. Identify the patient-centered option.

3   The majority of patients on the hospital's medical unit are older adults. When caring for older adults, the nurse understands that their developmental task according to Erikson is:
   ① Establishing trust
   ② Becoming dependent
   ③ Reconciling one's life
   ④ Assisting grown children
   TEST-TAKING TIP ◉ Identify the clue in the stem.

4   A mentally disadvantaged (retarded) adult patient is learning self-care. To increase learning, the nurse should:
   ① Verbally recognize when goals are met
   ② Set a variety of short-term goals to be met
   ③ Use candy as a reward when goals are met
   ④ Disregard the behavior when goals are not met
   TEST-TAKING TIP ◉ Identify opposites in options.

5   What should the nurse do to meet a patient's basic physiologic needs?
   ① Raise the side rails
   ② Provide a bed bath
   ③ Explain procedures
   ④ Converse with the patient
   TEST-TAKING TIP ◉ Identify the clue in the stem.

6 The nurse is teaching a patient with diabetes how to self monitor blood glucose levels. When predicting the success of a teaching program regarding the learning of this skill, the most important factor is the:
1. Learner's cognitive ability
2. Amount of reinforcement
3. Extent of family support
4. Interest of the learner

TEST-TAKING TIP ○ Identify the key word in the stem that sets a priority. Identify options that are patient centered.

7 In relation to Erikson's developmental theory, a question that can be asked that relates to the task of the school-age child is:
1. "Who am I?"
2. "What can I do?"
3. "Whom can I trust?"
4. "What have I done?"

TEST-TAKING TIP ○ Identify the clue in the stem. Identify opposites in options.

8 Patients draw pictures and sometimes hang them in their rooms. According to Maslow's Hierarchy of Needs, the specific human need being met is:
1. Physiologic
2. Self-esteem
3. Security
4. Love

9 The process of growth and development follows a pattern that is:
1. Uncertain
2. Nonpredictable
3. Based on motivation
4. Influenced by the previous step

TEST-TAKING TIP ○ Identify equally plausible options.

10 According to Erikson's developmental theory, a statement that can be associated with the task of generativity versus stagnation is:
1. "I want to do it myself."
2. "I will be getting married next week."
3. "I enjoy mentoring the new employees."
4. "I am pleased with the decisions I have made."

TEST-TAKING TIP ○ Identify the clue in the stem.

11 The nurse is assessing a patient with a severe sunburn. The nurse understands that in this situation, the sun is considered a:
1. Physical stress
2. Chemical stress
3. Physiologic stress
4. Microbiologic stress

12 An activity that promotes successful completion of the struggle associated with young adulthood is:
1. Going on a date
2. Raising children
3. Promoting a cause
4. Sharing knowledge

TEST-TAKING TIP ○ Identify the clue in the stem.

13 When planning to teach colostomy care to a young man who has just had a temporary colostomy, the nurse should *initially*:
1. Establish goals for the teaching plan
2. Follow the patient's usual bowel habits

③ Identify the patient's interest in self-care
④ Reinforce that the colostomy is only temporary
TEST-TAKING TIP ○ Identify the key word in the stem that sets a priority. Identify the specific determiner in an option. Identify the patient-centered options.

14 According to Maslow's Hierarchy of Needs, when planning care for several patients, the nurse should **first** assist the patient who needs to:
① Talk
② Void
③ Walk
④ Know
TEST-TAKING TIP ○ Identify the key word in the stem that sets a priority.

15 The nurse is interviewing an adolescent during a yearly physical. A patient activity that supports the developmental task of adolescence is:
① Reading a book
② Learning how to use a computer
③ Helping parents with household chores
④ Attending a high school basketball game
TEST-TAKING TIP ○ Identify the clue in the stem.

16 The process of growth and development within an individual can generally be described as:
① Plodding
② Unique
③ Simple
④ Even

17 Which word best describes the feelings associated with an infant in Erikson's stage of trust versus mistrust?
① Me
② We
③ You
④ They
TEST-TAKING TIP ○ Identify the key word in the stem that sets a priority.

18 The nurse is obtaining the psychosocial history of a patient. Considering theories about stress, which event generally precipitates the highest degree of stress?
① Retirement
② Relocation
③ Pregnancy
④ Marriage
TEST-TAKING TIP ○ Identify the key word in the stem that sets a priority.

19 When collecting information to prepare a teaching plan in the cognitive domain, the nurse asks a patient with diabetes:
① "How do you inspect your feet each day?"
② "Can you measure a serum glucose level?"
③ "What do you know about diabetes mellitus?"
④ "Are you able to perform a subcutaneous injection?"
TEST-TAKING TIP ○ Identify the clue in the stem. Identify the option that is unique.

20 The nurse is teaching a patient about self-injection with insulin. The most effective approach to use is through a:
① Book
② Video
③ Discussion
④ Demonstration
TEST-TAKING TIP ○ Identify the key word in the stem that sets a priority.

21 The nurse uses Maslow's Hierarchy of Needs to prioritize nursing care. According to Maslow's theory, which patient need takes priority?

① Security
② Belonging
③ Self-esteem
④ Self-actualization

TEST-TAKING TIP ⊙ Identify the key word in the stem that sets a priority.

22 An adult has a sense of inadequacy and inferiority at work. One could say that this person had the most difficulty resolving the conflict associated with which developmental age?

① Birth to 1 year
② 4 to 7 years
③ 8 to 12 years
④ 13 to 20 years

TEST-TAKING TIP ⊙ Identify the word in the stem that sets a priority. Identify the clue in the stem.

23 The stress of air pollution caused by wood-burning fireplaces in the home can be classified as a:

① Physical stress
② Chemical stress
③ Physiologic stress
④ Microbiologic stress

24 The nurse is interviewing a patient who is terminally ill. Which is an unexpected behavior associated with the usual process of grieving?

① Talking about the illness
② Becoming angry with people
③ Attempting to commit suicide
④ Seeking alternative therapies

TEST-TAKING TIP ⊙ Identify the word in the stem that indicates negative polarity.

25 When assessing patients coping with multiple stresses, the nurse understands that the general adaptation syndrome (GAS) primarily is controlled by the:

① Endocrine system
② Respiratory system
③ Integumentary system
④ Cardiovascular system

TEST-TAKING TIP ⊙ Identify the key word in the stem that sets a priority.

26 A patient asks the nurse, "What is health?" When considering an answer, the nurse identifies that one concept that is basic to most definitions is that health is:

① A progressive state
② The absence of disease
③ Relative to one's value system
④ An extreme of the wellness–illness continuum

TEST-TAKING TIP ⊙ Identify the clue in the stem. Identify the patient-centered option. Identify equally plausible options.

27 According to Maslow's Hierarchy of Needs, which most clearly demonstrates physiologic needs as a priority?

① Trauma
② Puberty
③ Restraints
④ Menopause

28 The nurse is observing a group of children playing in the child life center in the hospital. Which word best reflects the type of play associated with Erikson's stage of initiative versus guilt?

① Us

② Me

③ You

④ Them

TEST-TAKING TIP ◉ Identify the unique option.

29 The nurse is preparing a teaching plan for a patient who was just diagnosed with diabetes mellitus. The nurse identifies that the most effective teaching strategy that can be used in the cognitive domain is:

① Explanation

② Demonstration

③ Group discussion

④ Individual practice

30 The nurse is caring for a variety of patients on a medical unit in the hospital. Using Maslow's hierarchy as a basis for prioritizing care, in which order should the nurse perform the following actions?

① Administering 2 liters of oxygen via a nasal cannula

② Encourage a family member to visit as often as desired

③ Asking a patient about personal preferences before beginning care

④ Arranging the call bell within easy reach after a patient is transferred to a chair

Answer: _____

174 Common Theories Related to Meeting Patients'
Basic Human Needs
Answers and Rationales

1 **TEST-TAKING TIP** ⊙ The word *most* in the stem sets a priority. Options 3 and 4 are equally plausible.
 ① **Physiologic needs such as oxygen, food, fluid, rest, sleep, and elimination are basic for life.**
 ② Belonging needs are ranked third.
 ③ Security needs are ranked second.
 ④ Safety needs are ranked second.

2 **TEST-TAKING TIP** ⊙ Option 2 is unique and patient centered because it is the only one that seeks feedback from the patient. Options 1, 3, and 4 are similar because they all are concerned with how to send information to the patient.
 ① Using simple vocabulary helps to send a clearer message, but it does not inform the sender whether the receiver understood the message.
 ② **Seeking feedback enables the caregiver to know whether the message was understood as intended.**
 ③ Speaking distinctly when giving directions helps to send a clearer message, but it does not inform the sender whether the receiver understood the message.
 ④ Speaking slowly helps to send a clearer message, but it does not inform the sender whether the receiver understood the message.

3 **TEST-TAKING TIP** ⊙ The words "older adults" in the stem is a clue.
 ① Establishing trust is the major task of infants.
 ② Dependency is not a task for which one strives; dependency results if an 8- to 12-year-old is unable to resolve the conflict of industry versus inferiority.
 ③ **Older adults need to come to terms with the fact that the end of life is near; reviewing one's life is a step in this process.**
 ④ Middle-aged adults may help grown children; this is usually a task of this age group.

4 **TEST-TAKING TIP** ⊙ Options 1 and 4 are opposites.
 ① **Recognizing goals supports feelings of self-esteem and independence; it provides external reinforcement and promotes internal reinforcement.**
 ② A mentally disadvantaged person generally can focus on only one goal at a time; several goals may be overwhelming.
 ③ The routine ingestion of candy is not healthy; praise is a more acceptable reward.
 ④ A patient's behavior should never be disregarded; all behavior should be addressed in a nonjudgmental and supportive manner.

5 **TEST-TAKING TIP** ⊙ The word "physiologic" is a clue in the stem.
 ① Raising side rails relates to the patient's need for safety and security, the second level in Maslow's Hierarchy of Needs.
 ② **A bed bath supports the patient's physiologic need to be clean and is related to the first level, physiologic needs, in Maslow's Hierarchy of Needs.**
 ③ Explaining procedures relates to the patient's need for safety and security; patients have a right to know what is happening to them and why.
 ④ Conversing with a patient relates to the need for love and belonging, the third level in Maslow's Hierarchy of Needs.

6 **TEST-TAKING TIP** ⊙ The word "most" in the stem is a key word that sets a priority. Options 1 and 4 are patient centered.
 ① Although a teaching program must be designed within the patient's developmental and cognitive abilities, it is useless unless the patient recognizes the value of what is to be learned and has a desire to learn.
 ② Although reinforcement is important, self-motivation is the most significant factor in learning.
 ③ Although family support is important, the patient's interest and readiness to learn are the priorities for the successful learning of a skill; some patients do not have a family support system.
 ④ **The motivation of the learner to acquire new attitudes, information, or skills is the most important component for successful learning; motivation exists when the learner recognizes the future benefits of learning.**

7 **TEST-TAKING TIP** ⊙ The word "school-age" is a clue in the stem. Options 2 and 4 are opposites.
 ① "Who am I?" relates to the conflict of identity versus role confusion; the person aged 13 to 20 years seeks to develop peer relationships, defines goals, selects a vocation, gains independence, and seeks identity.

(2) **"What can I do?" relates to the conflict of industry versus inferiority; the child of 6 to 12 years is developing a sense of competence and perseverance.**

(3) "Whom can I trust?" relates to the conflict of trust versus mistrust. During the first year the infant depends on others to meet basic needs; the infant develops trust if these needs are met in a comfortable and predictable manner.

(4) "What have I done?" relates to the conflict of integrity versus despair; the person aged 60 years or more struggles to feel a sense of worth about past experiences and goals achieved and seeks a sense of integrity.

8 (1) "Physiologic" relates to meeting basic physical needs, such as the needs for oxygen, food, water, rest, sleep, and elimination.

(2) **The situation illustrated in the stem meets self-esteem needs; control, self-respect, and competence are reflected when a person hangs self-made pictures in a room for the enjoyment of self and others.**

(3) "Security" refers to shelter, clothing, and the need to feel comfortable with the rules of the society, community, and hospital.

(4) "Love" refers to the need for bonds of affection and a sense of belonging.

9 **TEST-TAKING TIP** ◎ Option 1 and 2 are equally plausible.

(1) Although growth and development progress through some stages faster than others, they still follow a certain predictable pattern.

(2) Stages of growth and development do follow a predictable pattern.

(3) Motivation may influence the achievement of tasks in some stages of growth and development; however, growth and development do not rely on motivation.

(4) **Success or failure of task achievement in one stage of development influences succeeding stages; failure to resolve a crisis at one stage damages the ego, which makes the resolution of the following stages more difficult.**

10 **TEST-TAKING TIP** ◎ The words "generativity versus stagnation" provide a clue in the stem.

(1) This statement relates to stage 2; this is the conflict of autonomy versus shame and doubt. The 2- to 4-year-old seeks a balance between independence and dependence and attempts to achieve autonomy.

(2) This statement relates to stage 6; this is the conflict of intimacy versus isolation. The young adult aged 20 to 30 years seeks to select a partner for a life relationship.

(3) **This statement relates to stage 7; this is the conflict of generativity versus stagnation. The person aged 30 to 60 years is interested in guiding younger individuals.**

(4) This statement relates to stage 8; this is the conflict of integrity versus despair. The person aged 60 years or older struggles to feel a sense of worth about past experiences and goals achieved and seeks a sense of integrity.

11 (1) **Physical stresses are stresses from outside the body and include light, environmental temperature, sound, pressure, motion, gravity, and electricity.**

(2) Chemical stresses relate to toxic substances such as acids, alkalines, drugs, and exogenous hormones.

(3) Physiologic stresses are disturbances in structure or function of any tissue, organ, or system within the body.

(4) Microbiologic stresses are organisms such as bacteria, viruses, molds, or parasites that can cause disease.

12 **TEST-TAKING TIP** ◎ The words "young adulthood" provide a clue in the stem.

(1) **The developmental task of the young adult is the establishment of intimacy with a relationship partner.**

(2) Raising children is related to the developmental task of generativity versus stagnation associated with middle adulthood.

(3) Promoting a cause is related to the developmental task of generativity versus stagnation associated with middle adulthood.

(4) Sharing knowledge is related to the developmental task of generativity versus stagnation associated with middle adulthood.

13 **TEST-TAKING TIP** ◎ The word *initially* is the key word in the stem that sets a priority. The word *only* in Option 4 is a specific determiner. Options 2 and 3 are patient centered.

(1) This is done after a readiness for learning is established. Words such as "establish" and "follow" are action words that are more appropriately related to planning or intervention than assessment.

(2) Same as #1.

(3) **Determining the patient's readiness for learning and point of reference are the priorities. Assessment is the first step in the nursing process.**

(4) Although the colostomy may be only temporary, the patient still needs to be taught self-care. Focusing on the "only temporary" nature of the colostomy may offer false reassurance. A colostomy may become permanent if the patient's condition does not improve as expected.

14 **TEST-TAKING TIP** ○ The word **first** in the stem is a key word that sets a priority.
① Although important, this is not the priority.
② **Elimination is a basic physiologic need. When setting priorities, the most basic physiologic needs should be met first.**
③ Same as #1.
④ Same as #1.

15 **TEST-TAKING TIP** ○ The word "adolescent" in the stem is a clue.
① Middle childhood (6 to 12 years), not adolescence, is concerned with developing fundamental skills in reading, writing, calculating, and using a computer; the school-age child is very industrious.
② Same as #1.
③ The childhood years, not adolescence, are related to helping behaviors; 3- to 5-year-olds like to imitate parents and 6- to 12-year-olds are developing appropriate social roles.
④ **Adolescents are concerned with developing new and more mature relationships with their peers; adolescents tend to associate with their peers rather than with their parents.**

16 ① Some stages are faster and some are slower.
② **Although a general pattern is followed, each individual grows and develops at a different rate or extent and therefore is unique.**
③ Growth and development is an extremely complex process based on many influencing variables.
④ Some stages of growth and development are faster and some are slower, not even, depending on the stage and the individual.

17 **TEST-TAKING TIP** ○ The word "best" is a key word in the stem that sets a priority.
① **The infant is egocentric and unaware of boundaries between the self and others; the infant is concerned with needs being met immediately.**
② The infant has not identified the difference between self and others.
③ Same as #2.
④ Same as #2.

18 **TEST-TAKING TIP** ○ The word "highest" is a key word in the stem that sets a priority.
① The mean stress unit for retirement is 45, which is less than the correct answer.
② The mean stress unit for a change in residence is 20, which is less than the correct answer.
③ The mean stress unit for pregnancy is 40, which is less than the correct answer.
④ **Holmes and Rahe (1967) determined stress units for life events based on the readjustment required by individuals to adapt to particular situations or events. The mean stress unit for marriage is 50, which is more than the other options presented.**

19 **TEST-TAKING TIP** ○ The word "cognitive" is a clue in the stem. Option 3 is unique because it is the only option that is concerned with "what is" rather than "how to." Options 1, 2, and 4 all relate to the performance of a skill.
① This statement focuses on the performance of a skill that relates to the psychomotor domain, not the cognitive domain.
② Same as #1.
③ **This is the cognitive domain because it deals with the comprehension of information.**
④ Same as #1.

20 **TEST-TAKING TIP** ○ The word "most" is the key word in the stem that sets a priority.
① Although a book can be used for learning a skill (psychomotor domain), it is not as effective as other methods; it is more appropriate for learning and comprehending information (cognitive domain).
② Although a video can be used for learning a skill (psychomotor domain), it is not as effective as other methods.
③ Learning via discussion is appropriate for the cognitive (knowing) and affective (feeling) domains.
④ **Demonstration uses a variety of senses such as sight, hearing, and touch. The opportunity to observe and manipulate the equipment promotes learning a skill.**

21 **TEST-TAKING TIP** ○ The word "priority" is the key word in the stem that sets a priority.
① **Safety and security needs, second-level needs according to Maslow, are ranked after basic physiologic needs and before the need for love and belonging; people need to feel physically and emotionally safe.**
② Belonging needs, third-level needs according to Maslow, are concerned with bonds of affection.
③ Self-esteem needs, fourth-level needs according to Maslow, are related to the need to feel competent and respected.
④ Self-actualization needs, fifth-level needs according to Maslow, are concerned with maximizing abilities and feeling content within the self.

22 **TEST-TAKING TIP** ○ The word "most" is a key word in the stem that sets a priority. The words "inadequacy and inferiority" in the stem provide a clue.

(1) Birth to 1 year of age is a time of concern with resolving the conflict of trust versus mistrust.

(2) During the ages of 4 to 7 years, the child is concerned with resolving the conflict of initiative versus guilt.

(3) **During the ages of 8 to 12 years, the child is concerned with resolving the conflict of industry versus inferiority. When a child is unable to develop physical, social, or cognitive skills well enough to perceive the self as competent, the child feels inadequate; these feelings of inferiority can be carried throughout adulthood.**

(4) During the ages of 13 to 20 years, the child is concerned with resolving the conflict of identity versus role confusion.

23 (1) Air pollution is not a physical stress; physical stresses include temperature, sound, pressure, light, motion, gravity, and electricity.

(2) **Burning wood releases toxic substances and gases into the air; these are considered chemical stresses. Acids, alkalines, drugs, and exogenous hormones are also considered chemical stresses.**

(3) Air pollution is not a physiologic stress; disturbances in the structure or function of any tissue, organ, or system of the body are considered physiologic stresses.

(4) Air pollution is not a microbiologic stress; bacteria, viruses, molds, and parasites are considered microbiologic stresses.

24 **TEST-TAKING TIP** ○ The word "unexpected" causes this stem to have negative polarity. You need to identify the behavior that is not usually associated with the grieving process.

(1) Although talking about the illness occurs throughout the grieving response, it is most expected during the early stage of disbelief (No, not me).

(2) Anger is expected and occurs when there is a developing awareness of the impending loss (Why me?).

(3) **Although some people who are terminally ill attempt suicide, it is not an expected response to loss.**

(4) Seeking alternative therapies occurs most often during the stage of bargaining (Yes me, but . . .).

25 **TEST-TAKING TIP** ○ The word "primarily" is the key word in the stem that sets a priority.

(1) **The GAS primarily involves the endocrine system and autonomic nervous system; the antidiuretic hormone (ADH), adrenocorticotropic hormone (ACTH), cortisol, aldosterone, epinephrine, and norepinephrine are all involved with the fight-or-flight response.**

(2) The respiratory system does not control the GAS. It is stimulated by a component of the GAS.

(3) The integumentary system does not control the GAS. It is stimulated by a component of the GAS.

(4) The cardiovascular system does not control the GAS. It is stimulated by a component of the GAS.

26 **TEST-TAKING TIP** ○ The words "basic to most" provide the clue that the answer is a common component of most definitions of health. Option 3 is patient centered. Options 1 and 4 are equally plausible.

(1) Health fluctuates on a continuum that has extremes of wellness to illness; movement can occur up or down the continuum, not only in one direction.

(2) The World Health Organization's definition of health is "A state of complete physical, mental, and social well-being, and not merely the absence of disease or infirmity;" some people who have a chronic illness consider themselves healthy because they are able to function independently.

(3) **A definition of health is highly individualized; it is based on each person's own experiences, values, and perceptions. Health can mean different things to each individual; people tend to define health based on the presence or absence of symptoms, their perceptions of how they feel, and their capacity to function on a daily basis.**

(4) Although high-level wellness is one extreme of the wellness–illness continuum and severe illness the other, where one plots a position on the continuum is based on the individual's value system. The perception of health is based on the individual's physical, emotional, social, mental, and spiritual senses of wellness.

27 (1) **Trauma can be life threatening and interfere with basic physiologic functioning.**

(2) Although physiologic changes are associated with the growth spurt and development of secondary sexual characteristics during puberty, self-identity and self-esteem often take priority at this time.

(3) Restraints meet safety and security needs because they protect the patient from harm.

(4) Although physiologic changes are associated with menopause, love, self-esteem, and self-actualization are often the priorities at this time.

28 **TEST-TAKING TIP** ○ The word "Us" in Option 1 addresses both sides of an interpersonal relationship. It is a word that reflects a united front. "Me," "You," and "Them" reflect just one side of an interpersonal relationship.

(1) **During the conflict of initiative versus guilt, the child aged 4 to 8 years strives to adjust to social spheres outside the home. The child begins to evolve as a social being seeking relationships with a small number of peers, with a focus on "Us."**

   (2) During the conflict of trust versus mistrust, the infant is egocentric, unaware of boundaries between the self and others, and concerned with the immediate satisfaction of needs. Therefore, the focus is on "Me."

   (3) During the conflict of intimacy versus isolation, the young adult aged 20 to 30 strives to select a relationship partner. A relationship partner in one's life is the important "You."

   (4) During the conflict of industry versus inferiority, the school-age child 7 through 12 years strives to become a productive group member. The school-age child joins a "gang," becomes less self-centered, and is more concerned with "Them."

29 **(1)** **An *explanation* is within the cognitive domain. An explanation defines, describes, and interprets information so that it is understood.**

   (2) A *demonstration* is most effective when dealing with skills, which are part of the psychomotor domain.

   (3) A *group discussion* is most effective when dealing with feelings, which are part of the affective domain.

   (4) *Practice* is most effective when dealing with skills, which are part of the psychomotor domain.

30 Answer: 1, 4, 2, 3.

   (1) **Administering 2 liters of oxygen via a nasal cannula—Meeting basic physiological needs (e.g., patent airway, nutrition, elimination) are first level needs according to Maslow.**

   (4) **Arranging the call bell within easy reach after a patient is transferred to a chair—Promoting a feeling of safety and security addresses second level needs according to Maslow.**

   (2) **Encourage a family member to visit as often as desired—Maintaining support systems provides for love and belonging needs, third level needs according to Maslow.**

   (3) **Asking a patient about personal preferences before beginning care—Promoting self-control supports self-esteem needs, fourth level needs according to Maslow.**

Communication and Meeting Patients' Emotional Needs

• • •

This section includes questions related to assessing and meeting patients' sociocultural, psychologic, and spiritual needs. It also includes questions that focus on the principles of communication, communication skills, interventions that support emotional needs, and communicating with the confused or disoriented patient. Additional questions focus on patterns of behavior in response to illness, nursing interventions that assist patients to adapt to illness, caring for the dying patient's emotional needs, defense mechanisms, and responding to the crying patient.

Questions

Please fill in the circle to mark your answer choice.

1   The nurse is conducting an intake interview with a patient. To provide the most therapeutic communication with this patient, the nurse should:
   ① Use probing questions
   ② Teach about hygiene
   ③ Ask direct questions
   ④ Listen attentively
   TEST-TAKING TIP ◎ Identify the key word in the stem that sets a priority. Identify the unique option.

2   A patient's son has just died. The patient states, "I can't believe that I have lost my son. Can you believe it?" The nurse's BEST response is to:
   ① Touch the patient's hand and say, "I am very sorry."
   ② Encourage a family member to stay and provide support.
   ③ Leave the room and allow the patient to grieve privately.
   ④ Assume a serious facial expression and say, "I can't believe it either."
   TEST-TAKING TIP ◎ Identify the key word in the stem that sets a priority. Identify the patient-centered options. Identify the option that denies the patient's feelings.

3   A patient is admitted to the hospital with multiple health problems. Which nursing intervention is least effective in meeting the patient's psychosocial needs?
   ① Addressing a patient by name
   ② Assisting a patient with meals
   ③ Identifying achievement of goals
   ④ Explaining care before it is to be given
   TEST-TAKING TIP ◎ Identify the key word in the stem that indicates negative polarity. Identify the clue in the stem.

4   When communicating with patients, it is important for the nurse to remember that:
   ① Progress notes are a form of nonverbal communication.
   ② Patients with expressive aphasia cannot communicate.
   ③ Touch has various meanings to different people.
   ④ Words have the same meaning for all people.
   TEST-TAKING TIP ◎ Identify specific determiners in options.

5   The nurse identifies that a usually talkative patient is withdrawn. The nurse's best response is:
   ① "You are very quiet today."
   ② "What is it that's bothering you?"
   ③ "Tell me what you're upset about."
   ④ "Why are you so withdrawn today?"
   TEST-TAKING TIP ◎ Identify the key word in the stem that sets a priority. Identify equally plausible options.

6 A patient's spouse died 1 week ago. When reminiscing about their life together, the patient begins to cry. The nurse's best response is to:
① Leave the patient alone to provide privacy
② Say, "Things will get better as time passes."
③ Encourage the patient to get grief counseling
④ Say, "This must be a very difficult time for you."

TEST-TAKING TIP ○ Identify the key word in the stem that sets a priority. Identify the options that deny the patient's feelings. Identify options that are patient centered.

7 A patient has a history of verbally aggressive behavior. One afternoon the patient starts to shout at another patient in the lounge. The most appropriate statement by the nurse is:
① "Stop what you are doing."
② "Let's go talk in your room."
③ "Please sit down until you are calm."
④ "Do not raise your voice in a hospital."

TEST-TAKING TIP ○ Identify the key word in the stem that sets a priority. Identify the unique option.

8 A patient is being discharged to a nursing home. While preparing the discharge summary, the patient says, "I feel that nobody cares about me." The nurse's *best* response is:
① "You feel as if nobody cares."
② "We all are concerned about you."
③ "It's hard to be angry at your family."
④ "Your family doesn't have the skills to care for you."

TEST-TAKING TIP ○ Identify the key word in the stem that sets a priority. Identify the clue in the stem that is a clang association in relation to an option. Identify the options that deny the patient's concerns.

9 A female patient talks about her children when they were young and states, "I was a very strict mother." A response by the nurse that reflects the technique of paraphrasing is:
① "It must have been difficult to be a disciplinarian."
② "Sometimes we are sorry for our past behaviors."
③ "You believe you were a firm parent."
④ "You were a very strict mother."

TEST-TAKING TIP ○ Identify the clue in the stem.

10 The nurse obtains a health history from a patient with a chronic illness. Which behavior supports the nurse's conclusion that the patient may be depressed?
① Wishing to attend a nephew's wedding
② Seeking multiple medical opinions
③ Evading activities of daily living
④ Being sarcastic to caregivers

TEST-TAKING TIP ○ Identify the clue in the stem.

11 A patient who has been withdrawn says, "When I have the opportunity, I am going to commit suicide." The *best* response by the nurse is:
① "You have a lovely family. They need you."
② "Let's explore the reasons you have for living."
③ "You must feel overwhelmed to want to kill yourself."
④ "Suicide does not solve problems. Tell me what is wrong."

TEST-TAKING TIP ○ Identify the key word in the stem that sets a priority. Identify the options that deny the patient's feelings. Identify the unique option.

12 A patient who is hearing impaired tells the nurse, "I cannot hear what people say to me." The nurse should:
① Provide pencil and paper for communication
② Ask questions that require a yes or no answer

③ Shout with a loud voice in the patient's better ear
④ Encourage the patient to use gestures and facial expressions when talking

13 A patient asks for advice regarding a personal problem. The <u>most</u> appropriate response by the nurse is to:
① Explain that nurses are not permitted to give advice to a patient
② Encourage the patient to speak with a family member
③ Ask the patient what would be the best thing to do
④ Offer an opinion after listening to the patient

TEST-TAKING TIP ○ Identify the key word in the stem that sets a priority. Identify the option that denies the patient's concerns. Identify opposites in options. Identify the patient-centered option.

14 A dying patient is withdrawn and depressed. The most therapeutic action by the nurse is:
① Explaining that the patient still can accomplish goals
② Assisting the patient to focus on positive thoughts
③ Accepting the patient's behavioral adaptation
④ Offering the patient advice when appropriate

TEST-TAKING TIP ○ Identify the key word in the stem that sets a priority. Identify the options that deny the patient's feelings. Identify the unique option.

15 When caring for dying patients, nurses must appreciate the fact that the sense that is most important to a person who appears to be in a coma is:
① Taste
② Smell
③ Touch
④ Hearing

TEST-TAKING TIP ○ Identify the key word in the stem that sets a priority.

16 A newly admitted patient appears upset and agitated. To best assist this patient, the nurse should:
① Arrange for the patient to remain on bed rest
② Encourage the patient to share feelings
③ Keep the patient as active as possible
④ Point out the behavior to the patient

TEST-TAKING TIP ○ Identify the key word in the stem that sets a priority. Identify the options that are opposites.

17 An older adult reminisces extensively and attempts to keep the nurse from leaving the room. The nurse's *most* therapeutic response is:
① Encouraging the patient to focus on the present
② Limiting the amount of time the patient talks about the past
③ Setting aside time to listen to the stories about the patient's past
④ Suggesting that the patient reminisce with other patients of the same age

TEST-TAKING TIP ○ Identify the key word in the stem that sets a priority. Identify the options that deny the patient's needs. Identify opposites in options.

18 A patient who is incontinent of urine becomes upset. When changing the gown and linens, the nurse's best intervention is to say:
① "I am a nurse. This is part of my job."
② "This doesn't bother me. It often happens."
③ "This occurs all the time. Try not to feel bad."
④ "I am your nurse. I will change your gown and linens."

TEST-TAKING TIP ○ Identify the key word in the stem that sets a priority. Identify the patient-centered option.

19 Nurses understand that psychosocial development is most influenced by:
① Food
② Society
③ Alcohol
④ Genetics

TEST-TAKING TIP ⊙ Identify a key word in the stem that is close to a clang association.

20 A patient has difficulty communicating verbally (expressive aphasia) because of a brain attack (stroke). To increase the patient's ability to communicate, the nurse should:
① Encourage the patient to elaborate with gestures
② Anticipate the patient's needs to reduce frustration
③ Talk to the patient without expecting a verbal response
④ Ask the patient questions that require a yes or no response

TEST-TAKING TIP ⊙ Identify the opposites in options.

21 Several times a day, every day, a patient who is experiencing short-term memory loss asks when medication is to be given. The patient receives medication at the same time every day. The most therapeutic nursing intervention is to:
① Inform the patient when medication has to be taken.
② Tell the patient to go to the nurse when it is time for medication
③ Encourage the patient to remember when it is time for medication
④ Make a sign for the patient's room indicating the time for medication

TEST-TAKING TIP ⊙ Identify the key word in the stem that sets a priority. Identify equally plausible options.

22 A patient is upset and rambles about an incident that occurred earlier in the week. The nurse should first:
① Ask the patient what is wrong
② Identify the patient's concerns
③ Recognize the patient is confused
④ Encourage the patient to focus on the present

TEST-TAKING TIP ⊙ Identify the key word in the stem that sets a priority. Identify the unique option. Identify the option that denies the patient's feelings.

23 When working with patients who are coping with multiple stresses, the nurse understands that defense mechanisms can be classified as:
① Relief behaviors
② Conscious behaviors
③ Somatizing behaviors
④ Manipulative behaviors

24 A dying patient says, "All my life I was fairly religious, but I am still worried about what happens after death." The nurse's best response is:
① "The unknown is often very frightening."
② "Religious people know that God is forgiving."
③ "People with near-death experiences say it is peaceful."
④ "You must feel good about being religious all your life."

TEST-TAKING TIP ⊙ Identify the key word in the stem that sets a priority. Identify equally plausible options. Identify the options that deny the patient's feelings.

25 A dying patient says to the nurse, "I was much more religious when I was young." The nurse's *best* response is:
① "Do you still believe in God?"
② "Do you want us to pray for you?"

③ "Would you like me to call a chaplain?"
④ "Are you concerned about life after death?"

TEST-TAKING TIP ○ Identify the word in the stem that sets a priority. Identify the unique option.

26 A female patient becomes upset whenever anyone mentions her upcoming birthday and does not want to talk about age. The nurse identifies this behavior as:
① Denial
② Sorrow
③ Loneliness
④ Suppression

27 A patient who usually is verbal appears sad and withdrawn. The nurse should:
① Describe the behavior to the patient
② Continue to observe the patient's behavior
③ Ensure that the patient has time to be alone
④ Attempt to engage the patient in cheerful conversation

TEST-TAKING TIP ○ Identify the unique option.

28 A patient is confused and disoriented. The route of communication used by the nurse that is most effective is:
① Touch
② Writing
③ Talking
④ Pictures

TEST-TAKING TIP ○ Identify the unique option.

29 A patient tells the nurse "The doctor just told me I have cancer" and then begins to cry. What is the best response by the nurse?
① "Sometimes it helps to talk about it."
② "I hope things will get better by tomorrow."
③ "Deep breathing may help you regain control."
④ "Crying is good because it gets it out of your system."

TEST-TAKING TIP ○ Identify the unique option.

30 The nurse understands that statements that provide false reassurance are nontherapeutic. Check all the statements that provide false reassurance.
① _____ "This is minor surgery."
② _____ "You're smiling this morning."
③ _____ "A lot of people hate injections."
④ _____ "It is difficult to cope with pain."
⑤ _____ "You'll walk better after you have physical therapy."

TEST-TAKING TIP ○ Identify the word in the stem that indicates negative polarity.

184 Communication and Meeting Patients' Emotional Needs

Answers and Rationales

1 **TEST-TAKING TIP** ○ The word "most" in the stem sets a priority. Option 4 is unique because it is a receptive, nonverbal action, whereas the other options are all active verbal interventions.

① Direct, not probing, questions might be asked later; probing questions violate a patient's right to privacy.

② Teaching self-care might be done later; it is not the priority.

③ Asking direct questions may be done later; it is not the priority.

④ **Reception of a message must occur before the nurse can intervene; by listening, the nurse collects information that influences future care.**

2 **TEST-TAKING TIP** ○ The word BEST in the stem is the key word that sets a priority. Options 1 and 4 are patient centered. Option 3 denies the patient's feelings.

① **Touch denotes caring; this statement is direct and supportive but does not reinforce denial.**

② Although this may be done later, the patient needs immediate support.

③ Leaving the room is a form of abandonment.

④ Although this statement identifies feelings, it supports denial.

3 **TEST-TAKING TIP** ○ The word "least" in the stem indicates negative polarity. The word "psychosocial" in the stem is a clue.

① Calling a patient by name individualizes care and supports dignity and self-esteem.

② **Usually eating is an independent ADL; for an adult, assistance with meals may precipitate feelings of dependence and regression.**

③ Identifying the achievement of goals is motivating and supports independence, self-esteem, and self-actualization.

④ Explaining care provides emotional support because it reduces fear of the unknown and involves the patient in the care.

4 **TEST-TAKING TIP** ○ In Option 2, the word "all" is understood; this option is really saying, "All patients with expressive aphasia cannot communicate." Option 4 contains the word "all," which is a specific determiner.

① Words, whether they are spoken or written, are verbal communication.

② Patients with expressive aphasia can often communicate using nonverbal behaviors, a picture board, or written messages.

③ **Touch is a form of nonverbal communication that sends a variety of messages depending on the person's culture, sex, age, past experiences, and present situation; touch also invades a person's personal space.**

④ People from different cultures and people in subgroups within the same culture place different values on words.

5 **TEST-TAKING TIP** ○ The word best is a key word in the stem that sets a priority. Options 2 and 3 are equally plausible because they make the assumptions that the patient is upset or bothered.

① **This statement identifies the behavior and provides an opportunity for the patient to verbalize further.**

② This statement is too direct; it may put the patient on the defensive and cut off communication. Also, the patient may not have the insight to answer the question.

③ Same as #2.

④ "Why" questions are too direct and often patients do not have the insight to answer them. Also, this statement draws the conclusion that the patient is withdrawn, which may be inaccurate.

6 **TEST-TAKING TIP** ○ The word "best" is the key word in the stem that sets a priority. Options 1 and 2 deny the patient's feelings. Options 3 and 4 are patient centered.

① Leaving abandons the patient at a time when emotional support may be beneficial. Abandonment is an ultimate form of denial.

② This statement is false reassurance and denies the patient's feeling.

③ This may eventually be done, but the patient needs immediate support.

④ **This statement identifies feelings, focuses on the patient, and provides an opportunity for the patient to share feelings.**

7 **TEST-TAKING TIP** ○ The word "most" in the stem sets a priority. Option 2 is unique because it is the only option that removes the patient from the room.

① This statement is a command that may demean the patient; it challenges the patient and may precipitate more abusive behavior.

② **This statement interrupts the behavior and protects the other patient; walking to another room uses energy, and talking promotes verbalization of feelings and concerns.**

③ This statement is judgmental; this implies the patient is not calm. An agitated patient has too much energy to sit quietly.

④ This statement is inappropriate because it challenges the patient and puts the patient on the defensive.

8 **TEST-TAKING TIP** ⊙ The word *best* is the key word in the stem that sets a priority. The words "nobody cares" appear in the stem and Option 1; this repetition is a clang association. Options 2 and 4 deny the patient's feelings.
   ① **Repeating the patient's statement allows the patient to focus on what was said, validates what was said, and encourages communication.**
   ② This statement may or may not be true and does not encourage verbalization of feelings.
   ③ This patient's statement reflects feelings of sadness and isolation, not anger.
   ④ Same as #2.

9 **TEST-TAKING TIP** ⊙ The word "paraphrasing" is the clue in the stem.
   ① This response uses reflective technique, not paraphrasing, because it identifies a feeling.
   ② The patient's statement does not reflect feelings of sorrow or guilt.
   ③ **This response restates the message using different words; paraphrasing focuses on content rather than the feeling or underlying emotional theme of the patient's message.**
   ④ Although some professionals consider a response that echoes the patient's statement as a form of paraphrasing, using the exact words used by the patient is not as effective as restating the patient's message in slightly different words.

10 **TEST-TAKING TIP** ⊙ The word "depressed" is the clue in the stem.
   ① This is future-oriented thinking and may be a form of bargaining for more time.
   ② This is associated with denial and bargaining.
   ③ **When patients are depressed, they may feel a loss of control, feel alone, and be withdrawn. With depression, there is little physical energy, a lack of concern about the ADLs, and a decreased interest in physical appearance.**
   ④ Sarcasm generally reflects feelings of anger.

11 **TEST-TAKING TIP** ⊙ The word *best* is the key word in the stem that sets a priority. Options 1, 2, and 4 deny the patient's feelings. Option 3 is unique because it is the only option that addresses feelings.
   ① This statement denies the patient's feelings. The patient is unable to cope, is selecting the ultimate escape, and is not capable of meeting the needs of others. This response may also precipitate feelings such as guilt.
   ② This statement denies the patient's feelings; the patient must focus on the negatives before exploring the positives.
   ③ **Open-ended statements identify feelings and invite further communication.**
   ④ This response is judgmental, denies the patient's feelings, and may cut off communication. In addition, this response is too direct and the patient may not consciously know what is wrong.

12 ① **Communication can be promoted in written rather than verbal form; this reduces social isolation and promotes communication.**
   ② Communication is a two-way process; the patient is not having difficulty sending messages; the patient is having difficulty receiving messages. This intervention is more appropriate for a patient with expressive aphasia.
   ③ Shouting is demeaning and unnecessary; enunciating words slowly and directly in front of the patient supports communication.
   ④ The patient is having difficulty receiving messages, not sending messages.

13 **TEST-TAKING TIP** ⊙ The word <u>most</u> is the key word in the stem that sets a priority. Option 1 denies the patient's concern. Options 3 and 4 are opposites. Option 3 is patient centered.
   ① This approach puts the focus on the nurse and cuts off communication.
   ② Although this might eventually be done, it is not the priority. Also, the patient may never want to talk about a particular concern with family members.
   ③ **This response provides an opportunity for the patient to explore concerns and alternative solutions without others influencing the decision making.**
   ④ Offering opinions is inappropriate; opinions involve judgments that are based on feelings and values that may be different from the patient's.

14 **TEST-TAKING TIP** ⊙ The word "most" is the key word in the stem that sets a priority. Options 1 and 2 deny the patient's feelings. Option 3 is unique because it is the only option that uses the word "patient's," the possessive form of the word "patient."
   ① This denies the patient's feelings.
   ② Same as #1.
   ③ **Depression is the fourth stage of dying according to Kübler-Ross; patients become withdrawn and noncommunicative when feeling a loss of control and recognizing future losses. The nurse should accept the behavior and be available if the patient wants to verbalize feelings.**
   ④ It is never appropriate to offer advice; people must explore their alternatives and come to their own conclusions.

15 TEST-TAKING TIP ◎ The word "most" is the key word in the stem that sets a priority.

(1) Although this sense is important, it is not the most important sense to an unconscious patient.

(2) Same as #1.

(3) Same as #1.

(4) Hearing is the most important sense to an unconscious patient because it is believed to be the last sense that is lost. The senses receive stimuli from the environment and hearing keeps one in contact with others.

16 TEST-TAKING TIP ◎ The word "best" is the key word in the stem that sets a priority. Options 1 and 3 are opposites and are distractors.

(1) Agitated patients may not be able to lie still. They need some outlet for energy expenditure.

(2) Agitation is a response to anxiety; the patient's feelings and concerns must be addressed to help relieve the anxiety and agitation.

(3) This may increase the agitation, particularly if the cause of the agitation is ignored.

(4) This is confrontational and may precipitate a defensive response by the patient.

17 TEST-TAKING TIP ◎ The word "most" is the key word in the stem that sets a priority. Options 1 and 2 deny the patient's needs. Options 2 and 3 are opposites.

(1) Avoiding reminiscing is inappropriate; the developmental task of older adults is to perform a life review.

(2) Same as #1.

(3) The nurse is responsible for assisting the older adult to explore the past and deal with the developmental conflict of integrity versus despair.

(4) Patients should not be responsible for meeting each other's needs.

18 TEST-TAKING TIP ◎ The word "best" is the key word in the stem that sets a priority. Option 4 is the only option that does not minimize the patient's feelings and focuses on the patient.

(1) This response cuts off communication and puts the focus on the nurse rather than on the patient.

(2) This response generalizes rather than individualizes care. It minimizes the patient's concern and may cut off communication.

(3) Same as #2.

(4) This response meets the patient's right to know who is providing care and what is to be done. This is a nonjudgmental, respectful response that reduces fears of the unknown. Although this response does not address the patient's feelings, it is the best response of the options offered.

19 TEST-TAKING TIP ◎ An important word in the stem is "psychosocial." When examining the options, you see that one of them contains the word "society." "Society" is closely related to "psychosocial." Carefully consider this option. More often than not, a clang is the correct answer.

(1) Food is only one aspect of a society and its culture; the primary purpose of food is to meet physiologic needs.

(2) A person's cultural environment, which includes the family and the community, has the greatest impact on psychosocial development.

(3) Although alcohol meets some individuals' psychologic needs and is served in social situations, it is not the factor that most influences psychosocial development.

(4) Although some theorists identify genetics as a factor related to personality and behavior, it is not the most influential factor in psychosocial development.

20 TEST-TAKING TIP ◎ Options 3 and 4 are opposites and are distractors.

(1) Communication can be both verbal and nonverbal. The use of gestures facilitates communication.

(2) Although anticipating needs may be done occasionally, it does not increase the patient's ability to communicate.

(3) Communication is a two-way process and the patient should be involved. The patient should be encouraged to respond in some way.

(4) Although this may be done occasionally, it does not increase the patient's ability to communicate; a yes or no response is too limited.

21 TEST-TAKING TIP ◎ The word "most" in the stem sets a priority. Options 2 and 3 are equally plausible.

(1) Although reminding the patient every time might be done, it is not the most therapeutic intervention because it addresses only the next dose.

(2) The patient probably is not capable of remembering. Too challenging a task can be frustrating.

(3) Same as #2.

(4) A sign promotes independence and does not demean the patient; the patient can refer to the schedule when necessary.

22 TEST-TAKING TIP ○ The word "first" is the key word in the stem that sets a priority. Option 2 is unique because it is the only option that uses the possessive form of the word patient (patient's). Option 4 denies the patient's feelings.

(1) This is too direct a statement; the patient may not be able to put into words what is wrong.

(2) **Active listening is necessary for data collection; after data are collected, the patient's feelings and concerns can be identified.**

(3) When people are anxious, their conversation may ramble, but it does not necessarily mean they are confused.

(4) This denies the patient's feelings; the patient must talk further about the situation to reduce anxiety.

23 (1) **Defense mechanisms are used to lower anxiety, manage stress, maintain the ego, and shelter self-esteem; although they can be productive or eventually detrimental, they do provide relief by releasing physical and emotional energy.**

(2) Most defense mechanisms are used on an unconscious level, except for suppression, which is used by the conscious mind.

(3) A somatizing behavior is identified when a patient experiences a psychologic conflict as a physical symptom; physical symptoms distract the patient from the actual emotional distress as the patient internally manages the anxiety physiologically.

(4) Manipulative behaviors are not known as defense mechanisms but rather as purposeful behaviors used to meet personal needs; manipulative behaviors can be adaptive or maladaptive; they are maladaptive when they are the primary method used to meet needs, the needs of others are ignored, or others are dehumanized to meet the needs of the manipulator.

24 TEST-TAKING TIP ○ The word "best" is the key word in the stem that sets a priority. Options 2 and 3 are equally plausible. Options 2, 3, and 4 deny the patient's feelings.

(1) **This statement uses reflective technique to identify the patient's feelings regarding fear of the unknown.**

(2) This statement denies the patient's feelings and cuts off communication; also, the patient's message did not indicate a need for forgiveness.

(3) This statement focuses on other people's experiences rather than the patient's feelings or concerns.

(4) This statement puts the emphasis on the wrong part of the message; it ignores the patient's concern about what happens after death.

25 TEST-TAKING TIP ○ The word "best" in the stem sets a priority. Option 3 is unique because it makes a referral to someone other than the nurse.

(1) This is inappropriate probing and violates the patient's right to privacy or may put the patient on the defensive.

(2) This is an inappropriate question; not all the nurses on the team may want to assume this intervention.

(3) **This response recognizes that the patient is considering personal spiritual needs; it provides an opportunity that the patient can accept or reject.**

(4) Same as #1.

26 (1) Denial is an unconscious defense mechanism; this patient consciously and voluntarily refuses to talk about the birthday.

(2) This is an assumption; there are insufficient data to reach this conclusion.

(3) Same as #2.

(4) **This is a conscious protective mechanism in which a person actively puts anxiety-producing feelings or concerns out of the mind.**

27 TEST-TAKING TIP ○ Option 1 is the only response that directly addresses the patient's behavior. The other options avoid the patient (Option 2), abandon the patient (Option 3), or deny the patient's feelings (Option 4).

(1) **Pointing out the patient's behavior brings it to the attention of the patient and provides an opportunity to explore feelings.**

(2) The patient's behavior needs to be addressed more fully than only by continued observation.

(3) This is a form of abandonment; sad, withdrawn patients need to know that they are accepted and that the nurse is available for support.

(4) This denies the patient's feelings.

28 TEST-TAKING TIP ○ Option 1 is unique. Touch is the only intervention that enters the patient's personal space.

(1) **Touch is a simple form of communication that is easily understood even by confused, disoriented, or mentally incapacitated individuals.**

(2) This requires interpretation of symbols, which is a more complex form of communication than touch.

(3) This requires an interpretation of words, which is a more complex form of communication than touch.

(4) Same as #2.

29 TEST-TAKING TIP ◯ Option 1 is unique. Options 2, 3, and 4 all imply that everything will get better; these are Pollyanna-like responses that deny the patient's feelings.

(1) **This recognizes the patient's behavior and provides an opportunity to verbalize feelings and concerns.**

(2) This is false reassurance.

(3) This implies that the patient is out of control. This interferes with the patient's coping mechanisms and may not help the patient regain control.

(4) This is false reassurance; crying may or may not help this patient. Also, the use of the word *good* is a value judgment.

30 TEST-TAKING TIP ◯ The word "nontherapeutic" in the stem indicates negative polarity.

(1) **_X_ This statement implies that there is no reason to worry, which is a form of false reassurance.**

(2) ____ This is an observation that invites the patient to explore feelings.

(3) ____ Although this statement does not provide false reassurance, it takes the focus away from the patient and cuts off further communication.

(4) ____ This is a supportive statement that focuses on what the patient may be thinking and invites an exploration of feelings and problem solving.

(5) **_X_ This statement supports an outcome that may or may not be accomplished by physical therapy; this is false reassurance.**

Physical Assessment of Patients

• • •

This section includes questions related to various aspects of physical and psychosocial assessment. Questions focus on temperature, pulse, respirations, blood pressure, level of consciousness, level of orientation, and principles related to specimens and the collection of specimens, such as wound cultures and stool specimens. Questions also address assessments common to infection, the general adaptation syndrome (GAS), and the inflammatory process. Additional questions focus on whether assessment data are subjective or objective in nature, whether sources are primary or secondary, the responsibilities of the nurse regarding data collected during assessment, the sources of data, and the use of common physical examination techniques.

QUESTIONS

Please fill in the circle to mark your answer choice.

1 The nurse identifies that the primary source for assessing how a patient slept is the:
   ① Nurse
   ② Patient
   ③ Physician
   ④ Roommate
   TEST-TAKING TIP ◦ Identify the clue in the stem. Identify the unique option.

2 When the nurse arrives in the room to take a patient's temperature, the patient is drinking a cup of coffee. How long should the nurse wait to take the patient's oral temperature?
   ① 5 minutes
   ② 7 minutes
   ③ 15 minutes
   ④ 30 minutes
   TEST-TAKING TIP ◦ Identify the clue in the stem.

3 The nurse is assessing the vital signs of several patients. Which signs of respiratory distress should the nurse report to the physician?
   ① Respiratory rate of 16 with an irregular rhythm
   ② Respiratory rate of 26 with an irregular rhythm
   ③ Respiratory rate of 18 with a regular rhythm
   ④ Respiratory rate of 20 with a regular rhythm
   TEST-TAKING TIP ◦ Identify the duplicate facts among the options.

4 When obtaining a radial pulse rate, the nurse understands that it reflects the function of the:
   ① Arteries
   ② Veins
   ③ Blood
   ④ Heart
   TEST-TAKING TIP ◦ Identify the clue in the stem. Identify the options that are opposites.

5 When assessing the vital signs of patients, the nurse understands that an individual's body temperature will be at its lowest at:
   ① 6 AM
   ② 10 AM
   ③ 6 PM
   ④ 9 PM
   TEST-TAKING TIP ◦ Identify the clue in the stem. Identify the options that are opposites.

6 When making rounds, the nurse finds a patient in bed with the eyes closed. The nurse should:
① Suspect that the patient is feeling withdrawn
② Return in 30 minutes to check on the patient
③ Collect more information about the patient
④ Allow the patient to continue sleeping

TEST-TAKING TIP ○ Identify the equally plausible options. Identify the options that are opposites.

7 When interviewing a patient, the nurse understands that an example of objective data is:
① Pain
② Fever
③ Nausea
④ Fatigue

TEST-TAKING TIP ○ Identify the clue in the stem. Identify the unique option.

8 The nurse in a long-term care facility is caring for a group of older adults. The nurse identifies that older adults tend to have higher blood pressures because they have:
① Aging hearts
② Thicker blood
③ Lifestyle stressors
④ Less elastic vessels

9 The nurse is assessing the patient's orientation times three. The nursing intervention that should be included in this assessment is:
① Asking the patient to state the time of day
② Inquiring if the patient remembers the nurse's name
③ Ascertaining if the patient can follow simple directions
④ Determining if the patient follows movement with the eyes

TEST-TAKING TIP ○ Identify the unique option.

10 The nurse takes the resting pulse rate of an older adult. The nurse identifies that the pulse rate within the expected range is:
① 50 beats per minute and irregular
② 90 beats per minute and regular
③ 105 beats per minute and irregular
④ 120 beats per minute and regular

TEST-TAKING TIP ○ Identify the clue in the stem. Identify the duplicate facts among the options.

11 The nurse obtains the rectal temperature of an adult. Which rectal temperature is within the expected range?
① 96.4°F
② 97.6°F
③ 99.8°F
④ 101.2°F

TEST-TAKING TIP ○ Identify the clue in the stem.

12 A patient has a history of heart disease. After walking to the lounge, the patient sits in a chair, places a fist against the chest, and complains of a severe upset stomach. The nurse should first:
① Take the patient's vital signs
② Walk the patient back to bed
③ Administer an antacid to the patient
④ Listen to the complaints of the patient

TEST-TAKING TIP ○ Identify the key word in the stem that sets a priority.

13 The nurse observes that a newborn's urine is very light yellow. The nurse understands that this occurs because infants:
① Ingest only fluids
② Cannot control urination
③ Are unable to concentrate urine
④ Always urinate more frequently than adults

TEST-TAKING TIP ○ Identify specific determiners in the options.

14 The nurse collects subjective data when the patient:
① Appears jaundiced
② Has a headache
③ Looks tired
④ Is crying

TEST-TAKING TIP ○ Identify the clue in the stem. Identify the unique option.

15 The physician orders a culture and sensitivity of a patient's urine. To ensure the most accurate results of a urine culture and sensitivity, the nurse should:
① Collect a midstream urine sample
② Use only the first voiding of the day
③ Obtain a double-voided urine specimen
④ Use a twenty-four hour urine collection

TEST-TAKING TIP ○ Identify the key word in the stem that sets a priority. Identify the option that contains a specific determiner.

16 When obtaining the vital signs of patients, the nurse understands that an accurate statement regarding blood pressure (BP) is:
① A BP differs 5 to 10 mm Hg between arms.
② A BP remains consistent regardless of the patient's position.
③ The arm must be kept at the level of the clavicles to obtain a correct BP.
④ The arm must be kept below the apex of the heart to obtain an accurate BP.

TEST-TAKING TIP ○ Identify the options that are opposites. Identify the option that is unique.

17 The nurse obtains the blood pressure of several patients. Which blood pressure reading is considered the most hypertensive?
① 90/70
② 130/86
③ 160/90
④ 150/115

TEST-TAKING TIP ○ Identify the key word in the stem that sets a priority.

18 A concern that is common to the collection of specimens, regardless of their source, for culture and sensitivity tests is that:
① The specimen should be collected in the morning
② Gloves, a gown, and a mask should be worn
③ Two specimens should always be obtained
④ Surgical asepsis should be maintained

TEST-TAKING TIP ○ Identify the phrase in the stem that is a clue. Identify the option that contains a specific determiner.

19 When assessing the pulse of a patient, the nurse identifies a change in rate from 88 to 56. The nurse should first:
① Wait 15 minutes and retake the patient's pulse
② Ask the patient about recent activity
③ Obtain the other vital signs
④ Alert the nurse in charge

TEST-TAKING TIP ○ Identify the key word in the stem that sets a priority.

20 The nurse is collecting a stool specimen for parasites. A consideration that is unique in comparison to other stool specimens is the need to:
① Wear protective gloves
② Obtain three successive daily specimens
③ Send the specimen to the laboratory while still warm
④ Take feces from several areas of the bowel movement
TEST-TAKING TIP ◉ Identify the clue in the stem.

21 The nurse needs to identify a patient's health beliefs before giving care. Therefore, the nurse must first assess the patient's:
① Level of wellness
② Acceptable values
③ Frame of reference
④ Use of defense mechanisms
TEST-TAKING TIP ◉ Identify the key word in the stem that sets a priority.

22 A nurse case manager from a nursing home is assessing an alert patient who is a candidate for the nursing home. The nurse manager understands that the *best* source of information about this patient is the:
① Patient's family
② Primary nurse
③ Physician
④ Patient
TEST-TAKING TIP ◉ Identify the key word in the stem that sets a priority.

23 To determine the presence of orthostatic hypotension, when is the most significant time for a patient's blood pressure to be assessed?
① After standing
② Between meals
③ During activity
④ Before standing
TEST-TAKING TIP ◉ Identify the options that are opposites.

24 The nurse is obtaining a patient's blood pressure. Which physiologic action is reflected by the diastolic blood pressure?
① Contraction of the ventricles
② Volume of cardiac output
③ Resting arterial pressure
④ Pulse pressure
TEST-TAKING TIP ◉ Identify the options with a clang association.

25 The nurse is obtaining a patient's pedal pulse. The nurse understands that this assessment reflects the function of the patient's:
① Veins
② Heart
③ Blood
④ Arteries
TEST-TAKING TIP ◉ Identify the options that are opposites.

26 Which principle of blood pressure physiology should the nurse understand when assessing a patient's cardiac function?
① A trough pressure occurs during systole
② The pulse pressure occurs during diastole

③ A peak pressure occurs when the ventricles relax
④ The blood pressure reaches a peak followed by a trough
TEST-TAKING TIP ○ Identify the options that are opposites.

27 Which adaptation indicates that the inflammatory response has entered the second phase?
① Pain
② A fever
③ Erythema
④ An exudate

28 When assessing the results of a culture and sensitivity report, the nurse understands that the sensitivity part of the report indicates:
① All of the microorganisms present
② Virulence of the organisms in the culture
③ Antibiotics that should be effective treatment
④ Extent of the patient's response to the pathogens
TEST-TAKING TIP ○ Identify the option that contains a specific determiner.

29 The primary nurse assesses all the patients in the district at the beginning of a shift. Which patient assessment requires the nurse to perform an immediate focused assessment?
① Edema of 2+ in the ankles
② Difficulty sleeping at night
③ Lack of a bowel movement in 3 days
④ Blanchable erythema in the sacral area
TEST-TAKING TIP ○ Identify the key word in the stem that sets a priority.

30 The nurse is obtaining an oral temperature with an electronic thermometer. What must the nurse do? Check all that apply.
① _____ Use the red probe
② _____ Take the temperature before breakfast
③ _____ Use a new probe cover for each patient
④ _____ Wipe the probe with alcohol after each use
⑤ _____ Assess if the route is appropriate for the patient

Physical Assessment of Patients
Answers and Rationales

1 TEST-TAKING TIP ○ The word "primary" is a clue in the stem. Option 2 is unique. Options 1, 3, and 4 involve people other than the patient.
① The nurse is a secondary source of data. The nurse may not be totally aware of how well the patient slept.
② **Patients are primary sources and the only sources able to provide subjective data concerning how they slept.**
③ The physician is a secondary source of information.
④ Patients should not be held responsible for other patients.

2 TEST-TAKING TIP ○ The word "oral" is a clue in the stem.
① This is too short a period of time for the mouth to recover from the hot fluid; the dilated vessels in the mouth and the warmth of the tissues from the hot fluid will cause an inaccurate elevation in the temperature reading.
② Same as #1.
③ **It takes at least 15 minutes for the vessels in the mouth and the mucous membranes to recover from the hot fluid and for the mouth to return to the patient's core temperature.**
④ This is too long a time period to wait.

3 TEST-TAKING TIP ○ Options 1 and 2 contain the duplicate fact that the patient's respirations are irregular. Options 3 and 4 contain the duplicate fact that the patient's respirations are regular. If you know that respirations should be regular, then Options 3 and 4 are distractors.
① This is within the expected range of 12 to 20 breaths per minute. An irregular rhythm without other signs of distress does not necessitate notifying the physician.
② **Tachypnea, a respiratory rate greater than 24 breaths per minute, along with an irregular rhythm, indicates that the body is in respiratory distress.**
③ Breathing is usually regular and within the range of 12 to 20 breaths per minute.
④ Same as #3.

4 TEST-TAKING TIP ○ The word "radial" is a clue in the stem. Options 1 and 2 are opposites and are distractors. Arteries carry blood away from the heart; veins carry blood to the heart. In this question, these options are distractors.
① Elasticity and rigidity of the vessel walls and the quality and equality of pulses provide data about the status of the arteries.
② A pulse is palpated in an artery, not a vein.
③ Blood is assessed through laboratory tests performed on blood specimens.
④ **The heart is a pulsatile pump that ejects blood into the arterial system with each ventricular contraction; the pulse is the vibration transmitted with each contraction of the heart.**

5 TEST-TAKING TIP ○ The word "lowest" is a clue in the stem. Options 1 and 3 are opposites.
① **A person's body temperature is at its lowest in the early morning. Core temperatures vary with a predictable pattern over 24 hours (diurnal or circadian temperature variations) because of hormonal variations.**
② Body temperature is not at its lowest at 10 AM; body temperature steadily rises as the day progresses.
③ Body temperature peaks between 5 and 7 PM.
④ Body temperature is not at its lowest at 9 PM; body temperature is still falling from its peak.

6 TEST-TAKING TIP ○ Options 2 and 4 are equally plausible. Options 3 and 4 are opposites.
① This is an assumption based on insufficient data.
② Waiting is unsafe.
③ **More information must be collected to make a complete assessment and reach an accurate conclusion.**
④ Same as #2.

7 TEST-TAKING TIP ○ The word "objective" is a clue in the stem. Option 2 is unique because it is measurable. Options 1, 3, and 4 are similar because the adaptations can be described only by the patient.
① Pain is subjective; subjective data are a patient's perceptions, feelings, sensations, or ideas.
② **Fever is objective because it can be measured with a thermometer.**
③ Nausea is subjective data based on a patient's feelings or perceptions.
④ Fatigue is subjective data, based on a patient's feelings or perceptions.

8 ① In aging hearts, there is decreased contractile strength of the myocardium that results in a decreased cardiac output. The body compensates for this by increasing the heart rate, not the blood pressure.
② Aging does not cause thicker blood. Polycythemia (greater concentration of erythrocytes to plasma), a pathologic condition, can cause a higher viscosity of the blood, resulting in hypertension.

(3) This is a generalization that may or may not be true. The older adult has physical, cognitive, and social changes, and how the person perceives them and adapts to them determines whether the individual's lifestyle is stressful and whether it influences blood pressure.

(4) **As people age, vascular changes and the accumulation of sclerotic plaques along the walls of vessels occur, making them more rigid. Vascular rigidity increases vascular resistance, which increases blood pressure.**

9 **TEST-TAKING TIP** ◉ Option 1 is unique. In Options 2, 3, and 4, the words "inquiring," "ascertaining," and "determining" are all followed by the phrase "if the patient."

(1) **Questions related to time, place, and person (assessing orientation in three ways) are essential when assessing a patient's level of orientation.**

(2) This assesses recent memory, not orientation.

(3) This can be done by confused, disoriented patients.

(4) Same as #3.

10 **TEST-TAKING TIP** ◉ The word "resting" is a clue in the stem. Options 1 and 3 relate to an irregular pulse rate. Options 2 and 4 relate to a regular pulse rate. If you know that a pulse rate should be regular, then Options 1 and 3 are distractors.

(1) A rate of 50 is below the expected range of a pulse rate in an older adult. The rhythm should be regular, not irregular.

(2) **The expected heart rate in an older adult is between 60 and 100 beats per minute and regular.**

(3) A rate of 105 is too high for a heart rate taken at rest; in older adults, a decreased contractile strength of the myocardium may cause the heart rate to increase to this rate during mild exercise. The rhythm should be regular, not irregular.

(4) A rate of 120 is too high for a heart rate taken at rest.

11 **TEST-TAKING TIP** ◉ The word "rectal" is a clue in the stem.

(1) This is below the expected range for a rectal temperature.

(2) Same as #1.

(3) **A temperature of 99.8°F is within the expected range of 98.6° to 100.6°F for a rectal temperature.**

(4) A temperature of 101.2°F indicates a fever.

12 **TEST-TAKING TIP** ◉ The word "first" is the key word in the stem that sets a priority.

(1) **A further assessment is necessary; vital signs reflect the cardiopulmonary status of the patient.**

(2) Activity at this time is unsafe because it will increase the demands on the heart.

(3) The nurse does not have enough information to conclude that the problem is gastritis; antacids require a physician's order.

(4) Although listening is important, it is not the priority at this time.

13 **TEST-TAKING TIP** ◉ The word "only" in option 1 and the word "always" in option 4 are specific determiners.

(1) Infants void very light yellow urine because of immature kidney function, not because they ingest only fluids.

(2) Although it is true that infants have not developed neuromuscular control of urination, the inability to control micturition voluntarily has no impact on the color of urine voided.

(3) **An infant's kidneys are unable to concentrate urine and reabsorb water efficiently. When the body is too immature to concentrate urine, urine is diluted and very light yellow in color.**

(4) Although this is a correct statement by itself, it is not related to the content in the stem. Infants' bladders are smaller than adults' bladders and they can retain only a small volume of urine. Frequency is not related to the color of urine.

14 **TEST-TAKING TIP** ◉ The word "subjective" is a clue in the stem. Option 2 is unique because the patient is the only one who can describe the headache. Options 1, 3, and 4 are similar because they include assessments that can be observed by another person.

(1) Jaundice is objective; objective data require the use of a sense to collect the data. Jaundice is a human response that is measured using the sense of vision and the assessment technique of inspection.

(2) **Subjective data are data that can be described or verified only by the patient; a patient's descriptions of pain, concerns, feelings, or sensations are additional examples of subjective data.**

(3) Looks tired is a conclusion based on observation.

(4) Crying is an objective datum because it can be observed by another person.

15 **TEST-TAKING TIP** ◉ The word "most" is the key word in the stem that sets a priority. The word "only" in Option 2 is a specific determiner.

(1) **A midstream urine sample contains a specimen that is relatively free of microorganisms from the urethra. After perineal care, cleansing of the urethral opening, and the initiation of urination, a specimen is collected during the midportion of the stream. This technique avoids collection of urine during the initial stream which may be contaminated with bacteria from the urethra.**

(2) Specimens collected from the first voiding of the morning should be avoided; stagnant urine does not reflect urine that is recently produced by the urinary system.

(3) A double-voided specimen is taken for the measurement of glucose and ketones in the urine; stagnant urine from the bladder does not reflect the current level of glucose and ketones found in the urine at the time of the voiding.

(4) Twenty-four hours of urine is needed for special tests such as the measurement of levels of adrenocortical steroids, hormones, and creatinine clearance tests, not for a urine culture and sensitivity.

16 **TEST-TAKING TIP** ◉ Options 3 and 4 are opposites and are distractors. Option 1 is unique because it is the only option that contains a number and it does not focus on the position of the arm when taking blood pressure measurements.

(1) **Because of variations in structure and distance, there might be 5 to 10 mmHg difference between arms; the arm with the higher blood pressure should be used for subsequent assessments.**

(2) The blood pressure is higher when the arm is below heart level and lower when the arm is above heart level. The patient's arm should be at the apex of the heart when taking blood pressure measurements.

(3) When the arm is above the apex of the heart, the resulting blood pressure will be abnormally low.

(4) When the arm is below the apex of the heart, the resulting blood pressure will be abnormally high.

17 **TEST-TAKING TIP** ◉ The word "most" is the key word in the stem that sets a priority.

(1) A blood pressure reading of 90/70 reflects hypotension.

(2) This is considered prehypertension, not hypertension. Blood pressure values of 120 to 139 systolic and 80 to 89 diastolic are considered prehypertensive.

(3) Although a systolic reading of 160 is high and needs to be reported to the physician, a blood pressure with a higher diastolic reading is more dangerous.

(4) **A blood pressure with a higher diastolic pressure is more hypertensive than a blood pressure with a higher systolic pressure but lower diastolic pressure. The diastolic pressure is the pressure exerted against the arterial walls when the ventricles are at rest; the higher the diastolic pressure, the more dangerous is the situation.**

18 **TEST-TAKING TIP** ◉ The phrase "common to" is a clue in the stem. Option 3 contains the word "always," which is a specific determiner.

(1) The time of day is irrelevant for the collection of most specimens for culture and sensitivity.

(2) Gloves may be worn when collecting specimens to protect the nurse, not to maintain sterility of the specimen; gowns and masks are generally unnecessary unless splashing of body fluids is likely.

(3) Generally, if a specimen is collected using sterile technique, one specimen is sufficient for testing for culture and sensitivity. However, blood cultures for a disease such as endocarditis may require several specimens over a 24- to 48-hour period.

(4) **The results of a culture and sensitivity will be inaccurate if the steps of the collection procedure and collection container are not kept sterile; a contaminated specimen container introduces extraneous microorganisms that falsify and misrepresent results.**

19 **TEST-TAKING TIP** ◉ The word "first" is the key word in the stem that sets a priority.

(1) Waiting is unsafe. The change in pulse may indicate an impending problem.

(2) Activity will increase, not decrease the heart rate.

(3) **Corroborative data should be obtained; the vital signs reflect cardiopulmonary functioning. When there is an alteration in one vital sign, there usually is a change in another.**

(4) Alerting the nurse in charge might be necessary after other more appropriate interventions.

20 **TEST-TAKING TIP** ◉ The word "unique" is the clue in the stem.

(1) Gloves should always be worn when dealing with body secretions or excretions.

(2) Three separate samples from stool are collected on consecutive days to screen for occult blood, not for parasites.

(3) **Stool specimens for ova and parasites should be sent to the laboratory while still warm; stool that is allowed to cool can alter the accuracy of the laboratory results.**

(4) Taking feces from several areas of the bowel movement is unnecessary; a 1-inch portion of stool provides an adequate sample for testing for parasites.

21 **TEST-TAKING TIP** ◉ The word "first" is the key word in the stem that sets a priority.

(1) Assessing a patient's level of wellness should be done later.

(2) Viewing a person's value system as acceptable or unacceptable is judgmental.

(3) **Attitudes and beliefs influence health practices and how one perceives self-health; the nurse must always "begin care where the patient is at."**

(4) Assessing the use of defense mechanisms should be done later.

22 **TEST-TAKING TIP** ○ The word *best* in the stem sets a priority.
① The patient's family members are secondary sources.
② The primary nurse is a secondary source.
③ The physician is a secondary source.
④ **The patient is the center of the health team and is the primary source for current objective and subjective data.**

23 **TEST-TAKING TIP** ○ Options 1 and 4 are opposites. These options should be given careful consideration. In this question, one of these options is correct.
① **When a patient moves from a lying-down to a sitting or standing position, an automatic vasoconstriction occurs in the lower half of the body; this prevents the pooling of blood and effectively maintains the blood pressure. When this vasoconstriction response is inadequate, the patient will experience orthostatic hypotension after moving from a horizontal to a vertical position.**
② This is unrelated to positional changes.
③ Assessment of blood pressure during activity is done during a stress test.
④ Although a patient's blood pressure is often taken before and after standing to assess for orthostatic hypotension, the result of the blood pressure taken after standing is more significant.

24 **TEST-TAKING TIP** ○ The word "pressure" appears in the stem and in options 3 and 4. Options 3 and 4 should be examined carefully. Option 3 is the correct answer.
① Contraction of the ventricles is reflected by the systolic pressure.
② The volume of cardiac output is computed by multiplying the stroke volume by the number of heartbeats per minute.
③ **Diastole is the period when the ventricles are relaxed and reflects the pressure in the arteries when the heart is at rest.**
④ Pulse pressure is the difference between the systolic and diastolic pressures.

25 **TEST-TAKING TIP** ○ Options 1 and 4 are opposites. Arteries carry blood away from the heart and veins carry blood to the heart. These opposites are more difficult to identify than most opposites.
① Veins do not have a pulse.
② Radial, carotid, or apical pulses, not pedal pulses, readily assess heart function.
③ Laboratory tests assess blood and its components.
④ **The presence, absence, or quality of pedal pulses reflects the adequacy of arterial circulation in the feet; peripheral pulses should be present, equal, and symmetrical.**

26 **TEST-TAKING TIP** ○ Options 1 and 3 are opposites. Consider these seriously or eliminate both of them. In this question, they are both distractors and can be eliminated.
① Peak pressures, not trough pressures, occur during systole.
② Pulse pressure is the difference between the systolic and diastolic pressures.
③ Peak pressures occur when the ventricles contract.
④ **Peak pressures occur when the ventricles contract, and trough pressures occur when the ventricles relax; these occur with each contraction and relaxation of the heart.**

27 ① Pain occurs during the first phase of the inflammatory response in reaction to the release of histamine at the injury site. Histamine promotes vessel permeability, which increases edema, causing pressure on nerve endings.
② Fever is a systemic, not a local, adaptation and is not indicative of phase 2 of the inflammatory response.
③ During the first phase of the inflammatory response, histamine is released, resulting in increased blood flow to the area. Dilation of capillaries causes the area to be flooded with blood, which makes the area appear red and warm to the touch.
④ **Phase 2 of the inflammatory response is characterized by the formation of an exudate; it consists of a combination of cells and fluids produced at the localized site of injury.**

28 **TEST-TAKING TIP** ○ Option 1 contains the word "all," which is a specific determiner. This option can be eliminated from consideration.
① Examination of a specimen under a microscope, not the sensitivity part of a culture and sensitivity test, identifies the microorganisms present.
② The ability to produce disease (virulence) is not determined by the sensitivity portion of a culture and sensitivity test; virulence is determined by statistical data concerning morbidity and mortality associated with the microorganisms.
③ **Areas of lack of growth of microorganisms surrounding an antibiotic on a culture medium indicates that the microorganism is sensitive to the antibiotic and the antibiotic is capable of destroying the microorganism.**
④ The clinical manifestation of the disease process reflects the extent of the patient's response to the microorganism present.

29 TEST-TAKING TIP ○ The word *immediately* in the stem sets a priority.

(1) **Dependent edema is an adaptation related to problems such as hypervolemia, a decreased cardiac output or impaired kidney functioning. The patient immediately should be assessed further because these medical conditions can be life threatening.**

(2) Although this should be explored further, it is not a life-threatening problem and therefore, is not the priority.

(3) Same as #2.

(4) Blanchable erythema in an area at risk for a pressure ulcer indicates that the area has been exposed to pressure. However, circulation to the area is not impaired. Pressure that produces non-blanchable erythema signals a potential ulceration and meets the criteria for a stage I pressure ulcer. The patient should be assessed further, but is not the priority.

30 (1) _____ The red probe is used for a rectal temperature.

(2) _____ This is unnecessary; however, daily temperatures should be taken at the same time for comparison purposes. Temperatures usually are lowest in the early morning and highest between 5 and 7 PM.

(3) _X_ **Because an electronic thermometer is used for multiple patients, a probe cover is a medical aseptic barrier technique used to prevent the spread of microorganisms.**

(4) _____ This is unnecessary.

(5) _X_ **The oral route should not be used for individuals who are unconscious, mouth breathers, cannot follow directions or who have just consumed cold or hot liquids or food.**

Meeting Patients' Physical Safety and Mobility Needs

• • •

This section includes questions related to maintaining patients' physical safety and mobility needs. In relation to patients' safety needs, this section emphasizes the concepts of the use of restraints, issues associated with smoking and fire, prevention of injury, electrical safety, protection of a patient experiencing a seizure, and safety related to oxygen use. In relation to patients' mobility needs, this section includes questions that address the maintenance and restoration of musculoskeletal function and the prevention of musculoskeletal complications. These questions focus on knowledge, principles, and devices related to the prevention of pressure (decubitus) ulcers, contractures, and other hazards of immobility. Additional questions test principles associated with body alignment, transfer, range of motion (ROM), ambulation, positioning, and dressing.

Questions

Please fill in the circle to mark your answer choice.

1   The nurse is aware that the main reason for accidents in hospitals is:
① People sneak in cigarettes
② Equipment breaks unexpectedly
③ Patients do not recognize hazards
④ Safety precautions always take extra time

TEST-TAKING TIP ◉ Identify the key word in the stem that sets a priority. Identify the option that contains a specific determiner.

2   When caring for patients, the nurse understands that restraints mainly are used to:
① Immobilize patients
② Reduce agitation
③ Limit movement
④ Prevent injury

TEST-TAKING TIP ◉ Identify the key word in the stem that sets a priority. Identify the equally plausible options.

3   The nurse identifies that a patient sitting in a wheelchair begins to have a tonic-clonic (grand mal) seizure. The patient should be:
① Wheeled to an empty room to a private area
② Secured in the wheelchair to prevent falling
③ Returned to bed to provide a soft surface
④ Moved to the floor to prevent injury

4   The nurse understands that disoriented, confused patients who are restrained often struggle against restraints primarily because they are:
① Attempting to gain control
② Responding to the discomfort
③ Trying to manipulate the staff
④ Unable to understand what is occurring

TEST-TAKING TIP ◉ Identify the key word in the stem that sets a priority. Identify the option that is unique.

5   The nurse is working in an assisted-living facility that is not "smoke free." The nurse can BEST prevent accidents associated with smoking by:
① Supervising patients when they smoke
② Taking away the cigarettes of patients who smoke

③ Encouraging patients to smoke in designated areas
④ Asking family members not to bring cigarettes for patients

TEST-TAKING TIP ○ Identify the key word in the stem that sets a priority. Identify options that deny patients' feelings, concerns, and needs.

6 A hospitalized patient dies after a long illness. As part of postmortem care, the nurse should:
① Slightly raise the head of the bed
② Carefully remove any dentures
③ Firmly tie the wrists together
④ Gently close the eyes

7 A nurse is responding to a fire alarm within the hospital. When transporting a fire extinguisher to a fire scene on a different level of the building than the one on which the nurse is working, the nurse should:
① Use the stairs
② Pull the safety pin
③ Keep it from touching the floor
④ Always run as quickly as possible

TEST-TAKING TIP ○ Identify the option that contains a specific determiner.

8 A primary nurse is orienting a newly admitted patient to the hospital. The first information the nurse should review with the patient is the:
① Use of the call bell
② Daily routine on the unit
③ Potential date of discharge
④ Name of the nurse in charge

TEST-TAKING TIP ○ Identify the key word in the stem that sets a priority.

9 The nurse on the evening shift in the hospital is caring for a slightly confused patient. To prevent disorientation at night, the most effective nursing intervention is to:
① Turn on a small light in the room
② Check on the patient regularly
③ Place a call bell in the bed
④ Describe the environment

TEST-TAKING TIP ○ Identify the key word in the stem that sets a priority. Identify the clues in the stem. Identify the unique option. Identify the equally plausible options.

10 While walking, a patient becomes weak and the patient's knees begin to buckle. What should the nurse do?
① Hold up the patient.
② Call for extra help quickly.
③ Walk the patient to the closest chair.
④ Lower the patient to the floor gently.

TEST-TAKING TIP ○ Identify the options that are opposites.

11 The nurse identifies that the electrical cord on a patient's radio is frayed near the plug. The nurse should:
① Report it to the supervisor
② Unplug it and put it in the patient's closet
③ Wrap the frayed area with nonconductive tape
④ Remove it and send it home with a family member

12 To provide for safety when administering oxygen, it is *most* important that the nurse first recognize that oxygen:
① Must have its flow rate adjusted
② Is drying to the nasal mucosa
③ Should be humidified
④ Supports burning

TEST-TAKING TIP ○ Identify the key words in the stem that set a priority. Identify the equally plausible options.

13 The nurse is caring for a patient with the potential for developing a pressure (decubitus) ulcer. The nurse places a synthetic sheepskin under the patient primarily to:
① Absorb urine
② Minimize friction
③ Eliminate shearing
④ Keep the skin warm

TEST-TAKING TIP ○ Identify the key word in the stem that sets a priority.

14 The nurse is caring for an older adult on bed rest. To best prevent a pressure (decubitus) ulcer in this patient, the nurse should provide:
① An air mattress
② A daily bed bath
③ A high-protein diet
④ An indwelling urinary catheter

TEST-TAKING TIP ○ Identify the key word in the stem that sets a priority.

15 When providing range-of-motion (ROM) exercises, touching the thumb to the small fifth finger of the same hand is called:
① Extension
② Abduction
③ Adduction
④ Opposition

TEST-TAKING TIP ○ Identify the options that are opposites.

16 What is the most therapeutic exercise that can be done by a patient on bed rest?
① Isometric exercises
② Active range of motion
③ Passive range of motion
④ Active-assistive exercises

TEST-TAKING TIP ○ Identify the key word in the stem that sets a priority. Identify the options that are opposites.

17 The physician orders that a patient with one-sided weakness (hemiparesis) be transferred out of bed to a chair twice a day. The nurse plans to:
① Pivot the patient on the unaffected leg
② Stand next to the patient's affected side
③ Stand next to the patient's strong side
④ Keep the patient's feet together

TEST-TAKING TIP ○ Identify the clue in the stem. Identify the unique option. Identify the opposites in options.

18 When the home care nurse places an egg-crate pad under a patient the spouse asks, "What is the purpose of that pad?" The home care nurse responds, "The primary purpose of an egg-crate pad is to:
① Absorb moisture."
② Limit perspiration."
③ Support the body in alignment."
④ Distribute pressure over a larger area."

TEST-TAKING TIP ○ Identify the key word in the stem that sets a priority. Identify the equally plausible options.

19 The nurse is transferring a patient from the bed to a chair using a mechanical lift. As the nurse begins to raise the lift off the bed, the patient begins to panic and scream. The nurse should:
① Lower the patient back onto the bed
② Quickly continue and say, "It's almost over"
③ Say, "Relax" and slowly continue with the transfer
④ Stop the lift from rising until the patient regains control

TEST-TAKING TIP ○ Identify the options that are opposites. Identify the options that deny the patient's feelings, concerns, and needs.

20 When planning a turning schedule for a patient with limited mobility, the nurse understands that the position that most contributes to the development of a pressure (decubitus) ulcer in the sacral area is the:
① Sims' position
② Prone position
③ Lateral position
④ High-Fowler's position
TEST-TAKING TIP ○ Identify the clue in the stem. Identify the option that is unique.

21 While a patient is lying in the dorsal recumbent position, the patient's leg externally rotates. What equipment should the nurse use to prevent external rotation?
① Bed cradle
② Trochanter roll
③ Elastic stockings
④ High-top sneakers
TEST-TAKING TIP ○ Identify the clue in the stem.

22 The nurse is caring for a group of patients. The patient with the greatest risk of developing a pressure (decubitus) ulcer is the patient who:
① Uses a reclining wheelchair
② Uses crutches to ambulate
③ Is ambulatory but is confused
④ Is on bed rest but able to move
TEST-TAKING TIP ○ Identify the key word in the stem that sets a priority. Identify the clue in the stem. Identify the unique option.

23 The action of moving a patient's lower extremity toward the midline and beyond during range-of-motion exercises is:
① Internal rotation
② Lateral flexion
③ Adduction
④ Inversion
TEST-TAKING TIP ○ Identify the clue in the stem.

24 A patient is afraid of falling and gets anxious when it is time to get out of bed to a chair. The best action by the nurse to reduce the patient's anxiety is to:
① Allow the patient to decide when to get up
② Transfer the patient using a mechanical lift
③ Explain to the patient that a fall will not occur
④ Permit the patient to set the pace of the transfer
TEST-TAKING TIP ○ Identify the key word in the stem that sets a priority. Identify the option that denies the patient's feelings, concerns, and needs. Identify the patient-centered options.

25 A patient who had a brain attack (stroke, cerebrovascular accident) 3 days earlier has left-sided hemiparesis. When dressing the patient, the nurse should plan to:
① Put the patient's left sleeve on first
② Encourage the patient to dress independently
③ Instruct the patient to wear clothes with zippers
④ Tell the patient to get clothes with buttons in the front
TEST-TAKING TIP ○ Identify the clue in the stem. Identify the equally plausible options. Identify the unique option. Identify the option that denies the needs of the patient.

26 When the nurse positions a patient, what is the *most* important principle of body mechanics?
① Elevating the arms on pillows
② Making the patient comfortable

③ Maintaining functional alignment
④ Keeping the head higher than the heart

TEST-TAKING TIP ⊙ Identify the key word in the stem that sets a priority.

27 The nurse understands that the main cause of pressure (decubitus) ulcers is:
① Pressure
② Desquamation
③ Skin breakdown
④ Cellular necrosis

TEST-TAKING TIP ⊙ Identify the word that is a clue in the stem. Identify the key word in the stem that sets a priority. Identify the equally plausible options.

28 The nurse is positioning a patient in a lateral position. Which action by the nurse MOST contributes to the patient's functional alignment?
① Using a bed cradle
② Utilizing a trochanter roll
③ Putting a pillow under the upper leg
④ Placing a small pillow under the waist

TEST-TAKING TIP ⊙ Identify the key word in the stem that sets a priority.

29 The physician orders warm, dry heat to be applied via an Aquathermia pad to a patient's lower back to ease muscle spasms resulting from a fall. The nurse should:
① Set the pad at 105° to 115°F
② Apply the pad directly to the skin
③ Remove the pad 30 minutes after it is applied
④ Place the pad under the patient who should be in the supine position

30 The range-of-motion exercise being performed in the following diagram is:
① Flexion
② Adduction
③ Supination
④ Opposition

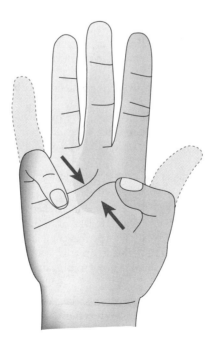

Meeting Patient's Physical Safety and Mobility Needs

Answers and Rationales

1 **TEST-TAKING TIP** ○ The word *main* in the stem is a key word that sets a priority. The word *always* in Option 4 is a specific determiner.
  ① Statistics do not support cigarette smoking as the most common cause of hospital accidents. Most hospitals are smoke free.
  ② Equipment usually is monitored for preventive maintenance; equipment generally shows wear and tear before it breaks.
  ③ **Patients can be cognitively impaired, deny their physical impairments, or have limited perception, which impedes their ability to recognize hazards.**
  ④ Usually it takes the same amount of time to do something correctly as it does to do it incorrectly.

2 **TEST-TAKING TIP** ○ The word "mainly" in the stem is a key word that sets a priority. Options 1 and 3 are equally plausible because they both focus on reducing movement.
  ① Immobilization is not the purpose of restraints. Restraints should be snug, yet loose enough for some movement.
  ② Restraints can increase agitation; if used when a patient is severely agitated, they can cause injury.
  ③ The purpose of restraints is not to limit movement.
  ④ **The primary reason for the use of restraints is to prevent patient injury; restraints are used only as a last resort to protect the patient from self- injury or from hurting others.**

3 ① The need for privacy is not the priority. Transporting a patient in a wheelchair during a tonic-clonic (grand mal) seizure can cause muscle strain, bone fractures, or other injury and is an unsafe action.
  ② Securing a patient in a wheelchair during a tonic-clonic (grand mal) seizure can cause muscle strain, bone fractures, or other injury and is an unsafe action.
  ③ Attempting to return a patient to bed during a tonic-clonic (grand mal) seizure can cause muscle strain, bone fractures, or other injury. Returning the patient to bed should be done after the seizure is over.
  ④ **Moving the patient to the floor is the safest action; it provides free movement on a supported surface.**

4 **TEST-TAKING TIP** ○ The word *primarily* is the key word in the stem that sets a priority. Option 4 is unique because it is the only option that does not contain an action verb ending in "-ing." The words *attempting, responding,* and *trying* in Options 1, 2, and 3 all end in "-ing" and therefore are similar.
  ① Confused, disoriented patients who are restrained may become agitated and respond in a reflex-like way; attempts to gain control require problem solving, which confused, disoriented patients usually are unable to perform.
  ② A restraint should not cause discomfort if it is applied correctly and checked frequently.
  ③ A patient usually struggles against a restraint to get free, not to manipulate staff.
  ④ **Disoriented and confused patients do not always have the cognitive ability to understand what is happening to them and often struggle against restraints.**

5 **TEST-TAKING TIP** ○ The word BEST is the key word in the stem that sets a priority. Options 2 and 4 deny patients' feelings, concerns, and needs.
  ① **If a facility allows smoking, supervision provides for patient safety because the nurse can intervene if the condition becomes unsafe.**
  ② Taking cigarettes away from patients who smoke is punitive and should be done only if attempts to teach safety precautions and policies fail to foster safe smoking behavior.
  ③ Although this should be done, this option does not take into consideration that patients who smoke should be supervised.
  ④ Asking family members not to bring in cigarettes for patients who smoke denies patients' feelings, concerns, and needs and is punitive.

6 ① A supine position is preferred; after rigor mortis sets in, it is difficult to reposition the body.
  ② Dentures should remain in the mouth to maintain facial structure and minimize facial distortion.
  ③ Firmly tying together the patient's wrists can cause permanent marks; wrists should be well padded and securely, yet loosely, tied so as not to cause permanent marks.
  ④ **The patient's eyelids should be gently closed to avoid injury; after rigor mortis sets in, it is difficult to reposition the eyelids.**

7 **TEST-TAKING TIP** ○ The word "always" in Option 4 is a specific determiner.
  ① **Using the stairs during a fire is safe practice; elevators must be avoided because they may break down and trap a person.**
  ② The safety pin is pulled only when the extinguisher is going to be used, not when en route to a fire.

(3) Often extinguishers are dragged along the floor en route to a fire because they are heavy; this is an acceptable practice.

(4) Running should be avoided; it can cause injury and panic.

8 **TEST-TAKING TIP** ⊙ The word "first" is the key word in the stem that sets a priority.

(1) **Explaining the use of a call bell meets basic safety and security needs; the patient must know how to signal for help.**

(2) Although this is important and should be done, safety needs come first.

(3) Identifying the potential date of discharge is the physician's, not the nurse's, responsibility.

(4) Although the patient should be told the name of the nurse in charge of the unit, this is not the priority intervention.

9 **TEST-TAKING TIP** ⊙ The word "most" is the key word in the stem that sets a priority. The words "night" and "minimally confused" are the clues in the stem. Option 1 is the only option that states an action that is unique to the nighttime. Options 2, 3, and 4 are equally plausible and are implemented regardless of the time of day or orientation of the patient.

(1) **A small light in the room provides enough light for visual cues for a minimally confused patient, which should help prevent or limit disorientation when the patient awakens at night.**

(2) Although checking on the patient regularly is something the nurse should do, it will not prevent disorientation.

(3) The patient has to be oriented enough to be aware of the presence of the call bell before it can be used.

(4) The patient may not remember the description of the environment on awakening and may become disoriented in the dark.

10 **TEST-TAKING TIP** ⊙ Options 1 and 4 are opposites.

(1) Trying to hold up the patient may injure the nurse and cause both the nurse and the patient to fall.

(2) By the time help arrives, the patient may already be on the floor; calling out can scare the patient and others.

(3) The patient is already falling; walking the patient to the closest chair is not an option.

(4) **Lowering the patient to the floor is the safest action; guiding the patient to the floor helps to break the patient's fall and minimize injury, particularly to the head.**

11 (1) Reporting the frayed wire is ineffective in preventing the risk of injury.

(2) Putting the radio in the patient's closet does not preclude that it may be taken out and used again.

(3) Attempting to repair an electrical cord is unsafe; it should be repaired by a trained person.

(4) **Removing the radio and sending it home with a family member is the safest option; this action removes it from use.**

12 **TEST-TAKING TIP** ⊙ The words "first" and "most" are the key words in the stem that set a priority. Options 2 and 3 are equally plausible because they both address the drying effects of oxygen therapy.

(1) Although the flow rate of oxygen must be adjusted, this is not the priority.

(2) Oxygen is drying to the nasal membranes, but this is not the priority.

(3) Oxygen should be humidified, but this is not the priority.

(4) **The nurse must recognize that oxygen supports burning. Although oxygen by itself will not burn or explode, it facilitates combustion; the greater the concentration of oxygen, the more rapidly fires start and burn.**

13 **TEST-TAKING TIP** ⊙ The word "primarily" in the stem sets a priority.

(1) Sheepskin is not designed to absorb urine; wet sheepskin will contribute to skin breakdown.

(2) **Soft tufts of sheepskin reduce friction and allow air to circulate under the patient.**

(3) A sheepskin will not eliminate shearing forces. Moving the patient with a pull sheet and avoiding a Fowler's position will limit shearing forces.

(4) Sheepskin helps to keep skin cool, not warm, by allowing air to circulate through the tufts of lamb's wool.

14 **TEST-TAKING TIP** ⊙ The word "best" in the stem sets a priority.

(1) **An air mattress distributes body weight over a larger surface and reduces pressure over bony prominences.**

(2) Although bathing removes secretions and promotes clean skin, it can be drying, which can compromise skin integrity.

(3) Protein does not prevent pressure (decubitus) ulcers. Protein is the body's only source of nitrogen and is essential for building, repairing, or replacing body tissue.

(4) An indwelling urinary catheter should never be used to prevent a pressure (decubitus) ulcer; however, a catheter may be used to prevent contamination of a pressure (decubitus) ulcer after it is present in a patient who is incontinent of urine.

15 **TEST-TAKING TIP** ○ Options 2 and 3 are opposites and are distractors.

① Straightening the finger joints is *extension*.

② Spreading the fingers out in relation to one another is *abduction*.

③ Bringing the fingers in alignment next to one another is *adduction*.

④ **Opposition is the correct term to describe touching the thumb to the tip of each finger of the hand.**

16 **TEST-TAKING TIP** ○ The word "most" is the key word in the stem that sets a priority. Options 2 and 3 are opposites.

① Isometric exercise involves contracting and relaxing a muscle without moving the joint; this improves muscle tone but does not put joints through the full ROM.

② **Active range-of-motion (ROM) exercise is preferable because it is an isotonic exercise that causes muscle contraction; active ROM exercise increases joint mobility, circulation, and muscle tone because the patient actively moves the joints through full ROM.**

③ Passive ROM exercise occurs when a joint is moved by a source other than the muscles articulating to the joint. Passive ROM exercise puts a joint through full range and prevents contractures but does not increase muscle tone because the muscles are not contracted.

④ In active-assistive ROM exercise, the patient attempts active ROM exercise and receives some support and assistance from the nurse. Active-assistive ROM exercise does not provide for as much isotonic exercise as does active ROM exercise.

17 **TEST-TAKING TIP** ○ The words *one-sided weakness* are a clue in the stem. Option 1 is unique because it does not use the possessive form of the word *patient* (i.e., patient's). Options 2 and 3 are opposites and are distractors.

① **Pivoting avoids unnecessary movement by transferring the patient to the chair while supporting body weight on the unaffected leg.**

② When transferring this patient, the nurse should stand in front of, not next to, the patient.

③ When transferring this patient, the nurse should stand in front of the patient, not next to the patient's strong side.

④ Keeping the patient's feet together narrows the base of support and decreases the patient's stability.

18 **TEST-TAKING TIP** ○ The word "primary" is the key word in the stem that sets a priority. Options 1 and 2 are equally plausible because they both address moisture.

① The purpose of an egg-crate pad is not to absorb moisture. A wet egg-crate pad should not be used because moisture against the skin can contribute to skin breakdown.

② The opposite may be true. Because egg-crate pads are made of synthetic materials, they often promote, rather than limit, perspiration.

③ Pillows and wedges, not an egg-crate pad, are used to keep the body in functional alignment.

④ **Intermittent raised areas on the egg-crate pad help to distribute body weight evenly over the entire body surface that is in contact with the pad.**

19 **TEST-TAKING TIP** ○ Options 1 and 2 are opposites. Options 2 and 3 deny the patient's feelings of fear.

① **Lowering the patient onto the bed recognizes the cause of the anxiety and responds to the source.**

② Continuing with the transfer denies the patient's fears and can intensify the anxiety.

③ Continuing with the transfer ignores the patient's concern. Telling a person to relax will not necessarily precipitate a relaxation response.

④ Leaving the patient up in the air can intensify the anxiety.

20 **TEST-TAKING TIP** ○ The phrase "sacral area" is the significant clue in the stem. Option 4 is unique because it is the only option with three words.

① The Sims' position avoids pressure on the sacral area; weight is on the anterior ilium, humerus, and clavicle.

② The prone position avoids pressure on the sacral area; prone is lying on the abdomen.

③ In the lateral position, pressure is off the sacral area; the body is side-lying with weight on the dependent hip and shoulder.

④ **In the high-Fowler's position, most of the weight is placed on the sacral area; this causes sacral pressure.**

21 **TEST-TAKING TIP** ○ The words "prevent external rotation" are the clue in the stem.

① A bed cradle keeps linen off the feet and legs; it supports patient comfort, but it does not prevent external rotation.

② **A trochanter roll prevents the hip and leg from externally rotating by positioning the leg in functional alignment.**

③ Elastic stockings do not prevent external rotation; they are used to increase venous return in the lower legs.

④ High-top sneakers prevent plantar flexion, not external rotation.

22 **TEST-TAKING TIP** ○ The word "highest" is the key word in the stem that sets a priority. The word "risk" is a clue in the stem. Option 1 is unique because it is the only option that does not mention that the patient is able to move independently.

(1) **A patient using a reclining wheelchair has minimal lower- or upper-body control. A reclining position places excessive pressure on the sacral area.**

(2) As long as a person can move, positioning can be changed to relieve pressure.

(3) A confused ambulatory patient is able to walk and therefore relieve pressure on bony prominences.

(4) As long as a patient on bed rest can move, pressure can be relieved by shifting the body weight or changing positions.

23 **TEST-TAKING TIP** ○ The word "toward" is a clue in the stem. One could say that the act of moving a body part "toward" another is like "adding" one to another. The first three letters of the word "adduction" in Option 3 are "add."

(1) *Internal rotation* is the act of rolling the leg and foot inward, thereby internally rotating the hip joint.

(2) *Lateral flexion* is when the head is tilted as far as possible to one shoulder and then the other shoulder.

(3) **The word *adduction* correctly represents the action of moving an extremity toward the midline of the body and beyond.**

(4) *Inversion* is when the sole of the foot is turned medially.

24 **TEST-TAKING TIP** ○ The word "best" is the key word in the stem that sets a priority. Option 3 denies the patient's feelings. Options 1 and 4 are patient centered.

(1) Waiting and thinking about the transfer can increase anxiety, not reduce it; the patient may decide never to get out of bed.

(2) Using a mechanical lift may contribute to feelings of dependence and loss of control. The question identifies a fearful patient, not an immobile patient.

(3) Explaining that a fall will not occur is false reassurance and denies the patient's fears.

(4) **Allowing the patient to set the pace of the transfer supports the need of the patient to be in control; the patient's anxiety generally is reduced in proportion to an increase in control.**

25 **TEST-TAKING TIP** ○ The phrase "3 days earlier" is a significant clue in the stem. Options 3 and 4 are equally plausible. Options 2, 3, and 4 are similar because they contain the verbs *encourage, instruct,* and *tell,* which all require verbal interaction with the patient. Option 1 is unique because it is the only option in which the nurse is actually dressing the patient and that uses the possessive form of the word "patient" (i.e., patient's). Option 2 denies the patient's need for assistance during the acute phase of this illness.

(1) **The extremity with the affected joints should be dressed first to avoid unnecessary strain; the unaffected side generally has greater joint range.**

(2) It is unreasonable to expect self-sufficiency during the acute phase.

(3) Zippers are difficult to close with one hand. Velcro closures may be more appropriate.

(4) Buttons are difficult to close with one hand. Velcro closures may be more appropriate.

26 **TEST-TAKING TIP** ○ The word *most* is the key word in the stem that sets a priority.

(1) The arms do not have to be elevated to be in alignment.

(2) A comfortable position for the patient may not provide the alignment necessary to prevent complications.

(3) **Anatomic alignment maintains physical functioning and minimizes strain and stress on muscles, tendons, ligaments, and joints.**

(4) The head can be at the same level as the heart; it does not have to be higher.

27 **TEST-TAKING TIP** ○ The word "pressure" in the stem and correct answer is a clang association. The word "main" is the key word in the stem that sets a priority. Options 3 and 4 are equally plausible.

(1) **Pressure ulcers occur when the pressure in the capillaries exceeds that of the arterioles (35 mm Hg). Pathologic changes begin within 1 to 2 hours when tissues are deprived of oxygen and nutrients. If pressure is not relieved, tissue breakdown and cellular death (necrosis) occur.**

(2) Desquamation (shedding of the epidermis) is seen in postmature infants. It is not a cause of pressure ulcers.

(3) Skin breakdown is the adaptation to pressure, not the cause of a pressure ulcer; also, skin breakdown may be caused by stressors other than pressure.

(4) Cellular necrosis is the death of tissues in response to prolonged pressure and oxygen deprivation; cellular necrosis is the adaptation to pressure, not the cause of a pressure ulcer.

28 **TEST-TAKING TIP** ○ The word MOST is the key word in the stem that sets a priority.

(1) A bed cradle is unnecessary when a patient is in the lateral position. In the lateral position a bed cradle keeps linen off the feet and legs only for comfort. It promotes functional alignment by preventing plantar flexion when the patient is in a back-lying, not lateral, position.

(2) A trochanter roll is used to prevent external rotation of the hip when the patient is in a back-lying position.

(3) **Putting a pillow under the upper leg positions the upper leg and hip in functional alignment and reduces stress and strain on the hip joint.**

(4) A pillow under the waist is used when a patient is positioned in the supine, not lateral, position.

29 (1) 105° to 115°F is the temperature required for the application of hot, dry heat. The Aquathermia pad should be set at 98° to 104°F for the application of warm, dry heat.

(2) A covering or towel should be placed between the pad and the patient to prevent burns.

(3) **This prevents the rebound phenomenon. Heat produces maximum vasodilation in 20 to 30 minutes; if left on beyond this, the blood vessels constrict, limiting the dissipation of heat via the blood circulation.**

(4) This is contraindicated because the heat cannot dissipate and may burn the patient.

30 (1) *Flexion* is movement that results in a decrease in the angle between the bones forming a joint

(2) *Adduction* is movement that results in drawing an extremity toward the central axis of the body.

(3) *Supination* is turning the forearm so that the palm of the hand faces upward.

(4) ***Opposition* of the thumb occurs when the thumb is touched to the tip of each finger on the same hand.**

Meeting Patients' Hygiene, Comfort, Rest, and Sleep Needs

• • •

This section includes questions related to meeting patients' hygiene, comfort, rest, and sleep needs. Questions focus on theories of pain; assessment of pain; pain relief measures; rest and sleep; the backrub; bedmaking; the use of heat and cold; principles associated with bed baths; preventing skin breakdown; perineal care; and care of the hair, feet, and oral cavity.

Questions

Please fill in the circle to mark your answer choice.

1 A patient has a high temperature, is diaphoretic, and did not sleep well during the night. When planning for this patient's hygiene needs, the nurse should:
① Do a complete bath
② Give a partial bed bath
③ Delay the bath until later
④ Provide only perineal care

TEST-TAKING TIP ◉ Identify the options that are opposites. Identify the equally plausible options. Identify the option that contains a specific determiner.

2 When the nurse is giving a patient a bed bath, the water temperature should be:
① 80° to 85°F
② 90° to 95°F
③ 100° to 105°F
④ 110° to 115°F

3 When administering perineal care, the nurse can *best* provide emotional comfort by:
① Placing the patient in the supine position
② Pulling a curtain around the bed
③ Using warm water for washing
④ Calling the patient by name

TEST-TAKING TIP ◉ Identify the key word in the stem that sets a priority. Identify the clues in the stem.

4 The nurse teaches a new Nursing Assistant to give a partial bed bath. The nurse identifies that the teaching is understood when the Nursing Assistant says, "When giving a partial bed bath, I should:
① Help the patient to wash the face, hands, underarms, back, and perineal area"
② Direct the patient to wash as much as possible and assist with the rest"
③ Instruct the patient to wash the face, hands, and perineal area"
④ Assist the patient to wash only one part of the body at a time"

TEST-TAKING TIP ◉ Identify the clue in the stem. Identify the option that contains a specific determiner.

5 The physician orders that a patient be kept NPO. The MOST important action by the nurse should be to:
① Allow the patient to sip clear fluids with medication
② Give the patient mouth care every 4 hours
③ Measure the patient's intake and output
④ Permit the patient to suck on ice chips

TEST-TAKING TIP ◉ Identify the key word in the stem that sets a priority. Identify the clue in the stem. Identify the equally plausible options. Identify the unique option.

6 When administering a bed bath, the nurse rinses the patient after applying soap and water mainly to:
① Increase circulation
② Promote rest and comfort
③ Minimize pressure ulcers
④ Remove residue and debris

TEST-TAKING TIP ○ Identify the key word in the stem that sets a priority.

7 The nurse identifies that a patient has an offensive mouth odor. The most effective nursing intervention is to encourage the patient to:
① Eat foods that do not generate odors
② Brush the teeth and tongue after meals
③ Rinse the mouth with mouthwash every shift
④ Flush the mouth with peroxide and baking soda

TEST-TAKING TIP ○ Identify the key word in the stem that sets a priority. Identify the option that contains a specific determiner. Identify the equally plausible options.

8 A female patient on bed rest asks the nurse what she can do to prevent her hair from becoming tangled and matted. The nurse bases a response on the fact that the action that is least effective in preventing hair from tangling and matting is:
① Conditioning the hair after shampooing
② Washing the hair with soap
③ Placing the hair in braids
④ Brushing the hair daily

TEST-TAKING TIP ○ Identify the key word in the stem that indicates negative polarity.

9 The nurse is changing the linens of a bed for a patient on bed rest. To prevent pressure (decubitus) ulcers, the bottom sheet should be:
① Covered by a draw sheet
② Made with a toe pleat
③ Kept free of wrinkles
④ Changed every day

TEST-TAKING TIP ○ Identify the option that contains a specific determiner.

10 The nurse makes the assessment that a patient's feet are dirty. When planning to clean this patient's feet, the *most* effective nursing intervention is to:
① Ask the patient to take a shower
② Lubricate the feet with lotion to soften dirt
③ Soak each foot in a basin with soap and water
④ Use an antiseptic to prevent a fungal infection

TEST-TAKING TIP ○ Identify the key word in the stem that sets a priority.

11 The nurse is washing the perineal area of a male patient. What is the most important action by the nurse when performing this procedure?
① Handling the penis always with a light touch
② Washing the scrotum before the shaft of the penis
③ Repositioning the foreskin after washing the penis
④ Cleansing down the length of the penis toward the glans

TEST-TAKING TIP ○ Identify the key word in the stem that sets a priority. Identify the option that contains a specific determiner.

12 A patient has a nasogastric tube. A daily nursing intervention that contributes to hygiene includes:
① Instilling the tube with thirty mL of water
② Replacing the tape on the nose
③ Suctioning the oral pharynx
④ Lubricating the nares

TEST-TAKING TIP ○ Identify the words that are clues in the stem.

13 The nurse is caring for a patient who is coping with chronic pain. A psychologic reaction to chronic pain that the nurse should monitor for is:
① Dyspnea
② Depression
③ Self-splinting
④ Hypertension
TEST-TAKING TIP ○ Identify the clues in the stem.

14 A patient says to the nurse, "Lately I've been having a hard time sleeping." To promote sleep, the nurse should encourage the patient to:
① Exercise daily
② Drink a cup of tea
③ Eat only light meals
④ Review the day's events
TEST-TAKING TIP ○ Identify the option that contains a specific determiner.

15 A behavioral response to moderate pain that the nurse should assess for is:
① Rapid, irregular breathing
② Increased muscle tension
③ Self-splinting
④ Fatigue
TEST-TAKING TIP ○ Identify the words that are clues in the stem.

16 During a clinic visit, an older adult complains about cold feet. The nurse should:
① Inform the patient that the feet should be kept elevated
② Teach the patient to place a heating pad over the feet
③ Instruct the patient in how to use a hot water bottle
④ Encourage the patient to wear socks
TEST-TAKING TIP ○ Identify the clue in the stem. Identify the equally plausible options.

17 The nurse is planning interventions to facilitate a patient's ability to sleep. Which action best minimizes the most common cause of insomnia?
① Decreasing environmental noise
② Exploring emotional concerns
③ Regulating room temperature
④ Promoting comfort
TEST-TAKING TIP ○ Identify the word in the stem that sets a priority. Identify the unique option.

18 The patient asks the nurse why the physician ordered cold compresses for a recent muscle sprain. The nurse should base a response on the fact that cold is effective in reducing the discomfort associated with a local inflammatory response because it:
① Anesthetizes nerve endings and causes vasoconstriction
② Stimulates nerve endings and causes vasoconstriction
③ Anesthetizes nerve endings and causes vasodilation
④ Stimulates nerve endings and causes vasodilation
TEST-TAKING TIP ○ Identify the duplicate facts among the options.

19 To best promote rest and sleep in the hospital for all patients, the nurse should:
① Administer a sleeping medication
② Provide a backrub before sleep
③ Turn the lights off at night
④ Encourage usual routines
TEST-TAKING TIP ○ Identify the word in the stem that sets a priority. Identify the clue in the stem.

20 When giving a backrub, the nurse understands that it promotes comfort and rest because it:
① Causes vasodilation
② Stimulates circulation
③ Relieves muscular tension
④ Increases oxygen to tissues

TEST-TAKING TIP ○ Identify the clue in the stem. Identify the unique option.

21 The physician orders the application of a warm soak for a patient's extremity. When applying heat, the nurse understands that it effectively reduces discomfort at a local inflammatory site because it:
① Decreases local circulation and limits capillary permeability
② Decreases tissue metabolism and increases local circulation
③ Increases local circulation and promotes muscle relaxation
④ Provides local anesthesia and decreases local circulation

TEST-TAKING TIP ○ Identify the duplicate facts among the options.

22 The nurse is providing oral hygiene for a patient with dentures. To support the patient's dignity, the nurse should:
① Provide a denture cup for the patient.
② Pull the curtain around the patient's bed.
③ Support the patient in a high-Fowler's position.
④ Resist looking at the patient while the dentures are out.

23 When providing physical hygiene the nurse identifies that the patient's hair is tangled and matted. The nurse should:
① Braid the hair in sections
② Use a comb instead of a brush
③ Comb a small section at a time
④ Brush from the roots toward the ends

24 The nurse is making an occupied bed. What is the most important nursing action?
① Use new linen
② Raise both side rails
③ Keep the patient covered
④ Place a pad on the draw sheet

TEST-TAKING TIP ○ Identify the key word in the stem that sets a priority. Identify the patient-centered option.

25 When assessing a patient who is experiencing pain, the nurse identifies that the most subjective characteristic of pain is:
① Intensity
② Duration
③ Location
④ Quality

TEST-TAKING TIP ○ Identify the key word in the stem that sets a priority. Identify the clue in the stem.

26 The school nurse is teaching a group of high school students about health promotion. The nurse includes the information that the individuals that require the least amount of sleep are:
① Adolescents
② Older adults
③ Young adults
④ Middle-age adults

TEST-TAKING TIP ○ Identify the key word in the stem that indicates negative polarity. Identify the options that are opposites.

27 The most important independent nursing intervention to reduce the incidence of a fungal infection of the feet is to:
   ① Increase circulation to the feet by encouraging exercise
   ② Soak the feet in an antiseptic solution during AM care
   ③ Apply body lotion to avoid cracks in the skin
   ④ Dry well between the toes after bathing

   TEST-TAKING TIP ⊙ Identify the key word in the stem that sets a priority. Identify the word in the stem that provides a clue.

28 The nurse is assessing a patient in pain. A concept that is important for the nurse to understand is that pain perception is MOST influenced by the:
   ① Duration of the stimulus
   ② Characteristics of the pain
   ③ Activity of the cerebral cortex
   ④ Level of endorphins in the blood

   TEST-TAKING TIP ⊙ Identify the key word in the stem that sets a priority.

29 The nurse is providing perineal care for a female patient. What should the nurse do during this procedure?
   ① Use a new area of the washcloth for each stroke
   ② Wash from the rectum toward the pubis
   ③ Clean the dirtiest area first
   ④ Use only warm tap water

   TEST-TAKING TIP ⊙ Identify the option that contains a specific determiner.

30 A patient has had difficulty sleeping and the physician orders zolpidem (Ambien CR) 12.5 mg at hour of sleep. The medication supplied by the pharmacy is 6.25 mg/tablet. How many tablets should the nurse administer?

   Answer: _____ Tablets

214 Meeting Patient's Hygiene, Comfort, Rest, and Sleep Needs
Answers and Rationales

1 **TEST-TAKING TIP** ⊙ Options 1 and 3 are opposites. Options 2 and 4 are equally plausible. Option 4 contains the word "only," which is a specific determiner.
  ① **Diaphoresis is a profuse secretion of sweat associated with an elevated body temperature, physical exertion, or emotional stress. The secretions must be removed from the entire body to limit the growth of microorganisms and promote comfort; evaporation during the bed bath may help lower the patient's temperature.**
  ② A partial bed bath is inadequate.
  ③ Delaying the bed bath is unsafe; the patient needs immediate physical hygiene.
  ④ Same as #2.

2 ① This temperature range is too cool; this will promote chilling.
  ② Same as #1.
  ③ Same as #1.
  ④ **The temperature of bath water should be between 110° and 115°F to promote comfort, dilate blood vessels, and prevent chilling.**

3 **TEST-TAKING TIP** ⊙ The word *best* is the key word in the stem that sets a priority. The words "perineal" and "emotional" are clues in the stem.
  ① Correct positioning provides for physical, not emotional, comfort.
  ② **Perineal care is a private activity, and measures should be taken to provide for privacy.**
  ③ Warm water provides physical, not emotional, comfort.
  ④ Although calling the patient by name is a respectful, individualized approach, it does not address the patient's right to privacy during a procedure that exposes the genitalia.

4 **TEST-TAKING TIP** ⊙ The word "partial" in the stem is a clue. Option 4 contains the word "only," which is a specific determiner.
  ① **These areas should be washed daily because they harbor the most microorganisms.**
  ② This intervention is considered a complete bed bath with assistance.
  ③ The axillary areas and the back must also be washed in a partial bed bath.
  ④ Same as #2.

5 **TEST-TAKING TIP** ⊙ The word MOST is a key word in the stem that sets a priority. "NPO" is the clue in the stem. Options 1 and 4 are equally plausible. Option 2 is unique because it is the only option including a number.
  ① Fluids of any kind are contraindicated; NPO *(non per os)* means "nothing by mouth."
  ② **When people are NPO, they tend to have dry mucous membranes and thick secretions on the tongue and gums; mouth care cleans the oral cavity.**
  ③ Although monitoring the patient's intake and output (I&O) may be done, the priority is direct physical care of the patient.
  ④ Same as #1.

6 **TEST-TAKING TIP** ⊙ The word "mainly" is the key word in the stem that sets a priority.
  ① Friction from firm, long strokes used during rinsing increases circulation; however, it is not the reason for rinsing.
  ② A backrub and positioning in functional alignment, not rinsing, promote rest and comfort.
  ③ Local massage and repositioning every 2 hours, not rinsing, prevent pressure ulcers.
  ④ **Rinsing flushes the skin with clean water, which removes debris and soap residue.**

7 **TEST-TAKING TIP** ⊙ The word "most" is the key word in the stem that sets a priority. Option 3 contains the word "every," which is a specific determiner. Options 3 and 4 are equally plausible.
  ① Although some foods can cause halitosis, it is more often caused by inadequate oral hygiene, a local infection, or a systemic disease.
  ② **Halitosis is often caused by decaying food particles and gingivitis; brushing the teeth and tongue cleans the oral cavity which promotes healthy teeth and gums.**
  ③ Rinsing or flushing will not remove debris caught between the teeth.
  ④ Same as #3.

8 **TEST-TAKING TIP** ⊙ The word "least" in the stem indicates negative polarity.
  ① Conditioners moisturize the hair, which makes the strands more supple, preventing tangles.
  ② **Soap is drying because it removes natural secretions, which keep the hair supple.**

(3) Braids organize the strands of hair, which limits movement of hair into mats and tangles because of friction and pressure.

(4) Brushing distributes oils along hair shafts, keeping them supple and preventing tangles and matting.

9 TEST-TAKING TIP ○ Option 4 contains the word "every," which is a specific determiner.

(1) A draw sheet is an additional sheet that can add to the number of wrinkles; the purpose of a draw sheet is to keep the bottom sheet clean.

(2) A toe pleat should be placed in the top sheet and spread, not the bottom sheet. A toe pleat prevents footdrop.

(3) **Wrinkles exert pressure and friction against the skin, promoting the formation of pressure (decubitus) ulcers.**

(4) The bottom sheet does not have to be changed every day unless the sheet is wet or dirty.

10 TEST-TAKING TIP ○ The word *most* is the key word in the stem that sets a priority.

(1) Showering is not as effective as submerging the feet in soapy water.

(2) A lubricant should be applied after the feet are clean.

(3) **Soaking in soap and water softens the debris on the skin, between the toes, and under the toenails, facilitating cleaning.**

(4) The application of an antiseptic requires a physician's order.

11 TEST-TAKING TIP ○ The word "most" is the key word in the stem that sets a priority. Option 1 contains the word "always," which is a specific determiner.

(1) A light touch is stimulating and may precipitate a penile erection; a firm but gentle touch should be used.

(2) This action violates the principle of working from clean to dirty. The tip of the penis at the urethral meatus is washed first; bathing should then progress down the shaft of the penis toward the perineum and then the scrotum.

(3) **Repositioning the foreskin protects the head of the penis and prevents drying and irritation; if it is allowed to remain retracted, it may cause local edema and discomfort.**

(4) Cleaning should occur in the opposite direction, starting at the urinary meatus and then progressing down the shaft of the penis away from the urinary meatus.

12 TEST-TAKING TIP ○ The words "daily" and "contribute to hygiene" in the stem are significant clues.

(1) After placement is verified, instillation of solution may be done to promote catheter patency, not hygiene.

(2) This is not necessary; the tape should be reapplied if the nares become irritated or the tape becomes soiled.

(3) Suctioning is not necessary; cleaning the oral cavity when necessary with a tooth brush, dental floss, and mouthwash and applying a lubricant to the lips are sufficient.

(4) **Lubricating the nares keeps the skin supple and prevents drying, which limits the development of encrustations.**

13 TEST-TAKING TIP ○ The words "psychologic" and "chronic" in the stem are clues.

(1) Dyspnea is a physiologic, not a psychologic, adaptation to a stress.

(2) **Patients with chronic pain commonly experience depression; this is a psychologic adaptation to lack of control over relentless pain.**

(3) Self-splinting is a physical attempt to minimize pain.

(4) Hypertension is a physiologic, not a psychologic, adaptation to a stress.

14 TEST-TAKING TIP ○ Option 3 contains the word "only," which is a specific determiner.

(1) **Exercise contributes to physical and mental relaxation, which reduces tension and promotes sleep.**

(2) Tea contains caffeine, which contributes to wakefulness.

(3) The opposite is true. Moderate to heavy meals promote sleep; the body's energy is engaged in the process of digestion.

(4) Reviewing the day's events can cause an increase in tension, which can prevent a person from falling asleep.

15 TEST-TAKING TIP ○ The words "behavioral" and "moderate" are clues in the stem.

(1) Rapid, irregular breathing is a physiologic response to pain; pain generally activates the fight-or-flight mechanism of the general adaptation syndrome (GAS).

(2) The GAS stimulates the sympathetic branch of the autonomic nervous system, which results in increased muscle tension; it is a physiologic response that prepares muscles for action.

(3) **Self-splinting is a behavioral attempt to protect the area in pain and minimize stress and strain to the area, such as supporting the area or leaning in the direction of the pain.**

(4) Fatigue is a physiologic response to pain; physical and emotional responses to pain can use a great deal of physical and emotional energy and leave a person fatigued.

16 TEST-TAKING TIP ⊙ The word "cold" in the stem is a clue. Options 2 and 3 are equally plausible.
1. Elevation will not alter the temperature of the feet.
2. Externally produced heat can burn the feet in older adults who have reduced peripheral sensation.
3. Same as #2.
4. **Wearing socks is the safest way to keep the feet warm; socks contain the heat generated by the body.**

17 TEST-TAKING TIP ⊙ The word **most** in the stem sets a priority. Option 4 is unique because it has 2 words and the other 3 options all have 3 words.
1. Although environmental noise can interfere with sleep, it is not the factor that has been proved most often to interfere with sleep.
2. Emotional concerns have not been proved to be the factor that most often interferes with sleep.
3. Room temperature has not been proved to be the factor that most often interferes with sleep.
4. **Inability to find a position of comfort is the main reason why patients have difficulty sleeping in the hospital.**

18 TEST-TAKING TIP ⊙ There are four hypotheses being tested in this option: cold anesthetizes nerve endings, causes vasoconstriction, stimulates nerve endings, and causes vasodilation. If you know that one of these hypotheses is wrong, then you can eliminate two distractors.
1. **Cold is a form of cutaneous stimulation that slows the nervous conduction of impulses, thereby anesthetizing nerve endings, which relaxes muscle tension and relieves pain. Vasoconstriction decreases the flow of blood to the affected area; this limits the development of edema, which puts pressure on nerve endings, resulting in pain.**
2. Cold anesthetizes rather than stimulates nerve endings; it does cause vasoconstriction.
3. Although cold does anesthetize nerve endings, it causes vasoconstriction, not vasodilation.
4. Cold anesthetizes, rather than stimulates, nerve endings and causes vasoconstriction.

19 TEST-TAKING TIP ⊙ The word "best" in the stem sets a priority. The words "all patients" in the stem are a clue.
1. Sleeping medication should not be administered until all nondrug approaches fail to achieve sleep.
2. A backrub invades personal space and should be administered according to a patient's need and preference; a backrub may be contraindicated in certain clinical situations such as myocardial infarction or back surgery.
3. In an unfamiliar environment, turning the lights off can precipitate confusion or disorientation; a small light provides visual cues if a person awakens at night.
4. **Usual routines meet self-identified needs and reduce anxiety because they provide a familiar pattern.**

20 TEST-TAKING TIP ⊙ The words "comfort and rest" are the clue in the stem. Option 3 is unique because it addresses muscles and what is decreased (relieves) rather than what is increased (causes, stimulates, increases). Options 1, 2, and 4 all refer to the circulatory system.
1. Vasodilation improves circulation by bringing oxygen and nutrients to the area, not by promoting comfort and rest.
2. Same as #1.
3. **Applying long, smooth strokes while moving the hands up and down the back without losing contact with the skin has a relaxing and sedative effect. Its effect may be related to the gate-control theory of pain relief; rubbing the back stimulates large muscle fiber groups, which close the synaptic gates to pain or uncomfortable stimuli, permitting a perception of relaxation.**
4. Same as #1.

21 TEST-TAKING TIP ⊙ The words "increases local circulation" in Options 2 and 3 and "decreases local circulation" in Options 1 and 4 are examples of duplicate facts.
1. Heat increases, rather than decreases, local circulation, capillary vasodilation, and permeability.
2. Although heat increases local circulation, it increases, rather than decreases, tissue metabolism. Heat causes vasodilation, facilitating the exchange of nutrients and waste products and increasing cellular metabolism.
3. **Heat increases circulation because of its vasodilating effect. Heat is known to relax muscle spasms and the discomfort associated with muscle spasm; this mechanism is unknown.**
4. Cold, not heat, provides local anesthesia and decreases local circulation.

22 1. This is used to store the dentures when the patient is sleeping and addresses the patient's safety and security needs.
2. **This provides privacy while the dentures are out of the mouth and supports the patient's dignity and self-esteem.**
3. This supports the patient's physical needs.
4. This is unsafe; the nurse must look at the patient to inspect the oral cavity.

23 (1) This should be done after the hair is combed and untangled. Not all patients want their hair to be braided.
    (2) Either a comb or brush can be used.
    (3) **Separating the hair into small sections promotes ease in combing and limits discomfort.**
    (4) When removing tangles, the hair should be grasped at the scalp and the loose ends combed; each stroke should start progressively higher than the preceding stroke up the shafts of hair strands.

24 **TEST-TAKING TIP** ○ The word "most" in the stem sets a priority. Option 3 is the patient-centered option because it focuses on the patient rather than on the steps in a procedure.
    (1) This is unnecessary unless the linens are wet or dirty.
    (2) This does not support correct body mechanics when working and puts excessive stress on the nurse; the side rail may be lowered on the side where the nurse is working.
    (3) **This supports privacy and dignity and prevents chilling.**
    (4) This promotes the formation of pressure ulcers; it should be used only during perineal care or for patients who are incontinent.

25 **TEST-TAKING TIP** ○ The word "most" in the stem sets a priority. The clue in the stem is the word "subjective," which modifies the word "characteristic." Options 2 and 3 are objective characteristics and can be eliminated from consideration.
    (1) **Intensity is the most subjective characteristic of pain; a patient's perception of pain influences the descriptive report of the severity of pain.**
    (2) This description is based on determining onset, periodicity, frequency, and duration; it is based on time frames, which can be objectively measured.
    (3) This description is based on anatomic landmarks in the patient's attempt to localize the pain.
    (4) Although subjective, quality is less subjective than intensity because there is more consistency in the language used to describe types of pain.

26 **TEST-TAKING TIP** ○ The word "least" in the stem indicates negative polarity. Option 2 is opposite to both options 1 and 3.
    (1) Adolescents go through a growth spurt and need more sleep than the age group addressed in other options.
    (2) **Studies demonstrate that the older adult requires less sleep than do people on any other developmental level.**
    (3) Young adults may still be growing and are active; they need more sleep than an age group addressed in another option.
    (4) These adults are usually involved with activities related to growing children and developing a career; this age requires more sleep than an age group addressed in another option.

27 **TEST-TAKING TIP** ○ The word "most" is the key word in the stem that sets a priority. The word "independent" is the clue in the stem.
    (1) Exercise does not minimize fungal growth.
    (2) Medicated footbaths generally are ordered for ingrown toenails, not fungal infections, and require a physician's order.
    (3) Moisturizers should be avoided between the toes because they keep the area moist, which supports fungal growth.
    (4) **Moist, dark, warm areas facilitate the growth of microorganisms, especially fungi in the area of the feet.**

28 **TEST-TAKING TIP** ○ The word MOST in the stem sets a priority. All of the options address factors that influence pain, but Option 3 is the MOST significant.
    (1) Duration is one component of a description of pain after it is perceived.
    (2) The characteristics of pain are the components of the description of pain after it is perceived.
    (3) **This controls the higher levels of the perceptual aspects of pain.**
    (4) Although endorphin levels influence pain perception, it is not the most influential factor that affects the perception of pain.

29 **TEST-TAKING TIP** ○ The word "only" in Option 4 is a specific determiner and can be eliminated from consideration.
    (1) **This is a basic principle of medical asepsis. This should be done so that contaminated material will not be carried by the washcloth to another area of the perineum.**
    (2) Cleaning from the pubis toward the rectum prevents contaminating the urinary meatus and vagina with fecal material.
    (3) The area closest to the urinary meatus and vagina is cleaned first because it is considered the cleanest area of the perineum.
    (4) Soap can be used on the perineal area.

30   Answer: 2 Tablets

Solve the problem using ratio and proportion.

$$\frac{\text{Desired}}{\text{Have}} \qquad \frac{12.5 \text{ mg}}{6.5 \text{ mg}} = \frac{x \text{ Tab}}{1 \text{ Tab}}$$

(Cross-multiply) $6.5 \, x = 12.5$

(Divide by 6.5) $\dfrac{6.5 \, x}{6.5} = \dfrac{12.5}{6.5}$

$$x = 12.5 \div 6.5$$

$$x = 2 \text{ Tablets}$$

Meeting Patients' Fluid and Nutritional Needs

• • •

This section includes questions related to basic fluid balance and nutrition. Specific questions focus on principles associated with therapeutic diets, enteral feedings, fluid and electrolyte balance, intake and output (I&O), dehydration, feeding patients, vitamins, parenteral nutrition, intralipids, and medications associated with meeting patients' nutritional needs.

Questions

Please fill in the circle to mark your answer choice.

1   A patient who is receiving chemotherapy is nauseated. When planning for the nutritional needs of this patient, the nurse should:
   ① Serve the ordered diet in small quantities frequently
   ② Withhold food by mouth until the nausea subsides
   ③ Obtain an order for a full liquid diet
   ④ Provide oral liquid supplements

2   To prevent burns during mealtime in patients with mental and physical impairments, the nurse should:
   ① Assist patients with warm drinks
   ② Use plastic instead of metal utensils
   ③ Serve unsteady patients only cold drinks
   ④ Wait until the food is cool before serving
   TEST-TAKING TIP ◦ Identify the options that deny the patient's feelings, concerns, and needs. Identify the option that contains a specific determiner. Identify the patient-centered option.

3   A patient drinks 9 oz of milk with breakfast. Which calculation should the nurse enter on the I&O record?
   ① 30 mL
   ② 90 mL
   ③ 240 mL
   ④ 270 mL

4   The nurse is caring for an obese patient who is on a 1000-calorie diet. Which action is LEAST therapeutic when providing nursing care?
   ① Telling the patient about low-calorie snacks that can be eaten
   ② Teaching the patient to avoid starches on the meal tray
   ③ Encouraging the patient to chew and eat slowly
   ④ Recognizing when the patient has lost weight
   TEST-TAKING TIP ◦ Identify the key word in the stem that indicates negative polarity.

5   The nurse is monitoring a patient's intake and output. What is the **most** accurate way for the nurse to measure the amount of urine in the patient's urinary retention catheter collection bag?
   ① With a urometer
   ② With a marked graduate
   ③ By the markings on the bag
   ④ By emptying it into a bedpan
   TEST-TAKING TIP ◦ Identify the key word in the stem that sets a priority.

6 When the amount of calories ingested is not sufficient for the patient's basal metabolic rate, the nurse understands that the patient will:
   ① Become dehydrated
   ② Develop edema
   ③ Lose weight
   ④ Sleep more

7 To avoid trauma to the oral mucous membranes from hot food being served to a cognitively impaired patient, the nurse should:
   ① Request a menu that includes many cold foods
   ② Always touch the food to test its temperature
   ③ Mix the hot food with appropriate cold food
   ④ Wait for the hot food to cool slightly
   TEST-TAKING TIP ○ Identify the option that contains a specific determiner. Identify the options that deny the patient's feelings, concerns, and needs.

8 The nurse is caring for an easily confused patient. To meet the nutritional needs of this patient, the most appropriate nursing intervention is:
   ① Feeding the patient each meal
   ② Providing supervision when the patient eats
   ③ Explaining to the patient where everything is on the tray
   ④ Encouraging family members to take turns feeding the patient
   TEST-TAKING TIP ○ Identify the key word in the stem that sets a priority.

9 How much fluid should the nurse give a patient during 24 hours to maintain *normal* fluid balance?
   ① 500 mL
   ② 1000 mL
   ③ 1500 mL
   ④ 2000 mL
   TEST-TAKING TIP ○ Identify the clue in the stem. Identify the options that are opposites.

10 A patient had a heart attack because of atherosclerotic plaques. The nurse should encourage the patient to include protein in the diet by primarily ingesting:
   ① White meats
   ② Whole milk
   ③ Legumes
   ④ Shrimp
   TEST-TAKING TIP ○ Identify the key word in the stem that sets a priority.

11 When caring for a patient with a vitamin K deficiency, the nurse should monitor for which adaptation?
   ① Muscle cramps
   ② Signs of infection
   ③ Cardiac dysrhythmias
   ④ Bleeding irregularities
   TEST-TAKING TIP ○ Identify the clues in the stem.

12 Which loss should be identified by the nurse as being most significant when caring for a patient with a draining pressure (decubitus) ulcer?
   ① Fluid
   ② Weight
   ③ Protein
   ④ Leukocytes
   TEST-TAKING TIP ○ Identify the clue in the stem. Identify the key word in the stem that sets a priority.

13 The nurse understands that all patients on a low-calorie diet will:
    ① Break down adipose tissue for energy
    ② Have a decreased body metabolism
    ③ Have decreased energy levels
    ④ Require vitamin supplements
    TEST-TAKING TIP ◉ Identify the equally plausible options.

14 When planning for the nutritional needs of patients, the nurse understands that the age group that
    has the highest energy requirements is:
    ① Birth to 1 year old
    ② 3 to 5 years old
    ③ 13 to 19 years old
    ④ Over 65 years old
    TEST-TAKING TIP ◉ Identify the options that contain opposites.

15 A patient with the diagnosis of dehydration is hospitalized for intravenous rehydration therapy. What
    should the nurse do immediately after the patient drinks 8 ounces of apple juice?
    ① Record 240 mL on the I&O flow sheet
    ② Assess the patient's skin turgor
    ③ Offer the patient a bedpan
    ④ Provide oral hygiene
    TEST-TAKING TIP ◉ Identify the option that is unique.

16 The nurse should encourage a patient on a low-sodium diet to ingest:
    ① Milk
    ② Fruit
    ③ Bread
    ④ Vegetables

17 A patient has a pressure (decubitus) ulcer. Which breakfast food should the nurse encourage the
    patient to eat?
    ① French toast and oatmeal
    ② Oatmeal and orange juice
    ③ French toast and poached eggs
    ④ Poached eggs and orange juice
    TEST-TAKING TIP ◉ Identify the duplicate facts among the options.

18 A patient has anemia. What vitamin should the nurse expect the physician to order?
    ① Ascorbic acid
    ② Riboflavin
    ③ Folic acid
    ④ Thiamin
    TEST-TAKING TIP ◉ Identify the clue in the stem.

19 When a patient is receiving total parenteral nutrition (TPN) and intralipids, the nurse MUST administer
    the intralipids:
    ① Via an infusion pump
    ② Through a separate line
    ③ Piggybacked into the proximal port of the TPN catheter
    ④ After the total parenteral nutrition (TPN) infusion is completed
    TEST-TAKING TIP ◉ Identify the key word in the stem that sets a priority. Identify the options that
    are opposites.

20 The nurse should not increase the ordered flow rate of total parenteral nutrition (TPN) because it can result in:
① Osmotic diuresis and hypoglycemia
② Hypoglycemia and dumping syndrome
③ Electrolyte imbalance and osmotic diuresis
④ Dumping syndrome and electrolyte imbalance

TEST-TAKING TIP ○ Identify the duplicate facts among the options.

21 After administering a gastrostomy tube-feeding formula, the nurse should:
① Instill 30 mL of water by gravity
② Insert 20 mL of air into the tube
③ Check the dressing site
④ Encourage activity

TEST-TAKING TIP ○ Identify the clue in the stem.

22 The nurse is caring for a group of patients. Which patient has the most need for supplemental iron?
① Menstruating women
② Active adolescents
③ Growing children
④ Older men

TEST-TAKING TIP ○ Identify the key word in the stem that sets a priority.

23 The nurse understands that to maintain life, the most important nutrients are:
① Carbohydrates
② Vitamins
③ Proteins
④ Fluids

TEST-TAKING TIP ○ Identify the key word in the stem that sets a priority.

24 The group of individuals with the GREATEST need for calcium is:
① Postmenopausal women
② School-age children
③ Pregnant women
④ Working men

TEST-TAKING TIP ○ Identify the key word in the stem that sets a priority.

25 The nurse identifies that a patient who has a fluid intake of 500 mL over 24 hours will:
① Produce urine with a low specific gravity
② Urinate small amounts at each voiding
③ Develop an atonic bladder
④ Have dark amber urine

26 The nurse is feeding a patient with hemiparesis as the result of a brain attack. What intervention by the nurse is most important when feeding this patient?
① Ensure that food is pureed.
② Provide foods that require chewing.
③ Offer fluids with each mouthful of food.
④ Allow time to empty the mouth of food between spoonfuls.

27 When urine output is less than fluid intake, the nurse can expect the patient to:
① Gain weight
② Void frequently
③ Become jaundiced
④ Experience nausea

28 The nurse is assessing a patient's pulse. What should the nurse do if the patient's pulse is full and bounding?
1. Check the flow rate of the patient's IV fluids
2. Measure the patient's urine specific gravity
3. Monitor the patient's serum glucose
4. Lower the head of the patient's bed

29 The physician orders iron supplements for a patient with the diagnosis of anemia. The nurse should teach the patient that the absorption of iron is facilitated by the ingestion of foods high in vitamin:
1. D
2. C
3. A
4. K

30 A patient is receiving a full-liquid diet. Which food should the nurse remove from the patient's tray?
1. Ice cream
2. Prune juice
3. Cream of Wheat
4. Raspberry gelatin

TEST-TAKING TIP ○ Identify the words in the stem that suggest negative polarity.

31 The nurse is working in a nursing home with a large population of older adults. Which factor related to aging influences the nutritional status of older adults?
1. Additional need for milk products
2. Greater production of gastric acid
3. Deterioration in taste perception
4. Increased need for kilocalories

TEST-TAKING TIP ○ Identify the unique option.

32 A patient is experiencing diarrhea and needs to replace potassium. The nurse identifies that additional teaching is necessary when the patient says, "I should increase my intake of:
1. Orange juice."
2. Warm tea."
3. Bananas."
4. Raisins."

TEST-TAKING TIP ○ Identify the phrase in the stem that suggests negative polarity. Identify the option that is unique.

33 A patient with cancer is concerned about having had a rapid weight loss and asks why this occurred. The nurse bases a response on the fact that:
1. Anabolism exceeds catabolism
2. Nutrients are unable to be absorbed
3. Cancer increases metabolic demands
4. Cell division causes an altered nitrogen balance

TEST-TAKING TIP ○ Identify the clang association in the stem.

34 Which patient statement indicates the need for nursing education about vitamins?
1. "Vitamins can be taken without the fear of toxic effects."
2. "I don't need vitamins because I eat a balanced diet."
3. "Some vitamins can be manufactured by the body."
4. "My need for vitamins will change as I get older."

TEST-TAKING TIP ○ Identify the phrase in the stem that reflects negative polarity.

35 When assessing a client for the extent of edema, the nurse depresses the edematous area as indicated in the drawing below. Place an X in front of the information that should be documented in the patient's progress notes when using the 4-point scale for grading edema.

① ____ Barely detectable
② ____ 1+ edema
③ ____ 2+ edema
④ ____ 3+ edema
⑤ ____ 4+ edema

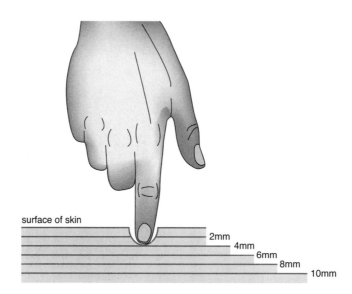

surface of skin
2mm
4mm
6mm
8mm
10mm

Meeting Patients' Fluid and Nutritional Needs
Answers and Rationales

1. (1) **Small quantities of food frequently offered establish small, realistic goals for the patient without being overwhelming.**
   (2) The patient may be nauseated for a long period of time; adequate food and fluid must be ingested to meet physiologic needs.
   (3) A full-liquid diet does not reduce nausea.
   (4) Supplements may interfere with the intake of regularly scheduled meals. Also, the patient may be too nauseated to ingest supplements.

2. **TEST-TAKING TIP** ◉ Options 3 and 4 deny the patient's right to have food and drinks served at warm temperatures. Option 3 contains the word "only," which is a specific determiner. Option 1 is patient centered.
   (1) **Patients with mental and physical deficits need assistance with warm drinks to prevent oral trauma or burns from spills.**
   (2) The use of plastic utensils does not prevent spilling hot liquids.
   (3) Patients have a right to have a variety of foods presented at different temperatures; serving only cold drinks violates a patient's rights.
   (4) Warm foods should be served warm and cold foods should be served cold.

3. (1) 30 mL is only 1 oz.
   (2) 90 mL is only 3 oz.
   (3) 240 mL is only 8 oz.
   (4) **270 mL is equal to 9 oz; 1 oz is equal to 30 mL.**

4. **TEST-TAKING TIP** ◉ The word LEAST is the key word in the stem that indicates negative polarity.
   (1) Identifying low-calorie snacks helps reduce caloric intake.
   (2) **The patient is receiving a special diet that has been carefully calculated, and all food on the tray should be eaten.**
   (3) This makes a meal take longer to eat and allows more time for the body to feel full.
   (4) Progress should be identified to provide motivation.

5. **TEST-TAKING TIP** ◉ The word **most** is the key word in the stem that sets a priority.
   (1) A urometer is used to measure the specific gravity of urine, not the volume of urine.
   (2) **A graduate is a special container with volume markings on the side for measuring fluid; of all the options offered, it is the most accurate way to measure urine.**
   (3) Using the markings on a urine collection bag is not accurate because the plastic that the bag is made of often stretches.
   (4) Bedpans are designed to collect excreta when a person cannot use a toilet or commode, not to measure urine volume.

6. (1) Dehydration occurs when fluid, not calorie, intake is insufficient.
   (2) Edema can occur if the patient experiences an inadequate intake of protein, not in response to a reduction in just caloric intake.
   (3) **When calories are insufficient to meet metabolic needs, the body catabolizes fat, resulting in weight loss.**
   (4) Sleeping is not related directly to a decreased caloric intake; however, a patient who is anemic may easily tire from an inadequate intake of iron or folic acid.

7. **TEST-TAKING TIP** ◉ The word "always" in Option 2 is a specific determiner. Options 1 and 3 deny the right of the patient to ingest foods of different temperatures.
   (1) Patients have a right to a variety of foods, textures, and temperatures within the ordered diet.
   (2) This will contaminate the food.
   (3) Foods should not be mixed; they should be served separately so that they retain their own flavor and texture.
   (4) **Waiting for hot foods to cool slightly is the safest and most practical action; food should be warm, rather than hot, to be safe to eat.**

8. **TEST-TAKING TIP** ◉ The word "most" is the key word in the stem that sets a priority.
   (1) Feeding the patient when only supervision is necessary contributes to feelings of dependence.
   (2) **Supervision best keeps the patient focused on the task of eating while supporting independence.**
   (3) Although this is something the nurse may do to orient the patient, the patient may forget or not understand the explanation.
   (4) Although family members can be helpful, it is the responsibility of the staff, not the family members, to care for the patient.

9 TEST-TAKING TIP ◉ The word *normal* is the clue in the stem. Options 1 and 4 are opposites among the volumes presented in the options.
1. This is an inadequate intake to maintain life.
2. Same as #1.
3. Same as #1.
4. **2000 mL is an average daily intake necessary to maintain fluid balance.**

10 TEST-TAKING TIP ◉ The word "primarily" is the key word in the stem that sets a priority.
1. White meat contains less fat than red meat but more fat than another option.
2. Whole milk contains fat, which contributes to plaque formation in atherosclerosis.
3. **Legumes, such as beans, peas, and lentils, contain the least amount of cholesterol and fat of the options presented and are high in protein, which is necessary for tissue regeneration.**
4. Although shrimp is a protein source, it is high in cholesterol, which should be avoided because it contributes to plaque formation.

11 TEST-TAKING TIP ◉ The words "deficiency" and "vitamin K" are significant clues in the stem.
1. Calcium contributes to neuromuscular excitability, and therefore lowered calcium levels can result in muscle cramps and tetany.
2. A deficiency in vitamin K does not contribute to the occurrence of infection. Vitamins A and C help build resistance to infection.
3. A deficiency of vitamin B_1 (thiamin) can result in tachycardia and cardiac enlargement; deficiencies in calcium, magnesium, and potassium can also contribute to cardiac problems.
4. **Vitamin K is essential for prothrombin formation and blood clotting; if a patient is deficient in vitamin K, the patient experiences a prolonged clotting time and is prone to bleeding.**

12 TEST-TAKING TIP ◉ The word "loss" is a significant clue in the stem. The word "most" is the word in the stem that sets a priority.
1. Although fluid is lost from a draining pressure ulcer, it does not have the most serious implication.
2. Weight loss is related to inadequate caloric intake, not the presence of a draining pressure ulcer.
3. **A patient can lose as much as 50 g of protein daily from a draining pressure ulcer; this is a large percentage of the usual daily requirement of 60 g of protein for women and 70 g of protein for men. Patients with draining pressure ulcers should ingest 2 to 4 times the usual daily requirements of protein to rebuild epidermal tissue.**
4. If a pressure ulcer is infected, the leukocyte count increases, not decreases.

13 TEST-TAKING TIP ◉ Options 2 and 3 are equally plausible because decreased energy levels are often associated with a decrease in the metabolic rate.
1. **When the number of calories ingested does not meet the body's energy requirements, the patient catabolizes body fat for energy and loses weight.**
2. Metabolism increases and decreases in response to the energy demands placed on the body, not as a result of a low-calorie diet.
3. Age, body size, body and environmental temperatures, growth, gender, nutritional state, and emotional state affect energy levels.
4. A well-balanced low-calorie diet should contain adequate vitamins, requiring no supplementation.

14 TEST-TAKING TIP ◉ Options 1 and 4 are opposites in relation to the age groups in the options offered.
1. **During the first year of life, the infant grows at a faster pace than at any other developmental stage; infants double their birth weight by 6 months and triple their birth weight during the first year.**
2. The preschool (3- to 5-year-old) child's growth rate is slower than the age identified in another option—namely, birth to 1 year old. The preschool child gains only another 7 to 12 pounds in addition to the 4 times the birth weight gained during the first 3 years.
3. Although the adolescent goes through a dramatic physical growth spurt that reflects significant changes in height, weight, dentition, and skeletal and sexual development, it is not as spectacular as the growth rate reflected in another option.
4. No physical growth occurs when a person is over 65 years of age; different parts of the body begin to degenerate, and function slowly.

15 TEST-TAKING TIP ◉ Option 1 is unique because it is the only option that has an abbreviation and numbers.
1. **Nursing care should be documented immediately after it is provided. There are 30 mL in each ounce; therefore, the patient ingested 240 mL.**
2. This is too early to evaluate the patient's response to fluid intake.
3. This is too early to expect the patient to void.
4. Mouth care usually is not required after drinking fluid; mouth care should be provided routinely on awakening, after meals, and at bedtime.

16 (1) Whole milk, depending on the brand, has approximately 6 to 130 mg of sodium per 8 oz.

(2) **Fresh fruits contain the least amount of sodium per serving of the options presented; most fresh fruits such as apples, pears, bananas, peaches, and cantaloupe contain less than 10 mg of sodium per serving.**

(3) White bread, depending on the brand, has approximately 55 to 225 mg of sodium per slice.

(4) Fresh vegetables, such as peas, beans, carrots, broccoli, cauliflower, corn, and celery contain approximately 40 mg of sodium per serving.

17 **TEST-TAKING TIP** ○ Five different foods are offered as foods that contribute to healing. If you can identify the one food that most contributes to healing (eggs), you have narrowed the correct answer to two options. If you can identify the one food that is the least beneficial to the healing process (oatmeal), you have narrowed the correct answer to two options.

(1) Although French toast contains some egg coating, which is protein, it does not contain the amount of protein in another option. Oatmeal does not contain protein or vitamin C.

(2) Although orange juice contains vitamin C, which contributes to wound healing, oatmeal does not contain protein or vitamin C.

(3) Each poached egg contains 6 to 8 g of protein; protein contains the amino acids necessary for building cells and therefore for wound healing. Although French toast contains some egg coating, which is protein, it does not contain vitamin C.

(4) **This is the best combination of foods in the options offered. Each egg contains 6 to 8 g of protein; protein contains the amino acids necessary for building cells and therefore for wound healing. Orange juice contains vitamin C, which promotes collagen formation, enhances iron absorption, and maintains capillary wall integrity.**

18 **TEST-TAKING TIP** ○ The word "anemia" is the significant clue in the stem.

(1) Ascorbic acid (vitamin C) promotes collagen formation, enhances iron absorption, and maintains capillary wall integrity.

(2) Riboflavin (vitamin B_2) functions as a coenzyme in the metabolism of carbohydrates, fats, amino acids, and alcohol.

(3) **Folic acid (vitamin B_9, folate) promotes the maturation of red blood cells. When red blood cells fall below the expected range of 4.2 million/mm³ for women and 4.7 million/mm³ for men, a person is considered anemic.**

(4) Thiamin (vitamin B_1) performs as a coenzyme in the metabolism of carbohydrates, fats, amino acids, and alcohol.

19 **TEST-TAKING TIP** ○ The word MUST is the word in the stem that sets a priority. Options 2 and 3 are opposites.

(1) Because an intralipid solution is a concentrated source of nonprotein kilocalories, it is desirable for an infusion pump to be used; however, an infusion pump does not have to be used because the solution can flow via gravity.

(2) **This action ensures that the intralipid solution is NOT mixed with a dextrose-amino acid solution. If they are mixed, the fat emulsion breaks down.**

(3) If an intralipid solution is mixed with a dextrose-amino acid solution, the fat emulsion breaks down; the solutions must not be administered through the same line.

(4) The solutions can be run at the same time but through different lines.

20 **TEST-TAKING TIP** ○ Four adaptations are offered as undesirable results associated with an increase in the flow rate of TPN above the prescribed rate: osmotic diuresis, hypoglycemia, dumping syndrome, and electrolyte imbalance. If you are able to identify one adaptation that is unrelated to an increased TPN rate, you eliminate two distractors. If you are able to identify the two adaptations that are unrelated to an increased TPN rate, you arrive at the correct answer. If you are able to identify one adaptation that is related to an increase in a TPN rate above the prescribed rate, you narrowed the correct answer to two options.

(1) Although osmotic diuresis does occur, hyperglycemia, not hypoglycemia, may result.

(2) Hyperglycemia, not hypoglycemia, may result. *Dumping syndrome,* the rapid entry of food from the stomach into the jejunum, can occur with an intermittent tube feeding, not TPN.

(3) **The hypertonic TPN solution pulls intracellular and interstitial fluid into the intravascular compartment; the increased blood volume increases circulation to the kidneys, raising urinary output (osmotic diuresis). Potassium and sodium imbalances are common among clients receiving TPN. Therefore, TPN rates must be carefully controlled.**

(4) Potassium and sodium imbalances are common among clients receiving TPN. However, dumping syndrome can occur with an intermittent tube feeding, not TPN.

21 **TEST-TAKING TIP** ○ The word "after" is the clue in the stem.

① **After administration of a tube-feeding formula, instilling 30 mL of water flushes the tube, preventing future blockage from a buildup of formula along the sides of the lumen of the tube.**

② Inserting 20 mL of air into the tube is part of the procedure that is done to determine if the tube is in the stomach before a tube feeding is initiated.

③ Checking the gastrostomy site is not necessarily part of the procedure for administering a gastrostomy tube feeding.

④ Activity is contraindicated immediately after a gastrostomy tube feeding to prevent aspiration. After a gastrostomy tube feeding, the patient should remain in a sitting or semi-Fowler's position for 30 to 60 minutes.

22 **TEST-TAKING TIP** ○ The word "most" is the key word in the stem that sets a priority.

① **Iron is essential to the formation of hemoglobin, a component of red blood cells, which is lost in menstrual blood.**

② Supplemental iron is unnecessary for active adolescents.

③ Supplemental iron is unnecessary in growing children (1 to 13 years). However, infants (birth to 1 year) who are breast fed need some iron supplementation from 4 to 12 months of age, and formula-fed infants need iron supplementation throughout the first year of life.

④ Supplemental iron is unnecessary for healthy older men.

23 **TEST-TAKING TIP** ○ The word "most" is the key word in the stem that sets a priority.

① Although carbohydrates are important, the body can survive longer without this nutrient than it can without the nutrient in the correct answer.

② Although vitamins are important, the body can survive longer without this nutrient than it can without the nutrient in the correct answer.

③ Although proteins are important, the body can survive longer without this nutrient than it can without the nutrient in the correct answer.

④ **The most basic nutrient needed is water because all body processes require an adequate fluid balance in the body.**

24 **TEST-TAKING TIP** ○ The word GREATEST is the key word in the stem that sets a priority.

① Although postmenopausal women can benefit from an increase in calcium to prevent osteoporosis, the need is not as high as the group of individuals in the correct answer.

② School-age children do not have the highest need for calcium. An adequate intake of milk and dairy products meets the minimum daily requirements of calcium for school-age children.

③ **Calcium should be increased 50 percent to an intake of 1.2 g per day to provide calcium for fetal tooth and bone development; this is essential during the third trimester when fetal bones are mineralized.**

④ Working men do not have the highest need for calcium. An adequate intake of milk and dairy products meets the minimum daily requirements of calcium for working men.

25 ① Reduced fluid intake produces a concentrated urine with a specific gravity higher than 1.030. The expected range for urine specific gravity is 1.010 to 1.030.

② The bladder still fills to the patient's usual capacity before there is a perceived need to void.

③ An atonic bladder is caused by a neurologic problem; it is a loss of the sensation of fullness that leads to distention from overfilling.

④ **Dark amber is the color of urine when fluid intake is below 1500 to 2000 mL per day; the urine is concentrated.**

26 ① Pureed food may not be necessary, but the patient may only need more time to thoroughly manage the food.

② This may be unsafe and possibly unreasonable because the patient has a reduced ability to move the muscles on one side of the face necessary for chewing. A mechanical soft diet may be necessary.

③ Fluids with each mouthful will increase the risk of aspiration; fluid is more difficult to control than food when swallowing.

④ **Allowing time to empty the mouth of food between spoonfuls minimizes food buildup in the mouth; also it does not rush the patient.**

27 ① **Fluid weighs 1 kg (2.2 lb) per liter. A patient can gain 6 to 8 pounds before edema can be identified through inspection.**

② The opposite is true; the patient will void infrequently.

③ Jaundice is related to impaired liver function, not fluid volume excess.

④ Nausea is not a common symptom of fluid volume excess.

28 ① **Intravenous solutions are administered directly into the intravascular compartment; if the intravenous flow rate is excessive, it will cause a full, bounding pulse related to hypervolemia.**

② The specific gravity of urine reflects the concentrating ability of the kidneys, not the cardiovascular system.

(3) A full, bounding pulse is not related to hyperglycemia or hypoglycemia; a weak, thready pulse is a late sign of diabetic ketoacidosis.

(4) A full, bounding pulse may indicate hypervolemia; in this compromised patient, lowering the head of the bed may impede respiration and is therefore contraindicated.

29 (1) Vitamin D is essential for adequate absorption and utilization of calcium in bone and tooth growth; it does not facilitate the absorption of iron.

(2) **Ascorbic acid (vitamin C) helps to change dietary iron to a form that can be absorbed by the body.**

(3) Vitamin A is essential for the growth and maintenance of epithelial tissue, maintenance of night vision, and promotion of resistance to infection.

(4) Vitamin K is essential for the formation of prothrombin, which prevents bleeding.

30 TEST-TAKING TIP ○ This question is really asking what food is NOT permitted on a full-liquid diet. Therefore this stem has negative polarity.

(1) Ice cream changes its state from a solid to a liquid at room temperature.

(2) Prune juice is a fluid and is permitted on a full-liquid diet.

(3) **Cream of Wheat is considered solid food and is not permitted on a full-liquid diet.**

(4) Raspberry gelatin changes its state from a solid to a liquid at room temperature.

31 TEST-TAKING TIP ○ Options 1, 2, and 4 have positive words (*greater, additional,* and *increased*). Option 3 includes the word "deterioration," which has a negative connotation.

(1) The need for food from all sections of the MyPyramid remains similar regardless of age; an increase in milk products is needed only by older adults who are at risk for osteoporosis.

(2) Gastric secretions decrease, not increase, with aging.

(3) **Taste perception decreases because of atrophy of the taste buds and a reduced sense of smell; sweet and salty tastes are lost first.**

(4) The need for kilocalories decreases because of the lower metabolic rate and the reduction in physical activity associated with older adults.

32 TEST-TAKING TIP ○ In the stem, the phrase "additional teaching is necessary" reflects negative polarity. This question is asking what food or drink contains the LEAST amount of potassium. Option 2 is unique because it is not a fruit. Options 1, 3, and 4 relate to fruit.

(1) One cup of orange juice contains approximately 475 mg of potassium.

(2) **One cup of tea contains approximately 35 mg of potassium.**

(3) One banana contains approximately 450 mg of potassium.

(4) One ounce (⅛ cup) of raisins contains approximately 200 mg of potassium.

33 TEST-TAKING TIP ○ The word "cancer" in both the stem and Option 3 is a clang association.

(1) With cancer, catabolism exceeds anabolism.

(2) The ability to utilize nutrients is not impaired with cancer.

(3) **The energy required to support the rapid growth of cancerous cells increases the metabolic demands 1.5 to 2 times the resting energy expenditure.**

(4) The byproducts of cell breakdown cause a negative nitrogen balance.

34 TEST-TAKING TIP ○ The phrase "the need for further teaching" indicates negative polarity. This question is asking which option contains inaccurate information.

(1) **This is an inaccurate statement. Megadoses of vitamins can cause hypervitaminosis and result in toxicity.**

(2) Ordinarily healthy persons who eat a variety of foods that reflect a balanced diet should not need vitamin supplements.

(3) Vitamin D can be synthesized by the body. In addition to dietary intake, vitamin D is manufactured in the skin.

(4) The National Academy of Sciences, National Academy Press, Washington, DC, publishes the Recommended Dietary Allowance (RDA) of vitamins. The list reflects age, gender, and physical status differences.

35 (1) _____ Barely detectable: Barely detectable and 1+ edema are synonymous and are characterized by a 2 mm or less depression when edematous tissue is compressed.

(2) _____ 1+ edema: 1+ and barely detectable are synonymous.

(3) **_X_ 2+ edema: 2+ edema is characterized by a 2 to 4 mm depression when compressing edematous tissue.**

(4) _____ 3+ edema: 3+ edema is characterized by a 5 mm to 10 mm depression when compressing edematous tissue depending on the reference source. Some sources say 5–10 mm and some say 6–8 mm.

(5) _____ 4+ edema: 4+ edema is characterized by more than 8 or 10 mm depression when compressing edematous tissue depending on the reference source. Some sources say more than 8 mm and some say more than 10 mm.

Meeting Patients' Elimination Needs

• • •

This section includes questions related to bowel and bladder needs. Topics associated with intestinal elimination include incontinence, constipation, diarrhea, enemas, bowel retraining, and medications. Questions also focus on patient needs associated with urinary elimination and include topics such as incontinence, bladder retraining, toileting, and external and indwelling urinary catheters.

Questions

Please fill in the circle to mark your answer choice.

1 The nurse is caring for a patient who has an indwelling urinary catheter (Foley catheter). The nurse teaches the patient that the urine collection bag should be:
① Carried at waist level when walking
② Kept below the level of the pelvis
③ Changed at least once a week
④ Clamped when out of bed
TEST-TAKING TIP ○ Identify the options that are opposites.

2 Which action should be included in all bladder-retraining programs?
① Toileting the patient before sleep
② Providing 3000 mL of fluids a day
③ Toileting the patient every 2 hours
④ Using adult incontinence underwear
TEST-TAKING TIP ○ Identify the clue in the stem. Identify the option that contains a specific determiner.

3 The nurse is applying a condom catheter (external catheter) after perineal care for an uncircumcised patient. The nurse must:
① Replace the foreskin over the glans
② Lubricate the distal penis and glans
③ Secure the condom directly behind the glans
④ Retract the foreskin behind the head of the glans
TEST-TAKING TIP ○ Identify the clues in the stem. Identify the options that are opposites.

4 A patient complains about being constipated. The nurse should encourage the patient to eat:
① Fresh fruit and whole wheat bread
② Baked chicken and plain yogurt
③ Whole wheat bread and chicken
④ Plain yogurt and fresh fruit
TEST-TAKING TIP ○ Identify the clue in the stem. Identify the duplicate facts among the options.

5 When administering a tap water enema, the nurse understands that its primary purpose is to:
① Minimize intestinal gas
② Cleanse the bowel of stool
③ Reduce abdominal distention
④ Decrease the loss of electrolytes
TEST-TAKING TIP ○ Identify the clue in the stem. Identify the key word in the stem that sets a priority.

6 A confused patient asks to use the bathroom even though the patient was toileted only 30 minutes earlier. The nurse should:
① Request a physician's order for an indwelling urinary catheter
② Persuade the patient to try to hold it for at least one hour
③ Remind the patient of the recent trip to the bathroom
④ Assist the patient to the bathroom

TEST-TAKING TIP ○ Identify the options that deny the patient's feelings, concerns, and needs. Identify the option that is patient centered.

7 The physician orders a 750-mL tap water enema. To best promote acceptance of the volume ordered, the nurse should:
① Administer the fluid slowly and have the patient take shallow breaths
② Place the patient in the left lateral position and slowly administer the fluid
③ Have the patient take shallow breaths and keep the fluid at body temperature
④ Keep the fluid at body temperature and place the patient in the left lateral position

TEST-TAKING TIP ○ Identify the key word in the stem that sets a priority. Identify the duplicate facts among the options.

8 The nurse understands that the patient at the highest risk for developing diarrhea is a patient who:
① Is physically active
② Drinks a lot of fluid
③ Eats whole-grain cereal
④ Is experiencing emotional problems

TEST-TAKING TIP ○ Identify the key word in the stem that sets a priority. Identify the clue in the stem.

9 When caring for a patient who is unable to tolerate a large amount of enema fluid, which solution should the nurse anticipate that the physician will order?
① Hypertonic fluid
② Normal saline
③ Soapy water
④ Tap water

TEST-TAKING TIP ○ Identify the key word in the stem that sets a priority.

10 Which patient identified by the nurse is at greatest risk for developing constipation?
① Toddler
② Adolescent
③ Middle-age man
④ Pregnant woman

TEST-TAKING TIP ○ Identify the key word in the stem that sets a priority.

11 The nurse makes the assumption that the patient may be experiencing urinary retention. Which adaptation supports this assumption?
① Concentrated urine
② Painful micturition
③ Abdominal distention
④ Functional incontinence

12 The nurse understands that a physiologic function of the body that helps prevent infection is:
① An elevated temperature
② A high pH of gastric secretions
③ The flushing action of urine flow
④ The rapid expulsion of stool from the intestine

TEST-TAKING TIP ○ Identify the clues in the stem.

13 The physician orders a tap water enema for a patient scheduled for surgery. When administering the enema, the nurse should position the patient in the:
① Dorsal recumbent position
② Right lateral position
③ Back lying position
④ Left Sims' position

TEST-TAKING TIP ○ Identify the equally plausible options. Identify the options that are opposites.

14 When planning for the elimination needs of a patient, the nurse understands that:
(1) Peristalsis increases after ingestion of food
(2) Emotional stress initially decreases peristalsis
(3) Enema solutions should be administered at room temperature
(4) Intrathoracic pressure decreases when straining during defecation

15 The nurse teaches a person to lean forward when attempting to defecate. Leaning forward specifically promotes fecal elimination because it:
(1) Relaxes the rectal sphincters
(2) Raises intra-abdominal pressure
(3) Uses gravity to facilitate elimination
(4) Elongates the curves of the sigmoid colon

TEST-TAKING TIP ○ Identify the clues in the stem.

16 A patient has a loose watery stool in the morning. To determine if the patient has diarrhea, the nurse should ask:
(1) "What did you have for dinner last night?"
(2) "Have you been drinking a lot of fluid lately?"
(3) "When was the last time you had a similar stool?"
(4) "Are you experiencing any abdominal cramping?"

17 When administering a soapsuds enema, the nurse understands that the primary action of the soapsuds is to:
(1) Increase pressure in the bowel
(2) Distend the lumen of the bowel
(3) Irritate the mucosa of the bowel
(4) Exert an osmotic effect in the bowel

TEST-TAKING TIP ○ Identify the key word in the stem that sets a priority. Identify the equally plausible options.

18 A patient has a full body cast and is experiencing diarrhea. The nurse concludes that this patient is at risk for developing:
(1) Pressure ulcers
(2) A wound infection
(3) Urinary incontinence
(4) A hip flexion contracture

19 The physician orders the nurse to begin a bladder-retraining program for a patient who has been incontinent. Which is the most important nursing intervention to promote a successful bladder-retraining program?
(1) Offering a full-liquid diet
(2) Washing the perineal area every shift
(3) Following the scheduled program exactly
(4) Maintaining a strict record of fluid balance

TEST-TAKING TIP ○ Identify the key word in the stem that sets a priority.

20 When differentiating among the types of urinary incontinence, the nurse understands that stress incontinence occurs:
(1) With a urinary tract infection
(2) In response to emotional strain
(3) As a result of increased intra-abdominal pressure
(4) When a specific volume of urine is in the bladder

21 The physician orders a rectal tube for a postoperative patient. Before inserting the rectal tube, the nurse teaches the patient that the main purpose of the tube is to:
(1) Administer an enema
(2) Dilate the anal sphincters

③ Relieve abdominal distention
④ Visualize the intestinal mucosa

TEST-TAKING TIP ○ Identify the key word in the stem that sets a priority.

22 The nurse understands that with a tap water enema, the:
① Volume of instilled water stimulates peristalsis
② Water can cause excessive interstitial fluid loss
③ Surface tension of water is reduced by soapsuds
④ Hypertonic nature of the water irritates the intestinal mucosa

TEST-TAKING TIP ○ Identify the clue in the stem.

23 What should the nurse assess for when establishing the patency of a urinary retention catheter (Foley)?
① Color
② Clarity
③ Volume
④ Constituents

TEST-TAKING TIP ○ Identify the option that is unique.

24 The nurse understands that the most common concern of patients who have a colostomy is:
① Maintenance of skin integrity
② Frequency of defecation
③ Ability to control odor
④ Consistency of feces

TEST-TAKING TIP ○ Identify the key word in the stem that indicates a priority.

25 Six hours after surgery, a patient has yet to void. The nurse should palpate which area of the abdomen to determine if the urinary bladder is becoming distended with urine? Place an X over the area that should be palpated.

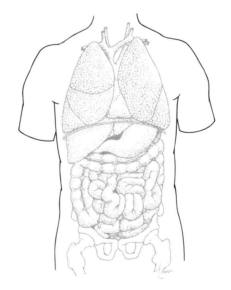

Meeting Patients' Elimination Needs
Answers and Rationales

1 **TEST-TAKING TIP** ○ Options 1 and 2 are opposites. The phrase "waist level" in Option 1 is opposite to "below the level of the pelvis" in Option 2. Waist level is above the pelvis.
① This will allow urine to flow back into the bladder, which can contribute to a urinary tract infection.
② **Positioning the catheter collection bag below the level of the pelvis prevents urine from flowing back into the bladder; urine flows out of the bladder by gravity.**
③ An indwelling urinary catheter and collection bag constitute a closed system and should be changed only every 4 to 6 weeks unless crusting or sediment collects on the inside of the tubing.
④ It is unnecessary to clamp an indwelling urinary catheter when a patient is out of bed; this is unsafe for some patients.

2 **TEST-TAKING TIP** ○ The word *all* is a clue in the stem. The word "every" in Option 3 is a specific determiner.
① **This is done for all patients; it contributes to less urine volume in the bladder during the night.**
② The volume of scheduled fluid intake is based on the individual needs of the patient.
③ Toileting is not automatically implemented every 2 hours but is based on the individual needs of the patient.
④ Incontinence pads are generally not encouraged when implementing a bladder-retraining program; however, devices used depend on the individual needs and preferences of the patient.

3 **TEST-TAKING TIP** ○ The words "uncircumcised" and "after perineal care" are the significant clues in the stem. Options 1 and 4 are opposites.
① **Perineal care should be provided when changing a condom catheter; in uncircumcised men, if the foreskin is not replaced to the normal position, it can tighten around the shaft of the penis, causing local edema and pain.**
② The distal end of the penis should not be lubricated; this will prevent the condom device from staying securely in place.
③ A condom catheter (external catheter) should be secured farther up the shaft of the penis, not immediately behind the glans.
④ If the foreskin is not returned over the glans, it can tighten around the shaft of the penis, causing local edema and pain.

4 **TEST-TAKING TIP** ○ The word "constipated" is a clue in the stem. Four different foods are offered as foods that help a patient who is constipated. If you are able to identify one food that contributes to increasing peristalsis and the relief of constipation, you can narrow the correct answer to two options. If you are able to identify one food that is not beneficial for the relief of constipation, you can delete two options.
① **Fresh fruit and whole wheat bread contain roughage, which adds bulk to stool, increasing peristalsis.**
② Chicken does not contain much roughage and plain yogurt contains yeast, not roughage.
③ Although whole wheat bread contains roughage, chicken does not contain much roughage.
④ Although fresh fruit contains roughage, plain yogurt contains yeast, not roughage.

5 **TEST-TAKING TIP** ○ The words "tap water" are a significant clue in the stem. The word "primary" is the key word in the stem that sets a priority.
① A Harris drip (Harris flush), not a tap water enema, helps evacuate intestinal gas.
② **A tap water enema introduces a hypotonic fluid into the intestinal tract; distention and pressure against the intestinal mucosa increase peristalsis and evacuation of stool.**
③ This is a secondary gain because flatus and stool are evacuated along with the enema solution.
④ A tap water enema increases, not decreases, the loss of electrolytes because it is a hypotonic solution.

6 **TEST-TAKING TIP** ○ Options 2 and 3 deny the patient's feelings, concerns, and needs. Option 4 is the patient-centered option.
① Indwelling urinary catheters should not be used to avoid incontinence or the inconvenience of frequently toileting a patient.
② The patient has a need to void now; 1 hour is too long to postpone urination.
③ Reminding the patient that voiding occurred 30 minutes earlier denies the patient's need to void now.
④ **Immediate toileting meets the patient's need to void and promotes continence. Regardless of whether or not the patient is confused, the patient should be taken to the bathroom.**

7 **TEST-TAKING TIP** ○ The word "best" is the word in the stem that sets a priority. Four different interventions are offered as actions that help a patient retain a 750-mL tap water enema. If you can identify one action that is based on a scientific principle associated with tap water enema administration, you can narrow the correct answer to

two options. If you can identify one action that is not based on a scientific principle associated with tap water enema administration, you can delete two options from consideration.

(1) Although the slow administration of enema fluid is appropriate, encouraging shallow breaths, versus deep breaths, may contribute to an increase in intra-abdominal pressure, which can interfere with the retention of enema fluid.

(2) **Both of these actions contribute to retention of enema fluid. In the left lateral position, the sigmoid colon is below the rectum, facilitating the instillation of fluid. The slow administration of enema fluid minimizes the probability of intestinal spasm and premature evacuation of the enema fluid before a therapeutic effect is achieved.**

(3) Encouraging shallow breaths and using a 98.6°F enema fluid interfere with the instillation and retention of enema fluid. Encouraging deep breaths, not shallow breaths, helps to prevent patients from holding their breath, which increases intra-abdominal pressure; increased intra-abdominal pressure can interfere with the instillation and retention of enema fluid. A water temperature of 98.6°F is too cool and can contribute to intestinal muscle spasm and discomfort.

(4) Although placing the patient on the left side is appropriate, a water temperature of 98.6°F is too cool and can contribute to intestinal muscle spasm and discomfort. Enema water temperature should be between 105° and 110°F because warm fluid promotes muscle relaxation and comfort.

8 **TEST-TAKING TIP** ⊙ The word "highest" is the key word in the stem that sets a priority. The word "diarrhea" in the stem is a significant clue.

(1) Being physically active helps to prevent constipation, but does not precipitate diarrhea.

(2) Drinking a lot of fluid helps to prevent constipation, but does not precipitate diarrhea.

(3) Eating whole-grain cereal helps to prevent constipation, but does not precipitate diarrhea.

(4) **Psychologic stress initially increases intestinal motility and mucus secretion, promoting diarrhea.**

9 **TEST-TAKING TIP** ⊙ The word "most" in the stem sets a priority.

(1) **A hypertonic enema solution uses only 120 to 180 mL of solution. Hypertonic solutions expend osmotic pressure that draws fluid out of the interstitial spaces; fluid pulled into the colon and rectum distend the bowel, causing an increase in peristalsis resulting in bowel evacuation.**

(2) A normal saline enema is isotonic and requires a volume of 500 mL to 750 mL to be effective; the volume of fluid, not its saline content, causes an evacuation of the bowel.

(3) A soapsuds enema requires a volume of 750 to 1000 mL of fluid to result in an effective evacuation of the bowel.

(4) A tap water enema usually requires a minimum of 750 mL of water.

10 **TEST-TAKING TIP** ⊙ The word "greatest" is the key word in the stem that sets a priority.

(1) A toddler usually drinks adequate fluids, eats a regular diet, and is very active; these activities contribute to bowel elimination.

(2) The adolescent usually eats more food than at earlier developmental stages and may complain of indigestion, not constipation; indigestion is a response to increased gastric acidity that occurs during adolescence.

(3) As people advance through middle adulthood, they are at risk for gaining weight, not developing constipation.

(4) **The growing size of the fetus exerts pressure on the rectum and bowel, which impinges on intestinal functioning, contributing to constipation; the decreased motility causes increased absorption of water, promoting constipation.**

11 (1) *Concentrated urine* is caused by inadequate fluid intake and indicates dehydration, not urinary retention.

(2) *Painful micturition (dysuria)* is generally caused by infection, inflammation, or injury, not urinary retention.

(3) ***Abdominal distention* occurs as a result of the buildup of urine in the bladder. Outlet obstruction, decreased bladder tone, neurologic dysfunction, opioids, and trauma can precipitate urinary retention.**

(4) *Functional incontinence* is unrelated to retention. Functional incontinence occurs when a person who is aware of the need to void is unable to reach the toilet in time.

12 **TEST-TAKING TIP** ⊙ The word "prevent" is an important clue in the stem.

(1) An elevated temperature results from released toxins in the presence of infection; it may help to limit an already existing infection, but it does not prevent an infection.

(2) Gastric secretions are acidic and have a low pH.

(3) **Microorganisms congregate at the urinary meatus because it is warm, moist, and dark; when urine flows down the urethra and out of the urinary meatus, the force of the urine carries away microorganisms, which minimizes ascending infections.**

(4) Rapid peristalsis results in diarrhea; this is not a usual physiologic function of the body but rather a response to an irritant or a pathogen.

13 **TEST-TAKING TIP** ⊙ Options 1 and 3 are equally plausible. Options 2 and 4 are opposites.

(1) This position will not use the natural curve of the rectum and sigmoid colon to facilitate instillation of the enema solution.

(2) Same as #1.

(3) Same as #1.

(4) **The left Sims' position permits the solution to flow downward via gravity along the natural curve of the rectum and sigmoid colon, promoting instillation and retention of the solution.**

14 (1) **Food or fluid that enters and fills the stomach or the duodenum stimulates peristalsis; this is called the "gastrocolic reflex" or "duodenocolic reflex."**

(2) Emotional stress initially increases peristalsis because the bowel evacuates its contents to prepare for the "fight." As the sympathetic nervous system increases its control in its response to stress, the action of the parasympathetic nervous system decreases. The parasympathetic nervous system stimulates peristalsis, and as its action decreases, peristalsis also decreases.

(3) Enema solutions should be administered slightly above body temperature (105° to 110°F). A solution that is warmer than this injures the mucosa, and one that is cooler than this causes muscle spasms.

(4) Straining at defecation increases, not decreases, intrathoracic pressure. Forcible exhalation against the closed glottis (Valsalva maneuver) raises the intrathoracic pressure, which impedes venous return. When the breath is released, blood is propelled through the heart, causing tachycardia and an increased blood pressure; a reflex bradycardia immediately follows. With an increase in intrathoracic pressure, immediate tachycardia and bradycardia occur in succession; patients with heart problems can experience a cardiac arrest.

15 **TEST-TAKING TIP** ⊙ The words "leaning forward" and "fecal elimination" are the clues in the stem.

(1) Relaxation of the internal and external rectal sphincters may result in response to this position; however, this relaxation of sphincters is in response to increased intra-abdominal pressure.

(2) **When a person leans forward, external pressure against the internal abdominal organs causes an increase in intra-abdominal pressure, facilitating fecal elimination.**

(3) The sitting position, not leaning forward, uses gravity to facilitate defecation.

(4) When a person is sitting and leaning forward, the curves of the sigmoid colon remain unchanged.

16 (1) Although this answer may help determine if food influenced the patient's intestinal elimination, it does not further assess the presence of diarrhea.

(2) Excessive fluid intake is excreted through the kidneys, not the intestinal tract.

(3) **Diarrhea is the defecation of liquid feces and increased frequency of defecation.**

(4) Cramping is not specific to diarrhea; it can also be associated with constipation and intestinal obstruction.

17 **TEST-TAKING TIP** ⊙ The word "primary" is the key word in the stem that sets a priority. Options 1 and 2 are equally plausible because they are both related to the effects of the volume of the enema solution, not the action of soapsuds, on the intestinal mucosa.

(1) Increasing pressure in the bowel is the rationale for using a high volume of fluid, not soapsuds.

(2) Distending the lumen of the bowel is the rationale for using a high volume of fluid, not soapsuds.

(3) **Soap is an irritant that stimulates the intestinal mucosa, precipitating peristalsis and the eventual evacuation of stool.**

(4) A hypertonic solution, not soapsuds, has an osmotic effect in the bowel.

18 (1) **In addition to being warm and moist, feces contain enzymes that promote tissue breakdown.**

(2) There is no wound present to become infected; fecal material may cause a vaginal or urinary tract infection, not a wound infection.

(3) Immobility may precipitate urinary retention rather than incontinence; diarrhea will not promote urinary incontinence.

(4) With a full body cast, the hips are usually in extension.

19 **TEST-TAKING TIP** ⊙ The word "most" in the stem sets a priority.

(1) A balanced diet plus adequate fluid is all that is necessary.

(2) Washing the perineal area does not contribute to a patient's ability to regain continence.

(3) **Toileting times are purposely scheduled in response to times of fluid intake and the patient's usual elimination pattern; to increase success, the schedule must be followed exactly.**

(4) The pattern of voiding relative to fluid intake is significant, not fluid balance.

20 (1) Urinary tract infections often cause frequency as a result of irritation of the mucosal wall of the bladder, not stress incontinence.

(2) Emotional strain may cause frequency, not stress incontinence.

(3) **When intra-abdominal pressure increases, the person with stress incontinence experiences urinary dribbling, or an approximate loss of 50 mL of urine or less.**

(4) This occurs in reflex, not stress, incontinence.

21 **TEST-TAKING TIP** ○ The word "main" in the stem sets a priority.
① An enema tube is used to administer an enema.
② This is not the purpose of a rectal tube.
③ **A rectal tube is inserted past the anal sphincters (6 inches in an adult and 2 to 4 inches in a child) and left in place for 30-minute intervals every 2 to 3 hours; rectal tubes are used to promote the passage of flatus, reducing abdominal distention.**
④ A rectal tube is not used to visualize the intestinal mucosa. A proctoscope is an instrument designed to visualize the rectum; a sigmoidoscope is an instrument designed to visualize the sigmoid colon and the rectum; and a colonoscope is an instrument designed to visualize the entire large intestine.

22 **TEST-TAKING TIP** ○ The words "tap water" modify the word "enema." This is the clue in the stem.
① **The large volume of instilled tap water distends the colon, which, in turn, stimulates peristalsis; it also softens feces.**
② Tap water is hypotonic, which can cause water intoxication and fluid and electrolyte imbalance, not excessive interstitial fluid loss.
③ Soap is not added to a tap water enema. Soapsuds enemas work by irritating the mucosa and distending the colon, which, in turn, stimulates peristalsis.
④ A tap water enema is hypotonic, not hypertonic.

23 **TEST-TAKING TIP** ○ Option 3 is the only option that does not begin with a "C."
① The color of urine reflects urine concentration or a reaction to a specific drug or food, not catheter patency.
② A cloudy urine indicates the presence of such products as red or white blood cells, bacteria, prostatic fluid, or sperm. Clarity will not indicate catheter patency.
③ **If urine volume is minimal or nonexistent, it indicates that the catheter is obstructed or the patient is not producing urine in the kidneys.**
④ Abnormal constituents of urine such as pus or blood indicates possible pathology, not catheter patency.

24 **TEST-TAKING TIP** ○ The word "most" modifies the word "common" indicating a priority.
① Maintenance of skin integrity is a physiologic, not a psychologic, concern.
② Frequency of defecation is a physiologic, not a psychologic concern.
③ **The ability to control odor is a major psychologic concern of people with a colostomy, because the odor can be offensive if not controlled.**
④ Consistency of the feces is not as major a concern as another factor. The consistency of feces varies according to the location of the stoma along the intestinal tract.

25 **Answer: Shaded area. Two transverse (horizontal) planes and two sagittal planes divide the abdomen into nine areas. When a urinary bladder fills with urine, it will rise upward into the abdominal cavity (shaded). In assessing a distended urinary bladder, palpation will reveal a round, firm mass above the symphysis pubis. Percussion will elicit a hollow, drumlike sound.**

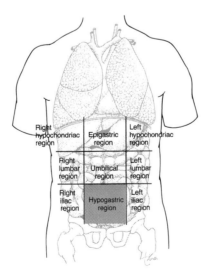

Meeting Patients' Oxygen Needs

• • •

This section includes questions related to assessments and interventions associated with expected and abnormal respiratory and circulatory function. Questions focus on topics such as preventing aspiration, providing emergency care for aspiration, techniques and devices that assess or increase respiratory or circulatory function, and assessments and interventions associated with the administration of oxygen.

Questions

Please fill in the circle to mark your answer choice.

1 The nurse is administering physical hygiene to a patient receiving a nasogastric tube feeding. To prevent aspiration when giving the bed bath, the nurse should:
   ① Obtain additional assistance
   ② Lower the height of the bag
   ③ Slow the rate of flow
   ④ Shut off the feeding
   TEST-TAKING TIP ◉ Identify the equally plausible options.

2 A patient walking in the hall complains of sudden chest pain. The initial intervention by the nurse should be to:
   ① Take the vital signs
   ② Get a chair so the patient can rest
   ③ Perform a detailed pain assessment
   ④ Walk the patient back to bed slowly
   TEST-TAKING TIP ◉ Identify the key word in the stem that sets a priority. Identify the options that are opposites.

3 The physician orders oxygen therapy via nasal cannula for a patient. The <u>first</u> action by the nurse is to:
   ① Post an oxygen in use sign on the door to the room
   ② Adjust the oxygen level before applying the cannula
   ③ Explain the rules of fire safety with oxygen use
   ④ Lubricate the nares with water-soluble jelly
   TEST-TAKING TIP ◉ Identify the key word in the stem that sets a priority.

4 A patient has dysphagia. To prevent aspiration after meals by this patient, the nurse should *first:*
   ① Position the patient in the low-Fowler's position
   ② Provide a pitcher of water at the bedside
   ③ Encourage mouth care when necessary
   ④ Inspect the mouth for pocketed food
   TEST-TAKING TIP ◉ Identify the key word in the stem that sets a priority. Identify the clue in the stem.

5 While assisting a patient to eat, the other patient in the room begins to choke on food and is unable to speak. What should the nurse do first?
   ① Initiate the abdominal thrust maneuver.
   ② Clap between the scapulae several times.
   ③ Instruct the patient to swallow forcefully.
   ④ Wait to see if the patient can cough up the obstruction.
   TEST-TAKING TIP ◉ Identify the key word in the stem that sets a priority.

6 A patient with a history of chronic respiratory disease begins to have difficulty breathing. For which two most serious adaptations should the nurse should assess?
   ① Orthostatic hypotension when rising and the need to sit in the orthopneic position
   ② Wheezing sounds on inspiration and the need to sit in the orthopneic position

③ Mucus tinged with frank red streaks and wheezing sounds on inspiration
④ Chest pain and mucus tinged with frank red streaks

TEST-TAKING TIP ○ Identify the key word in the stem that sets a priority. Identify the duplicate facts among the options.

7   What is the MOST important intervention by the nurse to increase both circulation and respiration in a patient?
①   Encourage the use of a spirometer
②   Reposition the patient every two hours
③   Massage the bony prominences with lotion
④   Teach the patient to cough and breathe deeply

TEST-TAKING TIP ○ Identify the key word in the stem that sets a priority. Identify the clue in the stem.

8   A patient is receiving oxygen through a nasal cannula. To prevent skin breakdown around the patient's nares, the nurse should:
①   Remove the tubing for 15 minutes every 2 hours
②   Provide oral hygiene whenever necessary
③   Adjust the cannula so it is comfortable
④   Reposition the patient every 2 hours

TEST-TAKING TIP ○ Identify the clue in the stem. Identify the specific determiners in the options.

9   While eating, a patient clutches the upper chest with the hands, appears unable to breathe, and has a frightened facial expression. The most appropriate initial nursing intervention is to:
①   Start artificial respirations
②   Perform abdominal thrusts
③   Slap the patient on the back
④   Ask the patient to attempt to speak

TEST-TAKING TIP ○ Identify the key word in the stem that sets a priority. Identify the unique option.

10   The nurse is monitoring a patient with a respiratory problem for the presence of cyanosis. Which are the most appropriate sites to assess?
①   Lower legs and around the mouth
②   Around the mouth and fingernail beds
③   Conjunctiva of the eyes and lower legs
④   Fingernail beds and conjunctiva of the eyes

TEST-TAKING TIP ○ Identify the key word in the stem that sets a priority. Identify the duplicate facts among the options.

11   To reduce anxiety related to the use of oxygen via a nasal cannula, the nurse should say to the patient:
①   "Your doctor ordered this treatment; it is important."
②   "Keep calm because everything will be fine."
③   "This is oxygen; it will help your breathing."
④   "It will be discontinued as soon as possible."

TEST-TAKING TIP ○ Identify the clue in the stem. Identify the option that denies the patient's feelings, concerns, and needs. Identify the option that contains a "clang."

12   A patient has moderate chronic impaired peripheral arterial circulation. The nurse should assess the patient for:
①   Yellow toenails and cool extremities
②   Cyanosis of the feet and yellow toenails
③   Cool extremities and continuous leg discomfort
④   Continuous leg discomfort and cyanosis of the feet

TEST-TAKING TIP ○ Identify the clues in the stem. Identify the duplicate facts among the options. Identify the unique option.

13 A protocol in the post anesthesia care unit is that all patients must have pulse oximetry monitoring. The nurse understands that pulse oximetry monitoring assesses the patient's:

① Heart rate
② Vital signs
③ Blood pressure
④ Oxygen saturation

TEST-TAKING TIP ◉ Identify the clue in the stem.

14 Which individual identified by the nurse is most likely to have life-threatening complications when experiencing a respiratory infection?

① Infant
② Adolescent
③ Older adult
④ School-age child

TEST-TAKING TIP ◉ Identify the key word in the stem that sets a priority.

15 The nurse identifies that the individual that has the most dramatic increase in the need for oxygen is a:

① Pregnant woman
② Person exercising
③ Patient with a fever
④ Patient receiving general anesthesia

TEST-TAKING TIP ◉ Identify the key word in the stem that sets a priority. Identify the clue in the stem.

16 Which intervention is most effective for maintaining a patent airway?

① Active coughing
② Incentive spirometry
③ Nebulizer treatments
④ Abdominal breathing

TEST-TAKING TIP ◉ Identify the key word in the stem that sets a priority.

17 When caring for a patient who is immobile, the nurse should specifically assess for signs of:

① Edema
② Ischemia
③ Orthopnea
④ Hypovolemia

TEST-TAKING TIP ◉ Identify the clues in the stem.

18 The nurse understands that the adequacy of tissue oxygenation is most accurately measured by:

① Hematocrit values
② Hemoglobin levels
③ Arterial blood gases
④ Pulmonary function tests

TEST-TAKING TIP ◉ Identify the key word in the stem that sets a priority. Identify the clue in the stem.

19 The nurse identifies that a patient with an infection has tachypnea. The nurse understands that this occurs because of the:

① Increase in the metabolic rate
② Need to retain carbon dioxide
③ Decrease in carbon dioxide levels
④ Attempt to compensate for respiratory alkalosis

TEST-TAKING TIP ◉ Identify the equally plausible options.

20 A hospitalized patient has difficulty swallowing. What should the nurse do during meals to help prevent this patient from aspirating?
① Allow enough time between spoonfuls for chewing.
② Encourage fluids before swallowing food.
③ Promote conversation during meals.
④ Mix cut up meat with gravy.

21 A patient comes to the emergency department in respiratory distress and the nurse identifies the presence of wheezing breath sounds. The nurse understands that wheezing breath sounds occur when:
① Fluid is in the lung
② Sitting in the orthopneic position
③ Air moves through a narrowed airway
④ Pleural surfaces rub against each other

22 The nurse documents that a patient has Kussmaul respirations when the respirations are:
① Rapid and deep
② Slow and regular
③ Slow and shallow
④ Rapid and irregular

TEST-TAKING TIP ◉ Identify the duplicates in the options. Identify the options that are opposites.

23 The nurse understands that the pathophysiology of anemia is associated with the ability to:
① Transport oxygen
② Exchange oxygen
③ Perfuse oxygen
④ Diffuse oxygen

TEST-TAKING TIP ◉ Identify the unique option.

24 A patient in respiratory distress is coughing excessively. The nurse assesses whether the cough is productive or nonproductive. The nurse understands that a productive cough is one that:
① Causes pain
② Results in sputum
③ Interferes with breathing
④ Gets progressively worse

25 A patient, with the diagnosis of pneumonia, is transferred from the emergency department to a medical unit at 4:30 PM. The patient arrives on a stretcher in the low-Fowler's position. The physician writes the following orders: chest x-ray, sputum for culture and sensitivity, oxygen via nasal cannula at 2 liters per minute, bed rest, regular diet, and ciprofloxacin (Cipro) 400 mg IVPB every 12 hours. In what order should the nurse perform the following activities?
① Obtain vital signs
② Administer the Cipro
③ Order a regular diet dinner
④ Place in the high-Fowler's position
⑤ Obtain sputum for culture and sensitivity
⑥ Begin oxygen via nasal cannula at 2 liters per minute

Answer: _____

Meeting Patients' Oxygen Needs
Answers and Rationales

1 **TEST-TAKING TIP** ○ Options 2 and 3 are equally plausible.
  ① Seeking additional assistance does not reduce the risk of aspiration.
  ② Lowering the height of the feeding bag only slows the rate of the feeding; it does not halt its flow. Continuing the feeding adds a volume of fluid that may be aspirated.
  ③ The administration of an additional volume of feeding may promote aspiration.
  ④ **Shutting off the feeding reduces the risk of aspiration by temporarily halting the administration of an additional volume of feeding.**

2 **TEST-TAKING TIP** ○ The word "initial" is the key word in the stem that sets a priority. Options 2 and 4 are opposites.
  ① This delays meeting the patient's immediate need. The patient's vital signs can be taken later.
  ② **Reducing activity decreases the oxygen demand on the heart; this in turn reduces the pain. After the activity is interrupted, the nurse should obtain the vital signs and conduct a thorough pain assessment.**
  ③ This delays meeting the patient's immediate need. A detailed pain assessment can be done later.
  ④ Walking should be avoided; activity increases the demand on the heart and increases the pain.

3 **TEST-TAKING TIP** ○ The word first is the key word in the stem that sets a priority.
  ① This is not as important as another intervention.
  ② Same as #1.
  ③ **Safety is a priority; patients must understand the rules related to oxygen use and that oxygen supports combustion.**
  ④ This is unnecessary; the nares should be cleaned only with soap and water daily and whenever necessary.

4 **TEST-TAKING TIP** ○ The word first is the key word in the stem that sets a priority. The words "after meals" are the clue in the stem.
  ① A high-Fowler's, not a low-Fowler's, position facilitates food retention by gravity.
  ② Fluids can be easily aspirated by a patient who has difficulty swallowing; fluid intake should be supervised.
  ③ Frequent mouth care provides comfort, but it does not reduce the risk of aspiration.
  ④ **Patients who have difficulty swallowing do not recognize that food can become trapped in the buccal cavity and eventually be aspirated.**

5 **TEST-TAKING TIP** ○ The word "first" is the key word in the stem that sets a priority.
  ① **The abdominal thrust maneuver pushes trapped air out of the lungs, forcing out the obstructing food.**
  ② This may cause aspirated food to lodge deeper in the respiratory passages.
  ③ Attempting to swallow may cause the food to move farther down the respiratory passages.
  ④ Waiting is unsafe because an inability to speak indicates that the person is experiencing a total obstruction. Letting the patient cough is appropriate if there is a partial obstruction.

6 **TEST-TAKING TIP** ○ The word "most" is the key word in the stem that sets a priority. Five adaptations are offered in different combinations for you to choose from as being the most serious in this situation. If you are able to identify one adaptation that appears in two options and that is most serious, you can narrow the choice to two options. If you can identify one adaptation that appears in two options and is least significant, you can eliminate two distractors from consideration.
  ① These are common adaptations of individuals with chronic respiratory disease and are not as serious as another option. Rising slowly permits the circulation to adjust to the change in position, thereby minimizing orthostatic hypotension. Elevating the head helps breathing by lowering the abdominal organs via gravity, which allows the diaphragm to contract more efficiently on inspiration.
  ② These are common adaptations to respiratory disease and are not as serious as another option. Raising the head of the bed helps breathing by lowering the abdominal organs by gravity, which allows the diaphragm to contract more efficiently on inspiration. Wheezing on inspiration is a response to an increase in airway resistance.
  ③ Although mucus tinged with frank red streaks is an uncommon adaptation to respiratory disease, wheezing is a common response.
  ④ **Mucus tinged with frank red streaks is a common response to chronic respiratory disease and chest pain may indicate a pneumothorax; these should be reported immediately.**

7 **TEST-TAKING TIP** ○ The word MOST is the key word in the stem that sets a priority. The word "both" in the stem is a clue. The intervention chosen must increase both circulation and respiration.
  ① The use of a spirometer helps only to prevent respiratory complications.

  ② Repositioning the patient every 2 hours helps prevent fluid from collecting in lung fields, which can contribute to infection and interfere with respiration. Repositioning the patient also relieves pressure and increases activity, thereby promoting circulation.

  ③ Massaging bony prominences with lotion only increases local circulation.

  ④ Coughing and deep breathing only help to prevent respiratory complications.

8 TEST-TAKING TIP ◉ The word "prevent" is a clue in the stem. The word "every" in Options 1 and 4 is a specific determiner.

  ① Fifteen minutes is too long to remove oxygen from a patient who needs oxygen.

  ② Although this is important, it is mainly pressure that causes skin breakdown; oral hygiene alone does not prevent skin breakdown.

  ③ If the cannula comfortably rests in the nares, it avoids pressure on the nares that can cause skin breakdown.

  ④ This prevents pressure ulcers of dependent areas of the body but does not prevent skin breakdown around the nares.

9 TEST-TAKING TIP ◉ The word "initial" is the key word in the stem that sets a priority. Option 4 is unique because it is the only option that is an assessment. Options 1, 2, and 3 are all actions.

  ① The patient is not in respiratory arrest; food is lodged in the respiratory passages.

  ② Abdominal thrusts may be done after it is determined that the patient cannot speak because of a totally obstructed airway.

  ③ Slapping the patient on the back may cause the aspirated object to lodge deeper in the respiratory passages.

  ④ If the patient can speak, the airway is partially obstructed. If the patient cannot speak, the airway is totally obstructed. Assessment is the priority because each of the situations requires a different intervention.

10 TEST-TAKING TIP ◉ The word "most" is the key word in the stem that sets a priority. Four different sites are presented as preferred sites to assess for the presence of cyanosis. If you are able to identify one site that is the least desirable to use for the assessment of cyanosis, you can dismiss two distractors and narrow the choice to two options. If you are able to identify one site that is desirable to use for the assessment of cyanosis, you can narrow the choice to two options.

  ① Although the lips and mucous membranes of the mouth are a primary site to assess for early signs of oxygen deprivation, the lower legs are not the first sites to assess for systemic oxygen deprivation.

  ② Nail beds, lips, and mucous membranes of the mouth are the primary sites to assess for signs of oxygen deprivation.

  ③ Pallor of the conjunctiva of the eyes, not cyanosis, reflects reduced oxyhemoglobin. The lower legs are not the first sites to assess for systemic oxygen deprivation.

  ④ Although the nail beds are a primary site to assess for signs of oxygen deprivation, pallor of the conjunctiva of the eyes, not cyanosis, reflects reduced oxyhemoglobin.

11 TEST-TAKING TIP ◉ The word "reduce" is a clue in the stem. Option 2 denies the patient's feelings because it is false reassurance. The use of the word "oxygen" in the stem and option 3 is a clang association.

  ① This statement does not address the fact that patients have a right to know what is being done and why.

  ② This statement is false reassurance and minimizes the patient's concerns.

  ③ This statement provides information and an explanation; this generally reduces fear and increases understanding and compliance. Oxygen therapy generally helps patients breathe more easily, and therefore the statement is not false reassurance.

  ④ This statement may intensify fear if the oxygen is not discontinued; also, it does not provide an explanation.

12 TEST-TAKING TIP ◉ The words "moderate chronic" and "peripheral arterial" are the clues in the stem. Four different adaptations are offered as common responses to prolonged impaired peripheral arterial circulation. If you are able to identify one adaptation that is common to this situation, you can narrow the choice to two options. If you are able to identify one response that is unrelated to prolonged impaired peripheral arterial circulation, you can eliminate two distractors and narrow the choice to two options. Option 1 is the only option that begins with the letter "Y."

  ① Yellow toenails and cool extremities both indicate impaired arterial circulation; there is a decrease in oxygen and nutrients to the area.

  ② Although yellow toenails indicate prolonged tissue hypoxia of the extremity, it is ascending pallor from the toes and descending rubor from the knees, not cyanosis, that reflect impaired peripheral arterial perfusion.

  ③ Although cool extremities reflect inadequate peripheral arterial perfusion, leg pain on activity (intermittent claudication), not continuous leg discomfort, is a clinical manifestation of chronic peripheral arterial disease.

  ④ Leg discomfort related to decreased peripheral arterial perfusion is usually intermittent and associated with activity (intermittent claudication). Pallor ascending from the toes and rubor descending from the knees, not cyanosis, reflect moderate chronic impaired peripheral arterial perfusion.

13 **TEST-TAKING TIP** ○ The "ox" in "oximetry" is a clue in the stem because it is similar to the word "oxygen" in Option 4. Both words begin with the letters "ox."
① The heart rate is obtained by palpating a peripheral pulse or auscultating the apical pulse.
② Temperature is measured by a thermometer, pulse by palpation, respirations by observation, and blood pressure by a sphygmomanometer.
③ Blood pressure is measured by a sphygmomanometer.
④ **Oxygen saturation via pulse oximetry measures the degree to which hemoglobin is saturated with oxygen; it provides some indication of the efficiency of lung ventilation.**

14 **TEST-TAKING TIP** ○ The word "most" is the key word in the stem that sets a priority.
① **Because of the small lumens of their respiratory passages, infants and toddlers are at serious risk for airway obstruction, which can develop as a result of respiratory tract infection.**
② Healthy adolescents usually do not encounter any serious event in response to respiratory infections.
③ Although the respiratory system undergoes changes during the aging process and there is a decline in respiratory function, complications related to infection usually are not as acute, sudden, or life threatening as an age group in another option.
④ Healthy school-age children usually do not encounter any serious event in response to respiratory infections; however, school-age children generally have respiratory infections more frequently because of exposure to other children.

15 **TEST-TAKING TIP** ○ The word "most" is the key word in the stem that sets a priority. The words "dramatic increase" are the clue in the stem.
① Although a pregnant woman's metabolic rate is increased, pregnancy does not place as high a demand on the body's need for oxygen as a factor in another option.
② **Most exercise dramatically increases the metabolic rate, which, in turn, increases the body's demand for oxygen.**
③ A fever causes an increase in a person's metabolic rate; however, a fever does not place as high a demand on the body's need for oxygen as a factor in another option.
④ General anesthesia relaxes the muscles of the body; and when muscles are relaxed, the metabolic rate decreases and the demand for oxygen also decreases.

16 **TEST-TAKING TIP** ○ The word "most" is the key word in the stem that sets a priority.
① **A cough forcefully expels air from the lungs and is an effective self-protective reflex to clear the trachea and bronchi of secretions.**
② An incentive spirometer is a device used to encourage voluntary deep breathing, not to clear an airway; it is used to prevent or treat atelectasis.
③ A nebulizer treatment does not clear an airway; it adds moisture or medication to inspired air to alter the tracheobronchial mucosa. After the respiratory passages are dilated or mucolytic agents have reduced the viscosity of secretions, the patient can cough more productively.
④ Abdominal breathing does not clear the air passages. It helps to decrease air trapping and reduce the work of breathing.

17 **TEST-TAKING TIP** ○ The words "immobile" and "specifically" are the clues in the stem.
① Edema is fluid in the interstitial compartment and is not specifically an adaptation to pressure.
② **Ischemia is a lack of blood supply to a body part (tissue ischemia) and is directly related to pressure, which can occlude blood vessels.**
③ Orthopnea is the ability to breathe only in an upright position, such as sitting or standing, and is not a local adaptation to pressure.
④ Hypovolemia is a reduction in blood volume and is not a local adaptation to pressure.

18 **TEST-TAKING TIP** ○ The word "most" is the key word in the stem that sets a priority. The word "accurately" is a clue in the stem.
① Although the hematocrit is the percentage of red blood cell mass in proportion to whole blood, it is not an accurate test for adequacy of tissue oxygenation; a low hematocrit may indicate possible water intoxication, and an elevated hematocrit may indicate dehydration.
② Although hemoglobin is the red pigment in red blood cells that carries oxygen, it is not an accurate test for adequacy of tissue oxygenation; a low hemoglobin is evidence of iron-deficiency anemia or bleeding.
③ **Arterial blood gases include the levels of oxygen, carbon dioxide, bicarbonate, and pH. Blood gases determine the adequacy of alveolar gas exchange and the ability of the lungs and kidneys to maintain the acid-base balance of body fluids.**
④ Pulmonary function tests measure lung volume and capacity; although these are valuable data, they do not provide specific data about tissue oxygenation.

19 **TEST-TAKING TIP** ○ Options 2 and 3 are equally plausible.
① **Because of the energy required to "fight" an infection, the basal metabolic rate increases, resulting in an increased respiratory rate.**
② The body has a need to exhale, not retain, carbon dioxide.
③ Tachypnea occurs in the presence of elevated levels of carbon dioxide and carbonic acid, not decreased carbon dioxide levels.
④ The patient with an infection is more likely to be in metabolic acidosis; tachypnea that progresses to hyperventilation causes respiratory alkalosis.

20 ① **Well-chewed food is broken down and mixed with saliva, forming a bolus of food; a bolus of food that is well chewed is easier to swallow causing less risk for aspiration.**
② Fluids before swallowing can flush food into the breathing passages rather than down the esophagus.
③ Talking while eating can increase the risk for aspiration. People should not talk with food in their mouths; people need to inhale before talking and this action may cause aspiration of food when food is in the mouth.
④ The patient has no difficulty chewing; food does not need to be cut up as long as the patient has the time to chew the food adequately before attempting to swallow.

21 ① Sounds caused by fluid in the alveoli of the lung are called *crackles* or *rales* and sounds caused by fluid or resistance in the bronchi of the lung are called *rhonchi* or *gurgles*.
② Positioning is unrelated to *adventitious sounds* (abnormal breath sounds).
③ ***Wheezes* occur as air passes through airways narrowed by secretions, edema, or tumors; these high-pitched squeaky musical sounds are best heard on expiration and are not usually changed by coughing.**
④ A *pleural friction rub* is a superficial grating sound heard particularly at the height of inspiration and not relieved by coughing; it is caused by the rubbing together of inflamed pleural surfaces.

22 **TEST-TAKING TIP** ○ This question focuses on the characteristics of respirations: rate, depth, and rhythm. If you know that Kussmaul respirations are rapid, Options 2 and 3 can be eliminated. Options 1 and 3 are opposites and Options 2 and 4 are opposites; consider these options in relation to each other.
① **Kussmaul respirations are rapid, deep, and regular; they are the body's effort to correct metabolic acidosis by blowing off excess carbon dioxide.**
② Slow (less than 12 breaths per minute), regular respirations are called bradypnea.
③ Slow respirations are called bradypnea. Biot's respiration and Cheyne-Stokes respiration have shallow breaths as part of their characteristics.
④ Rapid and irregular respiration is characteristic of Cheyne-Stokes respiration. The breathing cycle begins with shallow breaths that gradually increase to an abnormal depth and rate, and then the breaths gradually become slower and more shallow until there is a period of apnea, and then the cycle begins again.

23 **TEST-TAKING TIP** ○ The words *exchange, perfuse,* and *diffuse* all relate to actions that occur at particular sites within the body. The word *transport* refers to the movement of something from one place to another. The identification of Option 1 as the unique option was difficult because the interrelationship of these words was more obscure than most.
① **The hemoglobin portion of red blood cells carries oxygen from the alveolar capillaries in the lungs to distant tissue sites.**
② Exchange occurs in the capillary beds of the alveoli via the process of diffusion; this is unrelated to anemia.
③ Perfusion relates to the extent of inflow and outflow of air between the alveoli and pulmonary capillaries or the extent of blood flow to the pulmonary capillary bed; perfusion is not related to red blood cell levels.
④ Diffusion occurs at the alveolar capillary beds and is not related to anemia.

24 ① A productive cough may or may not produce pain, depending on the patient's underlying condition.
② **A productive cough is a cough accompanied by expectorated secretions. When a patient raises respiratory secretions and expectorates them, breathing usually improves.**
③ Although coughing does interfere with breathing, this is not the definition of a productive cough.
④ When a cough is productive, it does not indicate that it is progressive.

25 Answer: 4, 6, 1, 5, 2, 3.
④ **Place in the high-Fowler's position. The patient's respiratory status should be supported initially and then the other orders can be implemented in order of importance. The high-Fowler's position allows the abdominal organs to drop by gravity which promotes expansion of the thorax on inhalation.**
⑥ **Begin oxygen via nasal cannula at 2 liters per minute. The administration of exogenous oxygen increases the amount of oxygen being delivered to the alveoli.**
① **Obtain vital signs. Obtaining the vital signs collects information that provides critical baseline information about the patient. The time it takes to obtain the vital signs may compromise the patient's respiratory**

status and should be done after raising the head of the bed and administering oxygen. This follows the ABCs (Airway, Breathing, Circulation) of meeting a patient's basic needs.

(5) Obtain sputum for culture and sensitivity. After the patient's respiratory status is supported and assessed, then the sputum can be collected for the culture and sensitivity test. This specimen should be collected before the administration of any antibiotic that may alter test results.

(2) Administer the Cipro. Administering the Cipro after the sputum specimen is obtained prevents any erroneous test results.

(3) Order a regular diet dinner. Finally, the regular diet can be ordered; this is the least critical intervention for this patient.

Administration of Medications

• • •

This section includes questions related to the principles associated with the administration of medications via the oral, parenteral (intravenous, intramuscular, intradermal, and subcutaneous injections), topical, ear, eye, vaginal, and rectal routes. The questions focus on allergies, untoward effects, toxic effects, developmental considerations associated with medications, the Z-track method, peak and trough levels of medications, pain assessment before administering medication for pain, and computation of dosage.

Questions

Please fill in the circle to mark your answer choice.

1 Before administering a medication that is teratogenic, the nurse should ask the patient:
   ① "Have you ever had an anaphylactic reaction?"
   ② "Were you ever addicted to drugs?"
   ③ "Do you have any allergies?"
   ④ "Are you pregnant?"
   TEST-TAKING TIP ⊙ Identify the equally plausible options. Identify the unique option.

2 Which statement indicates to the nurse that the patient needs further teaching regarding care of the eyes and eye medications?
   ① "Excess medication on the eyelid can be wiped away."
   ② "I should gaze downward while instilling the eye drops."
   ③ "I should place one drop of the medication inside my lower eyelid."
   ④ "The risk of transmitting infection from one eye to the other is high."
   TEST-TAKING TIP ⊙ Identify the key word in the stem that indicates negative polarity.

3 The nurse changes the needle after drawing up the required dosage of a caustic drug. This is done primarily because the needle is:
   ① Too long for the required route
   ② Coated with the medication
   ③ No longer sterile
   ④ Not sharp
   TEST-TAKING TIP ⊙ Identify the key word in the stem that sets a priority. Identify the unique option.

4 The nurse must administer a 2-mL intramuscular injection to an adult patient who is in severe pain and lying in the supine position. The muscle that is the safest and most therapeutic is the:
   ① Deltoid
   ② Dorsogluteal
   ③ Ventrogluteal
   ④ Vastus lateralis
   TEST-TAKING TIP ⊙ Identify the key word in the stem that sets a priority. Identify the equally plausible options. Identify the clue in the stem.

5 When using an insulin syringe with a ½ inch needle to administer insulin, the nurse should insert the needle at an angle of:
   ① 30 degrees
   ② 45 degrees
   ③ 90 degrees
   ④ 180 degrees
   TEST-TAKING TIP ⊙ Identify the clue in the stem.

6 The nurse is administering oral medications to children. The nurse understands that the MOST important factor to consider is their:

① Age
② Weight
③ Level of anxiety
④ Developmental level

TEST-TAKING TIP ◉ Identify the key word in the stem that sets a priority. Identify the clue in the stem.

7 The physician orders ear drops for an adult patient. When instilling ear drops into the patient's ear, the nurse should:

① Press a cotton ball gently into the ear canal
② Pull the pinna of the ear upward and backward
③ Tug the pinna of the ear downward and backward
④ Hold the dropper approximately two inches above the canal

TEST-TAKING TIP ◉ Identify the clue in the stem. Identify the options that are opposites.

8 The nurse teaches a patient to self-administer eye drops. The nurse identifies that further teaching is needed when the patient says, "I should:

① Wipe my eye moving from the outer corner toward my nose."
② Hold the eyedropper about a half inch above my eye."
③ Close my eyes after putting the drops in my eyes."
④ Put the fluid in a pocket in the lower lid."

TEST-TAKING TIP ◉ Identify the key word in the stem that indicates negative polarity.

9 A patient is receiving an intravenous piggyback medication every 4 hours. Because the medication has a narrow therapeutic window, the physician orders a peak blood level. The nurse should plan to obtain a blood specimen:

① Halfway between two scheduled doses
② Three hours after administering a dose
③ One hour before administering a dose
④ One hour after administering a dose

TEST-TAKING TIP ◉ Identify the options that are opposites. Identify the options that are equally plausible.

10 Blood appears at the hub of the needle while the nurse is aspirating an intramuscular injection. The nurse should:

① Remove the syringe and attach a new needle
② Discard the syringe and prepare a new injection
③ Interrupt the procedure and notify the physician
④ Withdraw the needle slightly and inject the solution

TEST-TAKING TIP ◉ Identify the options that are opposites.

11 Besides inhibiting microbial growth, an antibiotic may also depress the bone marrow. The nurse understands that this response is classified as:

① An overdose
② A side effect
③ An habituation
④ An idiosyncratic effect

TEST-TAKING TIP ◉ Identify the unique option.

12 Because of the physiologic changes associated with aging, when administering drugs to older adults, the nurse should specifically assess for signs of:

① Toxicity
② Side effects

③ Drug interactions
④ Allergic reactions

TEST-TAKING TIP ○ Identify the clue in the stem.

13 Which route of administration is used only for its local therapeutic effect?
① Rectum
② Skin
③ Nose
④ Eye

TEST-TAKING TIP ○ Identify the clues in the stem.

14 The nurse plans to inject an intravenous medication via an existing intravenous line. What should the nurse do first?
① Select the port closest to the needle entry site.
② Pinch the tubing above the port being used.
③ Determine patency of the intravenous line.
④ Clean the injection port with an antiseptic.

TEST-TAKING TIP ○ Identify the key word in the stem that sets a priority.

15 The nurse is filling a syringe with medication from a multidose vial. What should the nurse do?
① Keep the needle above the level of the liquid and maintain sterile technique.
② Keep the needle below the level of the liquid and change the needle after withdrawing the solution.
③ Keep the needle below the level of the liquid and record the date and time on the vial when opened.
④ Keep the needle above the level of the liquid and inject air at 1.5 times the volume of the ordered dose.

TEST-TAKING TIP ○ Identify the duplicate facts among the options.

16 When administering an intradermal injection, the nurse understands that the patient is at the highest risk for exhibiting an:
① Overdose
② Allergic response
③ Idiosyncratic reaction
④ Interaction with other drugs

TEST-TAKING TIP ○ Identify the key word in the stem that sets a priority. Identify the clue in the stem.

17 The nurse is administering an oral medication to a patient. To best protect the patient from aspirating, the nurse should:
① Offer extra water
② Crush the medication
③ Position the patient in a sitting position
④ Inspect the mouth after the patient swallows

TEST-TAKING TIP ○ Identify the key word in the stem that sets a priority.

18 The nurse is preparing to instill a vaginal cream. What position should the nurse instruct the patient to assume?
① Dorsal recumbent position
② Low-Fowler's position
③ Left-lateral position
④ Supine position

19 The nurse evaluates that a mother correctly administered nose drops to her child when she:
① Told her child to sniff the medication into the lungs
② Allowed her child to sit upright after its administration
③ Put the remaining fluid in the dropper back into the bottle
④ Held the dropper slightly above the nares during instillation

TEST-TAKING TIP ○ Identify the clue in the stem.

20 The nurse recognizes that the most dangerous method of administering medication is via:
① Intravenous push
② Piggyback infusion
③ Subcutaneous injection
④ Intramuscular injection
TEST-TAKING TIP ◉ Identify the key word in the stem that sets a priority.

21 The nurse is administering medication via the Z-track injection method. Which action is unique to this procedure?
① The skin is pulled laterally before needle insertion.
② An air lock is established behind the bolus of medication.
③ The injection sites are rotated along a "Z" on the abdomen.
④ A "Z" is formed when dividing the buttocks into quadrants.
TEST-TAKING TIP ◉ Identify the clues in the stem.

22 Which route is considered to be the most accurate and safe when administering medications?
① Topical
② By mouth
③ Intravenous
④ Via injection
TEST-TAKING TIP ◉ Identify the key word in the stem that sets a priority. Identify the clues in the stem.

23 The physician orders peak and trough levels to monitor an antibiotic. To measure trough levels, the nurse should plan for a blood specimen to be drawn:
① First thing in the morning
② Halfway between scheduled doses
③ A half hour before a scheduled dose
④ A half hour after drug administration
TEST-TAKING TIP ◉ Identify the clue in the stem. Identify the options that are opposites.

24 Via what area should the nurse administer a medication in the form of a troche?
① Rectal route
② Buccal cavity
③ Vaginal vault
④ Auditory canal

25 The nurse understands that a transdermal patch for delivery of an analgesic is most effective because it:
① Has an immediate systemic effect
② Affects only the area covered by the patch
③ Releases controlled amounts of medication over time
④ Produces fewer side effects than other routes of administration
TEST-TAKING TIP ◉ Identify the key word in the stem that sets a priority. Identify the options that are opposites. Identify the specific determiner.

26 Which site should the nurse use for a subcutaneous injection to ensure its most rapid absorption?
① Abdomen
② Buttock
③ Thigh
④ Arm
TEST-TAKING TIP ◉ Identify the key word in the stem that sets a priority.

27 The physician orders a medication for an infant that must be administered via an intramuscular injection. What site is the best choice for the nurse to administer the injection?
① Deltoid
② Dorsogluteal

③ Ventrogluteal
④ Rectus femoris

TEST-TAKING TIP ○ Identify the key word in the stem that sets a priority. Identify the unique option.

28 The nurse plans to administer a medication via an intramuscular injection to an obese patient. The nurse understands that the least desirable site for an intramuscular injection in an obese adult is the:

① Vastus lateralis
② Rectus femoris
③ Dorsogluteal
④ Deltoid

TEST-TAKING TIP ○ Identify the word in the stem that indicates negative polarity.

29 Which route of delivery for medication should be questioned by the nurse if the patient is an older adult who is cachectic?

① Intradermal
② Intravenous
③ Subcutaneous
④ Intramuscular

TEST-TAKING TIP ○ Identify the unique option.

30 The physician orders ibuprofen 400 mg po twice a day. On hand is ibuprofen 200 mg per tablet. How many tablets should the nurse administer?

Answer: _____ **Tablets.**

Administration of Medications
Answers and Rationales

1   TEST-TAKING TIP ○ Options 1 and 3 are equally plausible. Option 4 is unique. Options 1, 2, and 3 discuss situations that relate to "prior" drug use.
(1) This question is unrelated to the concept of teratogenic. An anaphylactic reaction is a severe, systemic hypersensitivity to a drug, food, or chemical.
(2) This question is unrelated to the concept of teratogenic. Drug addiction refers to an uncontrollable craving for a chemical substance because of a physical or psychologic dependence.
(3) This question is unrelated to the concept of teratogenic. Allergies are unpredictable hypersensitive reactions to allergens such as drugs.
(4) **"Teratogenic," when used in the context of medication, refers to a drug that can cause adverse effects in a fetus or an embryo.**

2   TEST-TAKING TIP ○ The word "further" is the key word in the stem that indicates negative polarity. The correct answer is the option that is "not" an acceptable action when administering eye drops.
(1) Excess medication is unneeded and can be wiped away; also, it promotes comfort.
(2) **The reverse is true; gazing upward moves the cornea upward and away from the conjunctival sac where the medication is to be instilled.**
(3) The conjunctival sac, the correct location to instill eye drops, is inside the lower eyelid.
(4) Eye infections can be easily transmitted from one eye to the other; however, it must be stressed that if aseptic principles are followed, cross-infection can be minimized.

3   TEST-TAKING TIP ○ The word "primarily" is the key word in the stem that sets a priority. Option 2 is unique. Options 1, 3, and 4 are all negative statements. In Option 1, "too long" indicates that the needle is "not" the correct length.
(1) Any size needle can be used to draw up a caustic medication.
(2) **Changing to a new needle prevents tracking the medication through the subcutaneous tissue and skin.**
(3) If all of the principles of sterile technique are followed when preparing an injection, the needle is still considered sterile.
(4) Most needles are made of stainless steel with a beveled tip that makes them sharp; they do not need to be replaced due to dullness after drawing up medication because they remain sharp.

4   TEST-TAKING TIP ○ The word "most" is the key word in the stem that sets a priority. Options 2 and 3 are equally plausible because they both require repositioning the patient. The word "safest" is a clue in the stem.
(1) The deltoid is not well developed in many adults and children. The radial and ulnar nerves and brachial artery lie in the upper arm along the humerus. The deltoid should not be used for intramuscular injections unless other sites are unavailable.
(2) To access the dorsogluteal, the patient should be repositioned, which may increase pain. Historically, the dorsogluteal was the preferred site for an intramuscular injection; however, there is a higher risk of hitting the sciatic nerve, blood vessels, or greater trochanter. Hitting the sciatic nerve can cause partial or permanent paralysis of the leg.
(3) To access the ventrogluteal, the patient should be repositioned, which may increase pain. The ventrogluteal is the preferred site after the vastus lateralis; it is safe to use in cachectic patients and children older than 18 months.
(4) **The vastus lateralis is the preferred site for this patient because this muscle has no major nearby nerves and blood vessels and absorbs drugs rapidly. In addition, using this muscle does not require the patient, who is in pain, to be moved and repositioned.**

5   TEST-TAKING TIP ○ The words "½ inch needle" are a clue in the stem.
(1) A 30-degree angle is too shallow an angle for a subcutaneous injection.
(2) A 45-degree angle is too shallow for the administration of a subcutaneous injection with a needle that is only ½ inch long. A 45-degree angle is appropriate if the needle is ⅝ inch or 1 inch long.
(3) **A 90-degree angle is appropriate for a subcutaneous injection with a ½ inch needle; it injects the insulin into the loose connective tissue under the dermis.**
(4) To use a 180-degree angle for any injection is impossible. Various injection methods are from 15 degrees to 90 degrees, not 180 degrees.

6   TEST-TAKING TIP ○ The word MOST is the key word in the stem that sets a priority. The word "children" is a clue in the stem.
(1) Age is not reliable for calculating a pediatric dose of medication.
(2) **Children's body sizes are different, necessitating calculation of drug dosage by weight, rather than by age or developmental level. Weight is an objective, specific, and accurate way to calculate appropriate medication dosages for children.**

(3) Level of anxiety does not influence calculation of dosage of medication for a child.

(4) Developmental level does not influence calculation of dosage of medication for a child.

7 TEST-TAKING TIP ☉ The word "adult" is a clue in the stem. Options 2 and 3 are opposites.

(1) A cotton ball may be placed in the outermost part of the ear; it should not be pressed into the canal.

(2) **Pulling the pinna of the ear upward and backward straightens the ear canal of an adult. This action facilitates the distribution of the medication into the external ear canal.**

(3) The pinna of the ear should be pulled downward and backward to straighten the ear canal of a child less than 3 years of age, not an adult.

(4) The force exerted by a drop falling from the height of 2 inches can injure the eardrum. The dropper should be held ½ inch (1 cm) above the ear canal, and the drop should fall against the wall of the canal and then flow toward the eardrum.

8 TEST-TAKING TIP ☉ The word "further" is the key word in the stem that indicates negative polarity.

(1) **The eye should be wiped moving from the inner to the outer canthus; this promotes comfort, prevents trauma, and moves excess medication away from the nasolacrimal duct, minimizing systemic absorption and infection.**

(2) It is desirable to hold the dropper ½ to ¾ inch above the conjunctival sac. Holding it higher could injure the eye because of the force exerted by the drop; holding it lower increases the risk of contaminating the dropper or injuring the eye.

(3) Closing the eyes after administering eye drops is acceptable because it distributes the medication across the eye.

(4) This is appropriate because it permits the medication to remain in the eye and promotes an even distribution of the medication.

9 TEST-TAKING TIP ☉ Option 4 is opposite to both options 2 and 3. Options 2 and 3 are equally plausible because they are both one hour before administering a dose.

(1) A blood level specimen taken halfway between two scheduled doses will not provide an accurate result when testing for a peak blood level since most medications administered every 4 hours have a peak concentration about 1 hour after administration.

(2) A blood test taken 3 hours after administering a dose that is given every 4 hours will not provide an accurate peak blood level. A blood level 3 hours after administration of a drug given every 4 hours provides information about a trough level.

(3) A blood specimen taken one hour before administering a dose will not provide an accurate peak blood level. A blood level done at this time measures a trough level.

(4) **Most medications administered every 4 hours have a peak concentration about 1 hour after administration.**

10 TEST-TAKING TIP ☉ Options 2 and 4 are opposites.

(1) Removing the syringe and attaching a new needle is unsafe; the fluid in the syringe is contaminated.

(2) **The equipment should be discarded because a small vessel was pierced and the fluid and needle are contaminated. A new sterile syringe and medication should be prepared.**

(3) It is unnecessary to notify the physician.

(4) This is unsafe; the fluid in the syringe is contaminated.

11 TEST-TAKING TIP ☉ Option 2 is unique because it begins with the word "A" rather than "An." Options 1, 3, and 4 all begin with the word "An."

(1) An overdose occurs when a person receives a dose larger than the usual recommended dose; this is rarely planned and is usually an accident.

(2) **A side effect is a secondary effect; side effects can be harmless or can cause injury; if injurious, the drug is discontinued.**

(3) Habituation is an acquired tolerance from continued exposure to a substance.

(4) An idiosyncratic effect is an unexpected effect; it can be an overreaction, an underreaction, or an unusual reaction.

12 TEST-TAKING TIP ☉ The words "older adults" are the clue in the stem.

(1) **Biotransformation of drugs is less efficient in older adults than during younger developmental ages; when drugs are not fully metabolized, degraded, or excreted, toxic levels can accumulate.**

(2) Harmless or injurious side effects (secondary effects) are common to people of all ages, not just older adults.

(3) Drug interactions are common to people of all ages, not just older adults.

(4) Allergic reactions are common to people of all ages, not just older adults.

13 TEST-TAKING TIP ☉ The words "only" and "local" are the clues in the stem.

(1) Medication can be administered via the rectum for either a local or systemic effect; medications can be absorbed through the rich vascular bed in the mucous membranes.

(2) Medications can be administered via the skin for either a local or systemic effect.

(3) Medication can be administered via the nose for either a local or systemic effect.

(4) **Medications are instilled into the eye only for their local effect; part of the procedure for instillation of eye drops is to apply gentle pressure to the nasolacrimal duct for 10 to 15 seconds to prevent absorption of the medication into the systemic circulation.**

14 TEST-TAKING TIP ○ The word "first" is the key word in the stem that sets a priority.

(1) Selecting the port closest to the needle entry site is not the priority; it will be done later in the procedure.

(2) Pinching the tubing above the port being used is not the priority.

(3) **For medication to enter a vein, the intravenous line must be unobstructed; therefore, the nurse should determine the patency of the intravenous line. The nurse must also ensure that the medication is administered into a vein, not into subcutaneous tissue.**

(4) Cleaning the injection port is not the priority.

15 TEST-TAKING TIP ○ Options 1 and 4 contain a duplicate fact, and Options 2 and 3 contain a duplicate fact. If you know whether a needle should be kept above or below the level of fluid in a vial, you can reduce your final selection to two options.

(1) Although sterile technique should be maintained, the bevel of the needle should be kept below the level of the fluid to prevent the syringe from filling with air.

(2) Although the bevel of the needle should be kept below the level of the fluid, changing the needle is unnecessary. The needle needs to be changed only when the solution is caustic to tissues.

(3) **The bevel of the needle must be kept below the level of the fluid to prevent air from entering the syringe. Once opened, medications should be marked with the date and time of opening since medications generally have a recommended period of viability before they should be discarded.**

(4) The bevel of the needle should be kept below the level of the fluid or the syringe fills with air. The amount of air injected into the vial should equal the amount of solution to be withdrawn; extra air will result in excessive pressure within the closed space of the vial.

16 TEST-TAKING TIP ○ The word "highest" is the key word in the stem that sets a priority. The word "intradermal" is a clue in the stem.

(1) Overdoses are a risk with all types of injections, but the highest risk of overdose is via the intravenous, not the intradermal, route.

(2) **An intradermal injection is given under the skin to test for such things as tuberculosis and allergies; these drugs can cause an anaphylactic reaction if absorbed by the circulation too quickly or if the person has a hypersensitivity to the solution.**

(3) Idiosyncratic reactions are unpredictable effects; they are usually underreactions, overreactions, or reactions that are different from the expected reaction. Idiosyncratic reactions are less likely to occur than allergic reactions with intradermal injections.

(4) A drug interaction occurs when one drug alters the action of another drug; this is not a possible response to a singular intradermal injection.

17 TEST-TAKING TIP ○ The word "best" is the key word in the stem that sets a priority.

(1) Excessive water may promote aspiration.

(2) Although crushing the medication helps some people, it is not the consistency of medication but rather the amount of water taken with the medication that can promote aspiration. Also, multiple crushed particles taken with water can stimulate the gag reflex; crushed medications should be mixed in a soft food such as applesauce to increase safety.

(3) **The sitting position allows the patient to control the flow of fluid to the back of the oropharynx as well as promote the flow of fluid down the esophagus via gravity.**

(4) Inspecting the mouth is important after a patient swallows mediation, not when administering medication.

18 (1) **The dorsal recumbent position allows easy access to and exposure of the vaginal orifice. Lying in this position for 10 minutes after the administration of the vaginal cream prevents its drainage from the vaginal canal.**

(2) The low-Fowler's position does not thoroughly expose the vaginal orifice.

(3) The left-lateral position does not thoroughly expose the vaginal orifice. This position is used for the administration of enemas and rectal suppositories.

(4) The supine position does not expose the vaginal orifice.

19 TEST-TAKING TIP ○ The word "correctly" in the stem is a clue.

(1) Sniffing the medication is contraindicated because sniffing pulls the medication to the oropharynx, where it will be swallowed rather than inhaled into the upper respiratory tract. Nose drops should be directed toward the midline of the superior concha of the ethmoid bone as the patient breathes through the mouth.

(2) Sitting upright after administering nose drops is contraindicated because sitting up allows the fluid to drain from the nares rather than be inhaled into the upper respiratory tract. The patient should remain 1 minute with the head and neck hyperextended.

(3) Returning the remaining fluid in the dropper to the bottle is a violation of medical asepsis.

(4) **Holding the dropper approximately a half inch above the nares prevents touching the patient, which maintains cleanliness of the dropper; a half inch above the nares is not too high to cause trauma to the tissue by the falling drop.**

20 **TEST-TAKING TIP** ○ The word "most" is the key word in the stem that sets a priority.

(1) **An IV push or bolus administration of medication is the instillation of a medication directly into a vein; this rapid administration of an entire dose of medication places the patient at highest risk for adverse effects.**

(2) Although an intravenous piggyback is a dangerous route, the medication is diluted and it is infused over a longer time period than in an IV push.

(3) A solution injected into subcutaneous tissue or a muscle is absorbed over a longer period of time than an IV push.

(4) Same as #3.

21 **TEST-TAKING TIP** ○ The words "unique" and "Z-track" are clues in the stem. Be careful when assessing clang associations. In this question, Options 3 and 4 are distractors, even though they have a clang association with the "Z" in the stem.

(1) **The "Z" in the Z-track method refers to pulling the skin to the side before and during an intramuscular injection. This technique alters the position of skin layers so that after the skin is released and the needle is removed, the injected fluid is kept within the muscle tissues and does not rise in the needle tract, which can irritate subcutaneous tissues.**

(2) The air-lock technique also can be done with intramuscular injections. When air is injected behind the medication, the air clears the needle of medication. This technique is controversial and is being researched for evidenced-based practice.

(3) An intramuscular site, preferably the dorsogluteal, is used for Z-track, not the abdomen, which is used for subcutaneous injections.

(4) The buttocks are not divided by a "Z." When the buttocks (dorsogluteal) are used for intramuscular injections, the usual bony landmarks must be used to identify the correct insertion site.

22 **TEST-TAKING TIP** ○ The word "most" is the key word in the stem that sets a priority. The words "accurate" and "safe" are clues in the stem.

(1) Because absorption is affected by a variety of factors, such as the extent of the capillary network and condition of the skin, the topical route is not the most accurate method of administration.

(2) **Using the oral route is the safest way to administer medication because it is convenient, it does not require piercing the skin, it usually does not cause physical or emotional stress, and the medication is absorbed slowly.**

(3) The intravenous route carries the highest risk because a needle enters the skin and the medication is injected directly into the bloodstream.

(4) An injection carries a higher risk than medication administered via many other routes because the medication is rapidly absorbed and a needle enters the skin.

23 **TEST-TAKING TIP** ○ The word "trough" is a clue in the stem. Options 3 and 4 are opposites.

(1) The peak and trough of a blood plasma level depend on the time the last dose was administered.

(2) Halfway between scheduled doses will not be a time period when a drug is at its lowest concentration in the blood.

(3) **"Trough level" refers to when a drug is at its lowest concentration in the blood in response to biotransformation; this usually occurs during the time period just before the next scheduled dose.**

(4) Many variables affect the time when a drug reaches its peak plasma level within an individual; however, a half hour after the administration of an antibiotic, one can safely plot the antibiotic plasma level on the rising side of the curve of the plasma level profile, not within the trough.

24 (1) A suppository is designed for administering medication into the rectum.

(2) **A troche (lozenge) is placed in the space between the upper or lower molar teeth and gums (buccal cavity) so that it can dissolve and release medication.**

(3) A suppository, solution, or cream can be delivered to the vaginal vault by a vaginal applicator.

(4) Medication in a suspension can be administered via a dropper into the auditory canal.

25 **TEST-TAKING TIP** ○ The word "most" in the stem sets a priority. Options 1 and 2 are opposites and need to be considered carefully. The word "only" in Option 2 is a specific determiner.

(1) The systemic effect depends on the amount of time it takes for the drug to be absorbed through the skin; this takes longer than parenteral routes.

(2) Transdermal disks or patches deliver medications that produce systemic effects.

(3) **Transdermal disks or patches have semipermeable membranes that allow medication to be absorbed through the skin slowly over a long period of time (usually 24 to 72 hours).**

(4) The medication, not the route of delivery, produces side effects.

26 **TEST-TAKING TIP** ○ The word "most" in the stem sets a priority.

(1) **Medication injected into the abdomen is more rapidly absorbed than medication injected into the limbs of the body.**

(2) Medication injected into the buttocks is absorbed at a slower rate than medication injected into the abdomen.

(3) Medication injected into the thigh is absorbed at the slowest rate.

(4) Medication injected into the arm is absorbed at a slower rate than medication injected into the abdomen.

27 **TEST-TAKING TIP** ○ The word "best" in the stem sets a priority. Option 4 is unique because it is the only option with two words.

(1) The deltoid is contraindicated for intramuscular injections in infants and children. This site has a small amount of muscle mass and little subcutaneous fat, and it lies close to the radial nerve and brachial artery.

(2) The dorsogluteal muscle is contraindicated for an intramuscular injection in children younger than 18 months of age because the muscle mass is inadequate to allow a safe injection. Also, the sciatic nerve and gluteal artery lie close to the site.

(3) An infant or toddler should not receive an intramuscular injection into the ventrogluteal muscle; the muscle is not well developed until the child begins to walk.

(4) **The rectus femoris muscle, which belongs to the quadriceps muscle group, is the site of choice for intramuscular injections in infants and children. It is the largest and most well-developed muscle in infants, is easy to locate, and is away from major blood vessels and nerves.**

28 **TEST-TAKING TIP** ○ The word "least" in the stem indicates negative polarity.

(1) The vastus lateralis site is appropriate for an intramuscular injection in an obese individual as long as the amount of fluid injected is 3 mL or less.

(2) The rectus femoris is an appropriate site for an intramuscular injection in an obese individual as long as the amount of fluid injected is 3 mL or less.

(3) **The dorsogluteal muscle has a thick fat layer, and an intramuscular injection will deposit the medication into subcutaneous tissue.**

(4) The deltoid is an appropriate muscle for an intramuscular injection in an obese individual as long as the amount of fluid injected is 2 mL or less.

29 **TEST-TAKING TIP** ○ Options 1, 2, and 4 all have the prefix "intra-." Option 3 is unique.

(1) An intradermal injection is administered by inserting the needle of a syringe through the epidermis into the dermis where the fluid is injected. This is a safe procedure in an older adult who is cachectic.

(2) Intravenous medications can be administered safely to cachectic older adults.

(3) **Older adults and cachectic individuals have a decrease in subcutaneous tissue. When a subcutaneous injection is administered to a patient with insufficient subcutaneous tissue, the medication is usually absorbed faster; this may be unsafe.**

(4) Although muscle mass may be smaller in older adults and cachectic individuals, an intramuscular injection can be administered safely by using a 1 inch rather than a 1½ inch needle.

30 **Answer: 2 Tablets.**

Solve the problem using ratio and proportion.

$$\frac{\text{Desired}}{\text{Have}} \qquad \frac{400 \text{ mg}}{200 \text{ mg}} = \frac{x \text{ Tab}}{1 \text{ Tab}}$$

Cross-multiply $\qquad 200 \, x = 400$

Divide by 200 $\qquad \dfrac{200 \, x}{200} = \dfrac{400}{200}$

$$x = 400 \div 200$$

$$x = 2 \text{ Tablets}$$

Meeting the Needs of Perioperative Patients

• • •

This section includes questions related to meeting the needs of patients during the perioperative period. The questions focus on physical assessment and on prevention and care related to common complications associated with the perioperative period, such as hemorrhage, wound dehiscence, atelectasis, infection, and thrombophlebitis. The principles of perioperative teaching, meeting patients' emotional needs, sterile technique, and types of dressings and wounds are also tested. In addition, assessment and care of postoperative tubes and wound drainage systems are addressed.

Questions

Please fill in the circle to mark your answer choice.

1 Which nursing intervention is unrelated to the prevention of postoperative thrombophlebitis?
① Massaging the legs
② Ambulating regularly
③ Increasing fluid intake
④ Applying antiembolism stockings
TEST-TAKING TIP ○ Identify the word in the stem that indicates negative polarity.

2 When a patient is brought to the post anesthesia care unit, the nurse is told that the patient lost 2 units of blood during surgery. For which patient adaptations that are significant to this information should the nurse assess?
① Rapid, deep breathing and increased blood pressure
② Rapid, deep breathing and decreased blood pressure
③ Slow, shallow breathing and increased blood pressure
④ Slow, shallow breathing and decreased blood pressure
TEST-TAKING TIP ○ Identify the duplicate facts among the options. Identify the options that are opposites.

3 The nurse is caring for a postoperative patient who has a history of cigarette smoking. Initially, the nurse should monitor the patient for:
① Airway patency
② Dependent edema
③ Respiratory infection
④ Pulmonary hemorrhage
TEST-TAKING TIP ○ Identify the key word in the stem that sets a priority. Identify the clues in the stem.

4 While a preoperative patient is being transferred to a stretcher to be taken to the operating room, the patient states, "I do not want to be seen without my dentures in my mouth." The nurse should:
① Allow the patient to keep the dentures in the mouth
② Explore the patient's feelings regarding not wearing dentures
③ Explain that it is an important rule that preoperative patients must follow
④ Remove them before anesthesia and replace them as soon as the patient awakens
TEST-TAKING TIP ○ Identify the option that denies the patient's feelings, concerns, and needs.

5 Sterile technique is maintained when the nurse:
① Always holds a wet gauze upward until ready for use
② Changes the gloves if they are positioned below the waist
③ Wipes the wound in a circular motion from the outside inward
④ Cleans the edges of the wound before the center of the wound

TEST-TAKING TIP ○ Identify the specific determiner in an option. Identify the equally plausible options.

6 A patient is exhibiting difficulty coping with postoperative psychologic stress. What can the nurse do to best help this patient cope?
① Teach the use of imagery
② Encourage ventilation of feelings
③ Promote intellectual adaptive responses
④ Obtain an order for an antianxiety medication

TEST-TAKING TIP ○ Identify the key word in the stem that sets a priority. Identify the clue in the stem.

7 The nurse is caring for a group of patients in the post anesthesia care unit. Which intervention *best* prevents atelectasis after surgery?
① Oxygen via nasal cannula
② Diaphragmatic breathing
③ Progressive activity
④ Postural drainage

TEST-TAKING TIP ○ Identify the key word in the stem that sets a priority. Identify the clue in the stem.

8 The nurse on a surgical unit routinely assesses patients' incisions as part of postoperative care. After surgery, when should the nurse be alert for clinical signs of wound infection?
① Between days 3 and 5 after surgery
② Between days 1 and 2 after surgery
③ Within 24 hours after surgery
④ 7 days after surgery

9 Nursing care that is unique to a portable wound drainage system, such as a Hemovac or Jackson-Pratt, which is different from tubes such as a T-tube or an indwelling urinary catheter, is the need to:
① Maintain patency of the drainage tube
② Assess characteristics of the drainage
③ Ensure negative pressure
④ Measure output

TEST-TAKING TIP ○ Identify the clue in the stem.

10 The physician orders an enema for a patient scheduled for bowel surgery. The nurse understands that the enema is administered to this patient primarily to reduce:
① Preoperative peristalsis
② Postoperative constipation
③ Incontinence during surgery
④ Contamination of the operative field

TEST-TAKING TIP ○ Identify the key word in the stem that sets a priority.

11 When talking with a hospitalized preoperative patient, the nurse discovers that the patient has been smoking a pack of cigarettes daily. What should the nurse do?
① Inform the surgeon about the patient's smoking.
② Ask the patient to stop smoking until after surgery.

③ Remove the patient's cigarettes at midnight before surgery.
④ Advise the patient to join a Smoke Enders Club after discharge.

TEST-TAKING TIP ◉ Identify the options that deny the patient's feelings, concerns, and needs. Identify the unique option.

12 After a patient has a procedure that uses the femoral artery as an access, the physician orders a pressure dressing at the catheter insertion site. The nurse understands that the primary purpose of this pressure dressing is to:
① Prevent pain
② Limit infection
③ Decrease drainage
④ Promote hemostasis

TEST-TAKING TIP ◉ Identify the key word in the stem that sets a priority. Identify the unique option.

13 After concerns about pain, the nurse is aware that the question most commonly asked by preoperative patients is, "When will I be able to:
① Have visitors?"
② Go home?"
③ Shower?"
④ Eat?"

TEST-TAKING TIP ◉ Identify the key word in the stem that sets a priority.

14 The nurse is caring for a patient who has had thoracic surgery. The assessment that is MOST specific to this type of surgery is the:
① Blood pressure
② Urinary output
③ Intensity of pain
④ Rate and depth of respirations

TEST-TAKING TIP ◉ Identify the key word in the stem that sets a priority. Identify the clue in the stem. Identify the unique option.

15 The nurse is caring for patients with a variety of wounds. Which type of wound heals by primary intention?
① Surgical incision
② Excoriation
③ Deep burn
④ Abrasion

TEST-TAKING TIP ◉ Identify the clue in the stem. Identify the equally plausible options.

16 The nurse is caring for a patient with a nasogastric tube to low continuous suction. The MOST effective way for the nurse to prevent dislodging the placement of the nasogastric tube is by:
① Pinning it to the pillow
② Attaching it to the gown
③ Taping it to the patient's nose
④ Instructing the patient not to touch it

TEST-TAKING TIP ◉ Identify the key word in the stem that sets a priority. Identify the equally plausible options.

17 What should the nurse do when assessing for the presence of dehiscence after a patient had abdominal surgery?
① Monitor urine output.
② Assess for hypertension.
③ Observe the wound edges.
④ Palpate around the wound.

18 The nurse identifies that further preoperative teaching is needed when the patient says, "I should:
① Expect to be in the post anesthesia care unit after surgery."
② Apply pressure against the incision when coughing."
③ Ask for medication when I begin to have pain."
④ Lie still while I am on bed rest."

TEST-TAKING TIP ◉ Identify the word in the stem that indicates negative polarity.

19 What is the most therapeutic statement by the nurse when assessing a patient's knowledge of surgery?
① "Have you ever had surgery before?"
② "What are your concerns about surgery?"
③ "Surgery can be a frightening experience."
④ "Tell me about your experiences with surgery."

TEST-TAKING TIP ◉ Identify the key word in the stem that sets a priority.

20 The nurse is caring for a postoperative patient who had abdominal surgery. What should the nurse do to help prevent postoperative wound dehiscence?
① Keep the wound clean and dry
② Change the dressing every eight hours
③ Medicate the patient for pain regularly
④ Provide incisional support during activity

TEST-TAKING TIP ◉ Identify the equally plausible options. Identify the unique options

21 A postoperative patient has a history of heart disease. Which nursing assessment is *most* significant when monitoring this patient?
① Pain at the site of the incision
② Alterations in fluid balance
③ Irregular pulse rhythm
④ Dependent edema

TEST-TAKING TIP ◉ Identify the key word in the stem that sets a priority. Identify the equally plausible options.

22 Which adaptation identified by the nurse indicates mild postoperative laryngeal spasm after extubation?
① Rales
② Gurgles
③ Crackles
④ Wheezing

TEST-TAKING TIP ◉ Identify the equally plausible options.

23 A patient who received spinal anesthesia is transferred to the post anesthesia care unit. What is the most important postoperative nursing assessment of this patient?
① Peripheral circulation
② Level of consciousness
③ Sensation in the legs and toes
④ Orientation to time and place

TEST-TAKING TIP ◉ Identify the key word in the stem that sets a priority. Identify the equally plausible options.

24 Which factor places an older adult at greater risk during surgery than a younger person?
① Increased glomerular filtration rate
② Decreased rigidity of arterial walls
③ Higher basal metabolic rate
④ Reduced cardiac reserve

TEST-TAKING TIP ◉ Identify the key word in the stem that sets a priority.

25 A postoperative patient voids for the first time after surgery. The nurse measures the amount of urine in the urinal as indicated below. How many mL should the nurse document that the patient voided?

① 450 mL
② 550 mL
③ 575 mL
④ 600 mL

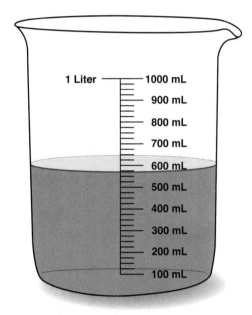

1 Liter — 1000 mL
900 mL
800 mL
700 mL
600 mL
500 mL
400 mL
300 mL
200 mL
100 mL

Meeting the Needs of Perioperative Patients
Answers and Rationales

1 **TEST-TAKING TIP** ○ The word "unrelated" in the stem indicates negative polarity. It is asking which option is not related to preventing thrombophlebitis.
   (1) **Massaging the legs can traumatize the vessels, contributing to the formation of thrombi.**
   (2) Ambulating increases circulation in the lower extremities, which helps prevent thrombus formation.
   (3) Increasing fluid intake promotes hemodilution, which limits thrombus formation.
   (4) Antiembolism stockings promote venous return, which prevents the formation of thrombi.

2 **TEST-TAKING TIP** ○ The question is testing your knowledge about the type of breathing and the type of blood pressure associated with hypovolemia secondary to blood loss. If you know just one of these facts related to hypovolemia, you can reduce your final selection to two options. Options 1 and 4 are opposites, and Options 2 and 3 are opposites. Although there are two sets of opposites in this item, it is easier and more productive to focus instead on the duplicate facts to help you eliminate distractors. The use of test-taking techniques should not become so complex that it makes the question more difficult to answer.
   (1) Although rapid, deep breathing is associated with hypovolemia, the blood pressure decreases, not increases.
   (2) **With a decrease in circulating red blood cells, respiration increases in rate and depth to meet oxygen needs. With a reduction in blood volume, there is a decrease in blood pressure.**
   (3) With hypovolemia, the breathing is rapid and deep, not slow and shallow, and the blood pressure decreases, not increases.
   (4) Although the blood pressure decreases with hypovolemia, the respirations are rapid and deep, not slow and shallow.

3 **TEST-TAKING TIP** ○ The word "initially" in the stem sets a priority. The words "postoperative" and "smokes" are clues in the stem.
   (1) **Smoking increases mucus production and destroys the protective action of cilia; a smoker is at risk for ineffective airway clearance.**
   (2) Dependent edema is related to heart and peripheral vascular diseases, not smoking.
   (3) Although the nurse should monitor the patient for signs of respiratory infection, this is not the priority.
   (4) Pulmonary hemorrhage is an unlikely occurrence; but it can occur with the erosion associated with lung cancer.

4 **TEST-TAKING TIP** ○ Option 3 denies the patient's feelings, concerns, and needs.
   (1) It is unsafe to allow dentures to be in the mouth during surgery because dentures may be aspirated while the patient is unconscious.
   (2) Although exploring the patient's feelings might be done, it does not address safety needs.
   (3) This response denies the patient's feelings and cuts off communication; care can be individualized while still meeting safety needs.
   (4) **Removing the dentures immediately before surgery and returning them as soon as possible after surgery meets the patient's self-esteem needs while providing for physical safety.**

5 **TEST-TAKING TIP** ○ Option 1 contains the word "always," which is a specific determiner. Options 3 and 4 are equally plausible.
   (1) Fluid from the wet gauze can run down the upraised hand. When the hand is repositioned with the fingers downward, the fluid that runs back down the hand may be contaminated, which in turn contaminates the gauze.
   (2) **When sterile gloves are accidentally positioned below the waist, they are considered out of the line of sight and must be changed because they may have inadvertently become contaminated.**
   (3) This action can move contaminated material from a more contaminated section to a less contaminated section of a wound. The center of a wound is considered less contaminated than the edges of the wound or the surrounding skin; therefore, the nurse should wipe a wound moving from the center outward using one gauze pad per stroke.
   (4) Same as #3.

6 **TEST-TAKING TIP** ○ The word "best" in the stem sets a priority. The word "psychologic" is a clue in the stem.
   (1) Teaching imagery may reduce anxiety temporarily, but it does not address the underlying concerns.
   (2) **This provides open-ended communication and allows the patient to explore concerns.**
   (3) Intellectual adaptive responses take place in the cognitive domain (addresses intellectual/knowledge needs), not the affective domain (addresses psychologic needs).
   (4) Medication may be unnecessary if the patient's psychologic needs are addressed effectively.

7 TEST-TAKING TIP ⊙ The word *best* is the key word in the stem that sets a priority. The words "prevent atelectasis" are a clue in the stem.

① Exogenous (originating outside the body) oxygen increases the partial pressure of oxygen; it does not prevent atelectasis.

② **Diaphragmatic breathing expands the alveoli, which prevents atelectasis; it also precipitates coughing, which prevents the accumulation and stagnation of secretions.**

③ Activity promotes cardiopulmonary and circulatory functioning in general; it does not specifically prevent atelectasis.

④ Postural drainage promotes the flow of mucus out of segments of the lung; it is not done routinely after surgery to prevent atelectasis.

8 ① **Microorganisms in a wound can precipitate an infection, which manifests itself in approximately 3 to 5 days; erythema, pain, edema, chills, fever, and purulent drainage indicate infection.**

② This is too short a time for an infectious process to develop from a surgical incision; a contaminated, traumatic wound may precipitate an infection this early.

③ Same as #2.

④ An infectious process generally manifests itself before 7 days; wound dehiscence or evisceration may occur 5 to 10 days after surgery before collagen formation occurs.

9 TEST-TAKING TIP ⊙ The word "unique" is a clue in the stem.

① All tubes must be patent for drainage to occur.

② All drainage must be assessed for quantity, color, consistency, and odor.

③ **Portable wound drainage systems work by continuous low pressure as long as the suction bladder is less than half full; T-tubes and indwelling urinary catheters work via gravity.**

④ The volume of fluid over specific time periods must be measured for all drainage.

10 TEST-TAKING TIP ⊙ The word "primarily" is the key word in the stem that sets a priority.

① An enema will increase, not decrease, peristalsis.

② Postoperative constipation is prevented by activity and adequate fluid intake.

③ Although an enema prevents incontinence during surgery, it is not the purpose of thorough bowel preparation for intestinal surgery.

④ **If feces are present in the bowel when the intestine is incised, the excrement spills into the abdominal cavity, causing contamination and increasing the risk of peritonitis.**

11 TEST-TAKING TIP ⊙ Options 2 and 3 deny the patient's feelings, concerns, and needs. Option 1 is unique because it involves communicating information to the surgeon. Options 2, 3, and 4 involve interacting with the patient.

① **The physician should be made aware of this fact because it may influence the type of anesthesia used and the perioperative medical regimen.**

② If the patient is willing to stop smoking, it should be discontinued before and after surgery to prevent respiratory complications. The nurse should recognize that the patient may need to continue to smoke because it may be a coping mechanism.

③ The nurse does not have a right to take a patient's belongings; the patient should be told where and when smoking is permitted or if the facility is "smoke free."

④ Discussing a Smoke Enders Club is inappropriate at this time because the patient is concerned with the present situation; this might eventually be done after surgery.

12 TEST-TAKING TIP ⊙ The word "primary" is the key word in the stem that sets a priority. Option 4 is unique because it comes from a positive perspective, expressed by the word "promote." Options 1, 2, and 3 come from a negative perspective, expressed by the words *prevent, limit,* and *decrease.*

① Although a pressure dressing may help prevent the accumulation of interstitial fluid, thereby limiting pain, it does not prevent pain; also, this is not the primary purpose of a pressure dressing.

② Surgical asepsis, not a pressure dressing, limits infection.

③ Dressings usually do not decrease drainage.

④ **Pressure causes the constriction of peripheral blood vessels, which prevents bleeding; it also eliminates dead space in underlying tissue so that healing can progress.**

13 TEST-TAKING TIP ⊙ The word "most" in the stem sets a priority.

① Although this may be important to some patients, it is not the most basic, common concern of the majority of patients.

② Same as #1.

③ Same as #1.

④ **Eating is a basic human need identified by Maslow and is considered very important by most postoperative patients.**

14 TEST-TAKING TIP ○ The word MOST is the key word in the stem that sets a priority. The word "thoracic" is a clue in the stem. Option 4 is unique because it is the only option with two assessments.
① Monitoring the blood pressure is important after any surgery and is not specific to thoracic surgery.
② Monitoring fluid intake and urinary output is important after all types of surgery; it is not unique to thoracic surgery.
③ Monitoring the characteristics of pain is required after all types of surgery and is not specific to thoracic surgery.
④ Thoracic surgery involves entering the thoracic cavity; respiratory function becomes a major priority.

15 TEST-TAKING TIP ○ The words "primary intention" are a clue in the stem. Options 2 and 4 are equally plausible.
① Primary intention is the healing process that consists of the stages of defensive, reconstructive, and maturative healing; it involves a clean wound that has edges that are closely approximated.
② An excoriation is an abrasion, a loss of superficial skin layers caused by trauma, friction, chemicals, and digestive enzymes.
③ A burn has wound edges that are not approximated, and the wound is usually wide and open. A burn heals by secondary intention.
④ An abrasion, like an excoriation, is the loss of superficial skin layers caused by trauma, friction, chemicals, and digestive enzymes.

16 TEST-TAKING TIP ○ The word MOST in the stem sets a priority. Options 1 and 2 are equally plausible.
① Pinning the tubing to the patient's bed linen is unsafe; tension on the tube will increase with patient movement, which may result in displacement of the tube.
② Attaching the tubing to the gown is unsafe. Patient movement will increase tension on the tubing and may result in displacement of the tube.
③ Taping a nasogastric tube to the patient's nose anchors the tube and helps prevent the tube from becoming dislodged.
④ Although the patient should be instructed not to touch the tube, this is not the most effective way to prevent dislodgment of the tube because patients tend to touch foreign objects that irritate the body.

17 ① Urine output is unrelated to dehiscence.
② Hypertension is unrelated to dehiscence.
③ Dehiscence is a separation of the wound edges at the suture line, which is evidenced by increased drainage and the appearance of underlying tissue. This most frequently occurs 5 to 12 days postoperatively. Dehiscence is precipitated by increased intra-abdominal pressure associated with coughing, vomiting, and distention; obesity is a risk factor.
④ Palpation assesses for edema and heat; if these signs occur 3 to 6 days postoperatively, infection, not dehiscence, is suspected.

18 TEST-TAKING TIP ○ The word "further" indicates negative polarity. The question is really asking which statement by the patient is "not correct."
① Patients are kept in the post anesthesia care unit until reactive and stable.
② Applying pressure against an incision is an acceptable practice to minimize incisional pain and help prevent dehiscence when performing any activity that raises intra-abdominal pressure.
③ Pain relief is more effective when analgesics are administered before pain becomes severe; this prevents excessive peaks and troughs in the pain experience.
④ Remaining immobile after surgery is unacceptable because it promotes cardiopulmonary, vascular, and gastrointestinal complications; the patient needs further preoperative teaching.

19 TEST-TAKING TIP ○ The word "most" is the key word in the stem that sets a priority.
① This statement is a direct question that can be answered with a "yes" or a "no."
② Concerns generally focus on feelings rather than knowledge; this statement is a direct question that the patient may be unable or unwilling to answer.
③ This statement may precipitate unnecessary anxiety; feelings should be raised by the patient, not by the nurse.
④ This statement is an open-ended question that invites the patient to discuss past experiences. The patient's past experiences may be less anxiety producing than the present situation, and they provide a data base for future teaching.

20 TEST-TAKING TIP ○ Options 1 and 2 are equally plausible; they both reflect actions that are associated with the dressing and prevent infection. Option 4 is unique; it does not contain the word "the."
① Keeping the wound clean and dry should prevent infection, not wound dehiscence.
② Changing the wound dressing every 8 hours should prevent infection, not wound dehiscence.
③ Pain medication promotes comfort; it does not limit the occurrence of dehiscence.
④ Pressure against the incision supports the integrity of the approximation of the edges of the wound.

21 **TEST-TAKING TIP** ☉ The word *most* in the stem sets a priority. Options 2 and 4 are equally plausible; they both relate to problems with fluid balance.

(1) Pain at the incisional site is common to postoperative patients and not specific to a postoperative patient with a history of heart disease.

(2) Although changes in fluid balance is an important assessment, an alteration in fluid balance is not immediately life threatening.

(3) **An irregular pulse rhythm may indicate a life-threatening dysrhythmia.**

(4) Although assessment of dependent edema is important, it is not as critical as another assessment.

22 **TEST-TAKING TIP** ☉ Options 1 and 3 are equally plausible.

(1) Rales, more commonly known as crackles, are sounds caused by air passing through respiratory passages containing excessive moisture.

(2) Gurgles, formerly known as rhonchi, are sounds caused by air moving through tenacious mucus or narrowed bronchi.

(3) Crackles, also known as rales, are sounds caused by air passing through respiratory passages containing excessive moisture.

(4) **Wheezing, which consists of high-pitched whistling sounds, is caused by air moving through a narrowed or partially obstructed airway.**

23 **TEST-TAKING TIP** ☉ The word "most" in the stem sets a priority. Options 2 and 4 are equally plausible if the patient had general anesthesia, not spinal anesthesia.

(1) Spinal anesthesia does not alter peripheral circulation.

(2) General anesthesia, not spinal anesthesia, acts on the cerebral centers to produce loss of consciousness.

(3) **Spinal anesthesia causes loss of sensation in and paralysis of the toes, perineum, legs, and abdomen. When motion and sensation of the legs and toes return, the patient is considered to have recovered from the effects of the spinal anesthetic.**

(4) General anesthesia, not spinal anesthesia, acts on the cerebral centers and alters orientation to time, place, and person.

24 **TEST-TAKING TIP** ☉ The word "greater" is the word in the stem that sets a priority.

(1) Older adults have a decreased, not increased, glomerular filtration rate.

(2) Older adults have an increased, not decreased, rigidity of arterial walls.

(3) Older adults have a lower, not higher, basal metabolic rate.

(4) **As one ages, cardiac output and strength of cardiac contractions decrease and the heart rate takes longer to return to the resting rate. Sudden physical or emotional stresses may result in cardiac dysrhythmias and heart failure.**

25 (1) This amount is too small.

(2) Same as #1.

(3) **575 mL is the correct volume. Each line represented 25 mL of urine.**

(4) This amount is excessive.

Meeting Patients' Microbiologic Safety Needs

• • •

This section includes questions on concepts and principles related to topics such as medical asepsis, surgical asepsis, types of isolation, and the chain of infection. Particular emphasis is placed on nursing actions that protect the nurse and the patient from microorganisms, including questions on handwashing and disposal of contaminated equipment and linen. The questions also address risk factors for infection, common adaptations to infection, and patient teaching/learning of infection control practices.

Questions

Please fill in the circle to mark your answer choice.

1 Which action breaks the chain of infection from a portal of exit from a reservoir?
① Washing the hands
② Disposing of soiled linen
③ Disinfecting used equipment
④ Avoiding talking over an open wound
TEST-TAKING TIP ○ Identify the clue in the stem.

2 The nurse is teaching a patient about ways to prevent infection. Which best increases a patient's defense against microorganisms?
① Intact skin
② Covering a cough
③ Changing bed linen daily
④ Using an antiseptic mouthwash
TEST-TAKING TIP ○ Identify the key word in the stem that sets a priority. Which option is unique?

3 What can the nurse do to prevent fungal infections in the hospitalized patient?
① Apply moisturizing lotion to the patient's body
② Dry the folds of the patient's skin well
③ Provide a daily bath for the patient
④ Keep the patient's room cool

4 The nurse identifies that further teaching about *standard precautions* is necessary when a nursing assistant caring for patients says, "Standard precautions apply when I:
① Clean up body fluids that contain blood."
② Provide perineal care."
③ Change soiled linen."
④ Wipe tears away."
TEST-TAKING TIP ○ Identify the key words in the stem that indicate negative polarity.

5 The nurse initiates *contact precautions* for a patient with a wound infection. What should the nurse do to best help the patient cope with the psychologic aspects of these precautions?
① Draw a smiley face on the mask
② Don gloves when providing direct care
③ Explain the importance of contact precautions
④ Wear a gown only when direct contact is expected
TEST-TAKING TIP ○ Identify the key word in the stem that sets a priority. Identify the option that contains a specific determiner. Identify the clang association.

6 The nurse irrigates the wound of a patient on contact precautions. What should the nurse do first to remove personal protective equipment when leaving this patient's room?
① Untie the gown at the waist
② Untie the gown at the neck
③ Remove the gloves
④ Remove the mask

TEST-TAKING TIP ◦ Identify the key word in the stem that sets a priority.

7 When planning care for patients who have acquired immune deficiency syndrome (AIDS), the nurse identifies that all these patients have the greatest risk for:
① Environmental disorientation
② Acquired infections
③ Secondary cancer
④ Pressure ulcers

TEST-TAKING TIP ◦ Identify the key word in the stem that sets a priority. Identify the word in the stem that is a clue.

8 Which factor identified by the nurse creates the greatest risk for a patient to develop a respiratory tract infection?
① Urinary catheter
② Long hospital stay
③ Painful chest injury
④ Nasogastric tube for decompression

TEST-TAKING TIP ◦ Identify the key word in the stem that sets a priority.

9 The nurse is caring for a patient with an infection. When assessing the patient, the nurse understands that the most common adaptation is:
① Dehydration
② Headache
③ Anorexia
④ Fever

TEST-TAKING TIP ◦ Identify the key word in the stem that sets a priority. Identify the word in the stem that is a clue.

10 Which question should the nurse ask a patient with an infection when taking a nursing history as opposed to a medical history?
① "Have you done any traveling lately?"
② "How long has the infection been present?"
③ "When did you first notice your symptoms?"
④ "How does the infection affect your daily routine?"

TEST-TAKING TIP ◦ Identify the equally plausible options.

11 A patient is admitted to the hospital with a medical diagnosis of fever of unknown origin. Which laboratory result should the nurse report to the physician?
① White blood cell count of 20,000
② Urine specific gravity of 1.020
③ Hemoglobin of 14.5 g/dL
④ Hematocrit of 42%

12 Which nursing action associated with handwashing is guided by a principle of *medical asepsis*?
① Washing with the hands held higher than the elbows
② Rinsing with the hands held lower than the elbows
③ Turning the water on with a clean paper towel
④ Adjusting the water to a hot temperature

13 The nurse observes a nursing assistant removing soiled gloves. The nurse identifies a violation of aseptic technique when removing the soiled gloves the Nursing Assistant:
① Grasps the outer surface of the left glove below the thumb with the gloved right hand
② Contains the removed glove from the left hand within the fingers of the gloved right hand
③ Discards the right glove that has been inverted containing the left glove into an appropriate waste container
④ Uses the left ungloved thumb and forefinger to grasp the inside and outside of the cuff of the gloved right hand

TEST-TAKING TIP ◉ Identify the key word in the stem that indicates negative polarity.

14 When removing the protective gloves that were worn to start an intravenous solution, a female nurse notices that there is a small amount of the patient's blood on her forearm. What should the nurse do first?
① Wash the exposed area with soap and water
② Wipe the blood with gauze moistened with alcohol
③ Flush the arm from the elbow to the fingers with hot water
④ Apply a new pair of gloves and absorb the blood with a paper towel

TEST-TAKING TIP ◉ Identify the key word in the stem that sets a priority.

15 The nurse is changing a patient's bed linens. Where should the nurse place the soiled linens when they are removed from the bed?
① In a soiled linen hamper
② On the overbed table
③ Into the linen chute
④ On a chair

TEST-TAKING TIP ◉ Identify the phrase that is a clue in the stem. Identify the equally plausible options.

16 The nurse is caring for a patient who is on contact precautions. Which nursing action is most appropriate when providing direct assistance with hygiene activites?
① Wearing a respirator device when giving direct care
② Washing the hands immediately after removing soiled gloves
③ Ensuring that negative air pressure in the room is maintained
④ Removing the gown before the gloves when leaving the room

17 The nurse understands that bacteria rapidly multiply in environments that are:
① Hot
② Cool
③ Cold
④ Warm

18 Linens that are still clean are often reused by the same patient. The article of linen that is *least* likely to be reused by the nurse when making the bed is the:
① Top sheet
② Bedspread
③ Pillowcase
④ Cotton blanket

TEST-TAKING TIP ◉ Identify the key word in the stem that indicates negative polarity. Identify the unique option.

19 A patient on contact precautions needs a blood pressure reading taken every shift. To keep the sphygmomanometer from spreading microorganisms, the most practical intervention by the nurse is to:
① Place it in a protective bag
② Keep it in the patient's room

③ Soak it in a germicidal solution
④ Store it in the dirty utility room

TEST-TAKING TIP ◉ Identify the key word in the stem that sets a priority. Identify the clue in the stem. Identify the unique option.

20 The nursing intervention that has the greatest impact on limiting the spread of microorganisms is:
① Using disposable equipment
② Double-bagging
③ Wearing gloves
④ Handwashing

TEST-TAKING TIP ◉ Identify the key word in the stem that sets a priority.

21 The physician orders airborne precautions for a patient with the diagnosis of tuberculosis. Which nursing action is specific to caring for the patient on airborne precautions?
① Keeping the patient's door closed
② Donning a gown when administering medications
③ Wearing disposable gloves when delivering a meal
④ Instructing the patient to wear a mask when receiving care

TEST-TAKING TIP ◉ Identify the words in the stem that are a clue.

22 Which action is an unacceptable technique when applying sterile gloves?
① Open the outer glove package, grasp the inner package, and lay it on a waist-high, clean surface.
② With the thumb and first two fingers of the nondominant hand, grasp the inside cuff of the glove of the dominant hand.
③ With the gloved dominant hand, pick up the nondominant glove from the inside of the cuff and insert the nondominant hand.
④ Apply the first glove with the fingers held toward the floor, and the second glove with the fingers held toward the ceiling.

TEST-TAKING TIP ◉ Identify the key word in the stem that indicates negative polarity.

23 The nurse is cleaning an emesis basin containing purulent material. What should the nurse do first?
① Wash the basin in hot, soapy water
② Rinse the basin with cold running water
③ Clean the basin with an antiseptic agent
④ Spray the basin with a disinfectant and let it work for several minutes

TEST-TAKING TIP ◉ Identify the word in the stem that sets a priority. Identify the equally plausible options.

24 After assessing a patient's wound, the nurse concludes that the wound may be infected because the exudate is:
① Serous
② Purulent
③ Sanguineous
④ Serosanguineous

TEST-TAKING TIP ◉ Identify the unique option.

25 A 75-year-old man is transferred from a nursing home to the emergency department of the hospital. After reviewing the transfer form supplied by the nursing home and the results of the initial physical assessment in the hospital, what type of isolation precautions should the nurse institute?
① Contact
② Droplet
③ Airborne
④ Protective

CHART/EXHIBIT

Laboratory: RBC 4.5×10^6
WBC 18,000/mm³
Hgb 16 g/dL
Hct 45%

History: MRSA Positive
Type 1 Diabetes
Brain attack with residual left hemiparesis

Physical Assessment: In the sacral area there is a full-thickness skin loss including sub-cutaneous tissue; area is 3 cm $\times$ 4 cm with a small amount of yellow drainage. Vital signs are T 100°F (oral route), P 92, and R 22. Patient is incontinent of urine and feces.

Meeting Patients' Microbiologic Safety Needs
Answers and Rationales

1 TEST-TAKING TIP ⊙ The words "portal of exit" provide a clue in the stem.
① This action is an important means of controlling the transmission of microorganisms from one person or object to another; it does not limit the number of microorganisms directly exiting from a reservoir.
② Same as #1.
③ Same as #1.
④ **Avoiding talking over an open wound limits the number of microorganisms that exit from a respiratory tract. The respiratory tract is one portal of exit from the human reservoir (source of microorganisms). Other human portals of exit include the gastrointestinal, urinary, and reproductive tracts and blood and body tissues.**

2 TEST-TAKING TIP ⊙ The word "best" in the stem sets a priority. Option 1 is unique. Options 2, 3, and 4 begin with a word ending in "-ing" and all involve an action.
① **The skin is a barrier to pathogens and, if pierced or broken, serves as a portal of entry.**
② Covering a cough protects others from the patient's microorganisms.
③ Although changing bed linen daily may reduce the number of microorganisms present, it does not best protect the patient from microorganisms.
④ Although using an antiseptic mouthwash may reduce the number of microorganisms present, it does not best protect the patient from microorganisms.

3 ① Moisturizers soften skin; they do not protect the skin from fungal infection.
② **Fungi multiply rapidly in places where moisture content is high, such as in skin folds. Careful drying of skin folds, especially under the breasts and arms, between the toes, and in the perineal area, helps prevent the development of fungal infections.**
③ Although bathing daily is helpful in preventing infection, it is not the best way to prevent the growth of fungi.
④ A cool room may reduce perspiration; however, it is not the best way to prevent the growth of fungi.

4 TEST-TAKING TIP ⊙ The words "further teaching . . . is necessary" indicate negative polarity.
① Standard precautions apply to blood, body fluids containing visible blood, semen and vaginal secretions, tissues, and cerebrospinal, pleural, synovial, peritoneal, pericardial, and amniotic fluid.
② Standard precautions should be followed when providing perineal care because the caregiver may come into contact with vaginal secretions, semen, or body fluids containing blood.
③ Soiled linen may be contaminated with semen, vaginal secretions, or body fluids containing blood. The caregiver should follow standard precautions when changing soiled linen.
④ **Additional teaching is necessary because, unless blood is present, it is not necessary to use standard precautions when coming into contact with tears.**

5 TEST-TAKING TIP ⊙ The word "best" in the stem sets a priority. Option 4 contains the word "only," which is a specific determiner. The words "contact precautions" appear in both the stem and Option 3.
① A mask is necessary only if splashing of blood or body fluids is expected. The patient may interpret a smiley face as an attempt to minimize the gravity of the illness; humor must be used carefully.
② This personal protective equipment must be worn by everyone who enters the room of a patient on contact precautions; it does not address the psychological needs of the patient.
③ **Explanations support understanding, acceptance, and compliance with isolation precautions. When people understand the reason for a procedure, fear of the unknown and anxiety are usually reduced.**
④ A gown is necessary if there is a possibility of contact with infected surfaces or items; in addition, it is necessary if the patient is incontinent or has diarrhea, a colostomy, or wound drainage not covered and contained by a dressing. Wearing a gown does not address the psychological needs of the patient.

6 TEST-TAKING TIP ⊙ The word "first" in the stem sets a priority.
① **The waist is considered contaminated and should be untied with a gloved hand.**
② Ties at the neck are considered clean and should be untied after the gloves are removed.
③ Gloves are removed after the contaminated waist ties are untied.
④ After the gloves are removed, the mask is removed by touching only the ties. This is done to prevent contamination of the nurse's head, hair, and hands.

7 TEST-TAKING TIP ⊙ The word "greatest" in the stem sets a priority. The word "all" in the stem is a clue. The correct answer must address something that is common to all patients with AIDS. Immunosuppression is common to all patients with AIDS.

① Not all patients who have AIDS have central nervous system involvement that may cause cognitive impairment.

② **Patients who have AIDS are immunosuppressed and have a decreased ability to fight infection; this places them at the greatest risk for acquired infections.**

③ Not all patients with AIDS develop cancer.

④ Not all patients with AIDS are bed-bound or cachectic, which places them at risk for pressure ulcers.

8 TEST-TAKING TIP ⊙ The word "greatest" in the stem sets a priority.

① A urinary catheter contributes to the risk for a urinary, not respiratory, tract infection.

② The hospital environment contains many pathogens; however, a person would have to be susceptible to contract an infection.

③ **Coughing and deep breathing are often avoided by people with painful chest injuries in an effort to self-splint and minimize pain; this allows pooling of respiratory secretions and contributes to an environment that supports the growth of microorganisms in the respiratory tract.**

④ A nasogastric tube decompressing the stomach removes fluid from the body, which does not increase the risk for a respiratory tract infection. A nasogastric tube used as a feeding tube may place the patient at risk for aspiration pneumonia.

9 TEST-TAKING TIP ⊙ The word "most" in the stem sets a priority. The word "common" modifies the word "adaptation" and is the clue in the stem.

① Although dehydration can occur in response to a fever or an inadequate intake of fluid, it is not as common a response to infection as an adaptation in another option.

② This is a nonspecific manifestation of infection and is not as commonly exhibited by a patient with an infection as an adaptation in another option.

③ Same as #2.

④ **Fever is the most common response of the hypothalamus (thermoregulatory center) to pyrogens that are released when phagocytic cells respond to the presence of pathogens.**

10 TEST-TAKING TIP ⊙ Options 2 and 3 both ask questions that identify a timeframe in relation to symptoms; these options are equally plausible.

① Although the nurse may ask this question, it is not the priority. This statement relates to the medical diagnosis and to planning of the medical treatment regimen.

② Same as #1.

③ Same as #1.

④ **The nurse is mostly concerned with how the infection affects a person's functional health patterns. Many nurse practice acts recognize that nurses diagnose and treat human responses.**

11 ① **A white blood cell count of 20,000 is higher than the expected range of 4,500 to 11,000/mL and generally indicates the presence of an infection.**

② This is within the expected range of urine specific gravity of 1.010 to 1.030 and is unrelated to infection.

③ This is within the expected range for hemoglobin, which is 12 to 18 g/dL

④ This is within the expected range for hematocrit, which is 40 to 54 percent for males and 37 to 47 percent for females and is unrelated to infection.

12 ① The hands should be held lower, not higher, than the elbows. The hands are more contaminated than the arms; water should flow from clean to contaminated surfaces.

② **Rinsing with the hands lower than the elbows is correct technique; the hands are more contaminated than the arms. Water washes away debris and microorganisms and prevents recontamination of the cleaner surfaces.**

③ The hands and the faucet are both considered contaminated and therefore it is not necessary to use a clean paper towel to turn on the faucet. A clean paper towel should be used to turn the faucet off after the hands are washed and dried.

④ The nurse should adjust the water to a warm, not hot, temperature; hot water removes protective oils from the skin, which causes chapping.

13 TEST-TAKING TIP ⊙ The word "violation" in the stem indicates negative polarity. The question is asking which action is not an acceptable practice when removing soiled gloves.

① The outer surfaces of both gloves are contaminated; this action keeps the soiled parts of the gloves from contaminating the skin of the left wrist or hand.

② This action contains the soiled glove within a small area and prevents inadvertent self-contamination.

(3) This action safely disposes of both contaminated gloves; the most contaminated surfaces are inside the inverted right glove and they are contained in an appropriate receptacle for removal from the patient's unit.

(4) **This is a violation of aseptic technique. The outer surface of a soiled glove is contaminated and should not be touched by an ungloved hand. While holding the removed left glove in the right hand, the individual should insert two fingers of the left, ungloved hand inside the cuff of the right glove. The individual then pulls the right glove off, turning it inside out, thereby containing the left glove inside the inverted right glove.**

14 TEST-TAKING TIP ⊙ The word "first" in the stem sets a priority.

(1) **Washing includes the action of wetting, rubbing, and rinsing; soap reduces the surface tension of water; friction mechanically disturbs microorganisms; and rinsing flushes microorganisms from the skin.**

(2) The disinfectant isopropyl alcohol can kill bacteria but cannot kill spores, viruses, or fungi.

(3) Hot water does not disinfect and is unnecessary; it also could injure the tissue.

(4) This action does not adequately remove the contaminated material from the surface of the skin.

15 TEST-TAKING TIP ⊙ The phrase "soiled linen" used in the stem and in Option 1 is a clang association. Options 2 and 4 are equally plausible because they are both furniture in the room and one is not better than the other.

(1) **This is a safe and acceptable way to contain microorganisms.**

(2) This contaminates the overbed table and is an undesirable practice; the overbed table is considered a clean surface and should not be used to hold soiled linen.

(3) This is an undesirable practice because it will contaminate the chute. Soiled linen should be bagged in an effort to contain microorganisms before it is deposited in a linen chute.

(4) This contaminates the chair and is an undesirable practice; a chair is considered a clean surface and should not be used to hold soiled linen.

16 (1) A respirator device is not necessary for a patient on contact precautions; a regular mask is necessary when the splashing of body fluids may occur.

(2) **The hands should be washed before donning and immediately after removing them.**

(3) A room with negative air pressure is not necessary for contact precautions; a room with negative pressure is necessary with airborne precautions.

(4) The gloves are removed before, not after, the gown.

17 (1) Hot temperatures are used to destroy bacteria (e.g., sterilization).

(2) Bacteria do not multiply rapidly in cool or cold environments.

(3) Same as #2.

(4) **Bacteria grow most rapidly in dark, warm, moist environments, particularly when the environment is close to body temperature (98.6°F).**

18 TEST-TAKING TIP ⊙ The word *least* is the key word in the stem that indicates negative polarity. Options 1, 2, and 4 are all similar because they are articles of linen that are generally placed over the patient. Option 3 is unique because it is the only article of linen in the options offered that is positioned under the patient.

(1) A top sheet is often used again if it is still clean.

(2) A bedspread is often used again if it is still clean.

(3) **The pillowcase comes in contact with the hair, exudate from the eyes, mucus from the nose, and saliva from the mouth. A pillowcase is easily soiled and usually needs to be replaced more often than other linens.**

(4) A cotton blanket is often used again if it is still clean.

19 TEST-TAKING TIP ⊙ The word "most" is the key word in the stem that sets a priority. The word "practical" in the stem is a clue. Option 2 is unique because it is the only option with the word "patient."

(1) This is unsafe. The outer surface of the bag is also contaminated and, if taken out of the room, will contaminate any surface on which it is placed.

(2) **This is the most practical action; when isolation is discontinued, all of the equipment can be terminally disinfected.**

(3) This is impractical and will harm the sphygmomanometer.

(4) The sphygmomanometer is contaminated and needs to be disinfected before it is removed from the patient's room.

20 TEST-TAKING TIP ⊙ The word "greatest" is the key word in the stem that sets a priority.

(1) This is not the most effective method to reduce the spread of microorganisms; not all equipment is disposable.

(2) Although double-bagging limits the spread of microorganisms, it is not the most effective method.

(3) Although the use of gloves protect the nurse and limit the spread of microorganisms, it is not the most effective method.

(4) **Handwashing is the most effective measure to reduce the spread of microorganisms because it removes them from the hands that come in contact with other patients and objects.**

21 TEST-TAKING TIP ○ The words "specific to" and "airborne precautions" are clues in the stem.

(1) **Keeping the door closed prevents the spread of microorganisms that can be transmitted via air currents.**

(2) When administering medications to a patient on airborne precautions, the nurse must wear a mask, not a gown.

(3) When delivering a meal tray to a patient on airborne precautions, the nurse must wear a mask, not gloves.

(4) The nurse, not the patient, wears the mask for self-protection.

22 TEST-TAKING TIP ○ The word "unacceptable" is the word in the stem that indicates negative polarity.

(1) This is acceptable technique. A clean, dry surface prevents contamination of the wrapper; objects below the waist are considered contaminated.

(2) The ungloved hand is permitted to touch the inner surface of a sterile glove; both surfaces are considered contaminated.

(3) **Attempting to put on the second glove by gripping the inner cuff of the second glove increases the risk of touching the gloved hand against the ungloved hand or wrist, resulting in contamination. The gloved hand should slip fingers underneath the outer surface of the folded cuff of the other glove. This sterile-to-sterile contact maintains sterility.**

(4) This is acceptable technique. It does not matter which direction the fingers are facing as long as the hands are kept above the waist, are in view, and do not become contaminated.

23 TEST-TAKING TIP ○ The word "first" in the stem sets a priority. Options 3 and 4 are equally plausible.

(1) Washing the basin in hot, soapy water should not be the initial intervention. Hot water coagulates the protein of organic material and causes it to stick to a surface.

(2) **Rinsing the basin with cold running water is a correct action because it does not coagulate the protein of organic material permitting it to be flushed from the surface of the basin.**

(3) Antiseptics are used to limit bacteria on the skin or in wounds, not for cleaning objects.

(4) Spraying the basin with a disinfectant is unnecessary.

24 TEST-TAKING TIP ○ The words in Options 1, 3, and 4 all begin with the letter "S." Option 2 is unique because it begins with a "P."

(1) Serous exudate is watery in appearance, is composed of mainly serum, and does not indicate an infection.

(2) **Purulent exudate contains material such as dead and living bacteria and dead tissue; it indicates the possibility of an infection.**

(3) Sanguineous exudate indicates damage to capillaries that allows escape of red blood cells from plasma.

(4) Serosanguineous exudate consists of clear and blood-tinged drainage as seen in surgical incisions.

CHART/EXHIBIT

Laboratory: RBC 4.5 × 10⁶
WBC 18,000/mm³
Hgb 16 g/dL
Hct 45%

History: MRSA Positive
Type 1 Diabetes
Brain attack with residual left hemiparesis

Physical Assessment: In the sacral area there is a full-thickness skin loss including sub-cutaneous tissue; area is 3 cm × 4 cm with a small amount of yellow drainage. Vital signs are T 100°F (oral route), P 92, and R 22. Patient is incontinent of urine and feces.

ANSWER AND RATIONALE: **1** **The patient needs to have contact precautions because of the history of the patient's being methicillin-resistant *Staphylococcus aureus* (MRSA) positive, and having incontinence and a wound with drainage. Contact precautions prevent the spread of pathogens from the patient to the nurse and others. The WBCs are elevated above the expected range indicating an infectious/inflammatory process. Patients with diabetes are at risk for infection because of a decreased immune response and the high glucose in tissues which supports the growth of microorganisms. Yellow drainage from a pressure ulcer is suspicious of an infection. The elevation in vital signs above the expected range reflect the stimulation of the general adaptation syndrome in response to the presence of a pathogen (e.g., MRSA).**

2 There is no sputum culture result indicating a respiratory infection that requires airborne or droplet precautions. The elevated vital signs indicate an infection, but there are no adaptations (e.g., dyspnea, cough, increase in respiratory secretions, labored breathing, crackles/rhonchi) indicating a respiratory infection that requires a need for airborne or droplet precautions.

3 Same as #2.

4 Protective precautions are necessary if the WBCs were low, not high, putting the patient at risk for infection. The brain attack is insignificant related to the need for isolation precautions. There are no adaptations (e.g., dyspnea, cough, increase in respiratory secretions, labored breathing, crackles/rhonchi) indicating a respiratory infection other than the elevated vital signs that requires a need for airborne or droplet precautions.

Meeting the Needs Of Patients in the Community Setting

• • •

This section encompasses questions related to caring for an individual, a family, a subgroup, or the population within a community. The questions include topics such as health-care delivery settings (e.g., nursing homes, day-care centers, assisted-living residences, occupational settings, and private homes), the focus of nursing actions (e.g., prevention of illness, health promotion, maintenance of safe environments, protection and restoration of health), and specific nursing activities (e.g., screening, health education). The questions also focus on levels of health-care services (e.g., primary, secondary, and tertiary health-care delivery), levels of disease prevention (e.g., primary, secondary, and tertiary levels of prevention), and community-focused examples related to nursing intervention (e.g., developmental stresses, common health problems, crisis intervention, and the needs of individuals in the community based on Maslow's Hierarchy of Needs).

Questions

Please fill in the circle to mark your answer choice.

1 The nurse is caring for a patient recently discharged from the hospital. Which nursing intervention takes priority?
① Exploring the need to modify the environment to prevent falls
② Teaching a family member how to feed a client who has a decreased gag reflex
③ Encouraging the client to ventilate negative feelings about loss of independence
④ Providing opportunities for the client to make choices concerning the plan of care
TEST-TAKING TIP ◉ Identify the key word in the stem that sets a priority.

2 The trend in health care that received the most attention in the 1990s was:
① Tertiary care
② Early diagnosis
③ Health promotion
④ Restorative rehabilitation
TEST-TAKING TIP ◉ Identify the key word in the stem that sets a priority. Identify the clue in the stem.

3 Community health nursing mainly is associated with:
① Delivering home health-care services
② Assisting economically disadvantaged high-risk groups
③ Addressing the nursing needs of a specific individual or group within the community
④ Providing interventions that help people on the health end of the health–illness continuum
TEST-TAKING TIP ◉ Identify the key word in the stem that sets a priority. Identify the clue in the stem.

4 The community health nurse can expect which population to experience a maturational/developmental crisis?
① Homosexual adolescents
② Recently divorced men
③ Critically ill children
④ Unemployed adults
TEST-TAKING TIP ◉ Identify the clue in the stem.

5 The nurse understands that an essential aspect of community health nursing is its:
① Emphasis mainly on health promotion
② Focus on the needs of individuals
③ Practice within the home setting
④ Interdisciplinary nature
TEST-TAKING TIP ◉ Identify the key word in the stem that sets a priority.

6 Which group is covered by Medicare?
① People who receive Aid to Families with Dependent Children
② People who need nurse midwife services
③ People with just a low income
④ People 65 years and older
TEST-TAKING TIP ◦ Identify the option that contains a specific determiner.

7 "Upstream thinking" is a conceptual approach used in public health efforts. A community health nurse is demonstrating "upstream thinking" when:
① Convincing parents of children with asthma that continued medical supervision is necessary
② Teaching a person with diabetes how to perform self-monitoring of blood glucose
③ Conducting screening programs for the presence of hypertension in older adults
④ Encouraging parents who live in old buildings to test for lead-based paint

8 A soon-to-be-discharged patient who has respiratory medications states, "Whenever I have difficulty breathing, I'll just take extra puffs on my inhaler." What should be the first response by the nurse?
① "If you cannot breathe, you should call for help."
② "How often do you have difficulty breathing?"
③ "If you cannot breathe, don't you think you should call your physician?"
④ "Let's review why it's dangerous to take medications more frequently than ordered."
TEST-TAKING TIP ◦ Identify the key word in the stem that sets a priority.

9 A person is exposed to an individual diagnosed with severe acute respiratory syndrome (SARS). The nurse should expect which method to be implemented to control the spread of infection?
① Isolation
② Quarantine
③ Segregation
④ Surveillance

10 Which statement most accurately reflects the principle of providing for a patient's nutritional needs in the home?
① The patient should eat whatever is preferred as long as adequate amounts of protein is ingested.
② The patient should plan to eat meals at the same time as other family members.
③ Supplements should be taken whenever the patient is hungry between meals.
④ Support groups may be used to ensure adequate nutrition for the patient.
TEST-TAKING TIP ◦ Identify the key word in the stem that sets a priority.

11 Which is a priority when the nurse cares for an older adult in the community?
① Encouraging interaction within the family
② Helping with bureaucratic paperwork
③ Supporting rehabilitation needs
④ Maintaining quality of life
TEST-TAKING TIP ◦ Identify the key word in the stem that sets a priority. Identify the global option.

12 Which categories of health-care delivery are mainly associated with community-based nursing?
① Primary and tertiary
② Secondary and primary
③ Tertiary and rehabilitation
④ Rehabilitation and secondary
TEST-TAKING TIP ◦ Identify the key word in the stem that sets a priority. Identify duplicate facts among the options.

13 Which nursing action provides support during a situational stress?
① Counseling a parent experiencing the empty nest syndrome
② Encouraging an older adult to visit the senior center
③ Providing sex education classes to adolescents
④ Providing pain relief for a woman with cancer
TEST-TAKING TIP ◦ Identify the clue in the stem.

14 Which statement is most accurate about health perception and health status?
①　Disability is related to the extent to which one is able to carry out the behaviors of the role chosen.
②　Anticipation of the future has minimal impact on the understanding of one's health.
③　The ability to tolerate illness and disability is the same for one person as for another.
④　Assuming the sick role is generally maladaptive and harmful to recovery.

TEST-TAKING TIP ⊙ Identify the key word in the stem that sets a priority.

15 Which sociologic trend in the United States is predicted to have the most impact on the delivery of health care in the community in the next 20 years?
①　Increase in the graying population
②　Decrease in the number of immigrants
③　Increase in the number of multiple-birth deliveries
④　Decrease in the number of people living in poverty

TEST-TAKING TIP ⊙ Identify the key word in the stem that sets a priority.

16 Which nursing activity in the community addresses the most basic need according to Maslow's Hierarchy of Needs?
①　Arranging for Meals on Wheels
②　Exploring the meaning of one's life
③　Teaching the client to remove throw rugs
④　Encouraging the client to visit with friends

TEST-TAKING TIP ⊙ Identify the key word in the stem that sets a priority. Identify the clues in the stem. Identify the unique option.

17 Which phrase is most accurately associated with the concept of community coalition?
①　Wellness programs
②　Growing diversity
③　Shared purpose
④　Home care

TEST-TAKING TIP ⊙ Identify the key word in the stem that sets a priority. Identify the clue in the stem.

18 The visiting nurse is caring for a bed-bound patient with a pressure ulcer. Which nursing intervention associated with providing pressure ulcer care in the home is often different from providing pressure ulcer care in the acute-care setting?
①　Measuring a wound weekly versus daily
②　Changing dressings daily versus three times a day
③　Employing medical asepsis versus sterile technique
④　Using a bulb syringe versus a piston syringe when irrigating

19 Which action by the nurse in the occupational setting reflects the lowest-level need according to Maslow?
①　Identifying hazards in the environment
②　Assessing the health status of employees
③　Initiating an ordered immunization program
④　Promoting employees' social adaptation to the job

TEST-TAKING TIP ⊙ Identify the clues in the stem.

20 Which population variable is being assessed in a community profile inventory when the nurse asks, "How many people live within a square mile in the community?"
①　Size
②　Density
③　Mobility
④　Composition

21 Which statement reflects the concept of prevalence?
① "On Monday morning, the school nurse identified that six children had measles."
② "During the last 5 years, 1 percent of the population of the United States had tuberculosis."
③ "On the first day of June this year, 10 percent of the population of Middletown had heart disease."
④ "Last year, of the people at risk for developing breast cancer, 9 percent actually developed the disease."

22 The nurse is conducting a screening program for the leading cause of death associated with adults 60 years or older. Which assessment by the nurse is most appropriate?
① Apical pulse
② Breath sounds
③ Liver palpation
④ Respiratory rate

TEST-TAKING TIP ◉ Identify the key word in the stem that sets a priority. Identify the options that are equally plausible.

23 The nurse is assessing adolescents in the community. Which problem is most commonly associated with this age group?
① Mumps
② Measles
③ Child abuse
④ Substance abuse

TEST-TAKING TIP ◉ Identify the key word in the stem that sets a priority. Identify the word that is a clue in the stem. Identify the equally plausible options.

24 An older adult, who needs minimal help with ADLs and who takes prescription medication twice a day, is to be discharged from the hospital. Which facility most appropriately meets this individual's needs?
① Group home
② Nursing home
③ Day-care center
④ Assisted-living facility

TEST-TAKING TIP ◉ Identify the key word in the stem that sets a priority. Identify the clue in the stem.

25 When the nurse is caring for patients in the home, it is important to incorporate principles related to community health nursing. Place the following principles in order of priority.
① Listen attentively
② Examine own beliefs and values
③ Remain open to other peoples' views
④ Elicit the support of community resources
⑤ Assist patients and family members to problem solve

Answer: _____.

280 Meeting the Needs of Patients in the Community Setting
Answers and Rationales

1 TEST-TAKING TIP ○ The word "priority" in the stem requires the nurse to identify what should be done first.

① This addresses safety, which is not as great a priority as physiologic needs according to Maslow's Hierarchy of Needs.

② Preventing aspiration and meeting a client's physiologic need to ingest adequate nutrition take priority over higher-level needs according to Maslow.

③ Feelings of acceptance are related to Maslow's category of love and belonging. Love and belonging are higher-level needs than physiologic needs, which are more basic according to Maslow.

④ This supports self-esteem and the need to feel more empowered over one's situation. According to Maslow, this is a higher-level need than physiologic needs.

2 TEST-TAKING TIP ○ The word "most" is the key word in the stem that sets a priority. The clue in the stem is "1990s."

① *Tertiary care* involves helping patients adapt to limitations caused by illness; historically, this always has been a focus of health care.

② Early diagnosis and treatment to prevent complications of illness is a part of secondary care; historically, this always has been a focus of health care.

③ Health promotion activities, including exercise programs and low-cholesterol diets, that assist patients to maintain their present levels of health or to enhance their health in the future is a focus of primary care. Primary care received increased importance in the 1990s.

④ Restorative rehabilitation services are a part of tertiary care; historically, this always has been a focus of health care.

3 TEST-TAKING TIP ○ The word "mainly" in the stem sets a priority. The word "community" in Option 3 is directly associated with the words "community health nursing" in the stem. The word "community" in the stem and in Option 3 is a clang association.

① The home setting is traditionally associated with the concept of community nursing. However, in the current health-care environment, the community includes settings such as schools, work environments, community centers, neighborhood clinics, and even mobile units that bring services directly to people in a neighborhood.

② Community-based health activities are designed to help individuals and groups across all economic levels and low- as well as high-risk groups.

③ Community health nursing reaches out to people and groups outside of acute-care facilities. Services are provided in neighborhoods, which includes the home.

④ Community-based nursing assists individuals and groups from one end of the health–illness continuum to the other, not just the health end of the continuum.

4 TEST-TAKING TIP ○ The word "developmental" modifies the word "crisis" and is the clue in the stem.

① Maturational crises are changes that occur during a period of growth that often require the assumption of a new role. Adolescents experience rapid bodily changes, have a need to be accepted and to be part of a group, and attempt to become independent. Most important, the adolescent is striving to establish sexual identity. This maturational crisis is compounded in adolescents who recognize that they are homosexual. Many schools and parents are unprepared to deal with this situation, which can often have lifelong emotional effects on the individual.

② A recent divorce is a situational, not a maturational, crisis. A situational crisis is an external event that is not part of everyday living. It causes a high degree of anxiety and generally requires learning new coping mechanisms.

③ Being critically ill is not an expected part of normal growth and development. It is a situational crisis for the child and the parents.

④ Unemployment is a situational crisis.

5 TEST-TAKING TIP ○ The word "essential" in the stem sets a priority.

① Community health nursing focuses on illness prevention, health education, providing support services, hospice care, and rehabilitation, not just health promotion.

② Community health nursing focuses on the health-care needs of groups and families within the community, not just individuals.

③ Community nurses practice in many different settings, including clinics, schools, centers of all kinds, mobile units, and places of employment, not just in the home.

④ Community health nurses must develop collaborative relationships with other health professionals as well as with individuals and groups in the community.

6 **TEST-TAKING TIP** ⊙ The word "just" in Option 3 is a specific determiner.
(1) Aid to Families with Dependent Children is unrelated to Medicare. It provides assistance to people during the childbearing years, particularly divorced or single women with children.
(2) Midwife services is unrelated to Medicare.
(3) Income is unrelated to Medicare. In 1965, Medicaid was established under Title 19 of the Social Security Act. Medicaid is a federal public assistance program for people who require financial assistance, such as low-income groups.
(4) **In 1965 the Medicare amendments (Title 18) to the Social Security Act provided a national and state health insurance program for people 65 years and older.**

7 (1) This is providing care after a person has a disease, which reflects "downstream thinking."
(2) Same as #1.
(3) Same as #1.
(4) **"Upstream thinking" challenges providers to look "upstream" to identify the etiology of disease and intervene to prevent illness rather than to provide care "downstream," when the person is in the "river of illness."**

8 **TEST-TAKING TIP** ⊙ The word "first" in the stem sets a priority.
(1) Although the concept in the statement may be true, it should not be the nurse's first response to the patient's statement.
(2) This should not be the initial response. This question might be asked later.
(3) This delays the arrival of help. When it gets to the point where a person cannot breathe, 911 should be called.
(4) **When a patient makes a statement that includes inaccurate information, the person is exhibiting an opportunity for learning. The nurse has a responsibility to teach appropriate self-care. The old adage "Strike when the iron is hot" supports this teaching/learning concept.**

9 (1) *Isolation* is used to separate an infected person during the time the person is communicable. The person in the question has been exposed to the SARS pathogen but is not yet infected.
(2) ***Quarantine*** **is used to prevent further transmission of the disease in case the person should become infected as a result of exposure to the SARS pathogen. The exposed person is kept separate for the duration of the longest incubation period known for the disease.**
(3) *Segregation* is used to keep separate a group of infected individuals to control the spread of a disease. In the early 1900s, sanitariums were established to separate infected individuals with tuberculosis from the general population. In China, in the spring of 2003, a separate hospital was built to segregate and treat individuals diagnosed with SARS.
(4) *Surveillance* is associated with either personal or disease surveillance. Personal surveillance is supervision without limitations on movement. Disease surveillance is the continuing investigation of the incidence and spread of disease relevant to effective control.

10 **TEST-TAKING TIP** ⊙ The word "most" in the stem sets a priority.
(1) Although a diet should be designed with a patient's food preferences in mind, the diet chosen needs to address all nutritional components associated with the patient's needs, not just protein.
(2) Although eating is considered a social activity and patients may be encouraged to eat with family members, this may not meet the nutritional needs of the patient. A variety of issues should be considered: a family meal may be too confusing and distracting; the patient may be on a restricted diet that may make the patient feel uncomfortable when eating with the family; the patient may be receiving a tube feeding and prefer not to be with the family at meal time; or the odor of food may be difficult to tolerate.
(3) Supplements should be taken only if nutritional needs cannot be met with the prescribed diet. Supplements are rich in calories, vitamins, and/or minerals and, if taken whenever a patient is hungry, they may exceed the patient's metabolic needs. This may contribute to complications such as excessive weight gain.
(4) **Meeting the nutritional needs of a patient living at home requires the nurse to consider all phases of achieving adequate nutritional intake, such as the patient's and family's knowledge about nutrition and the ability to shop for, buy, prepare, cook, and eat food. Community support such as home-delivered meals, senior center lunch programs, meals provided by missions and shelters, school lunch programs, and community food pantries help people in need.**

11 **TEST-TAKING TIP** ⊙ The word "primary" in the stem sets a priority. Option 4 is a global option that inherently includes the interventions identified in Options 1, 2, and 3.
(1) This is only one part of caring for an older adult.
(2) Same as #1.
(3) Same as #1.
(4) **This option is broad in scope and addresses improvement in all aspects of the life of the older adult.**

12 **TEST-TAKING TIP** ⊙ The word "mainly" in the stem sets a priority. Four concepts of health-care delivery are being associated with community-based nursing: primary, secondary, tertiary, and rehabilitation. If you know one concept (either primary or tertiary) that is associated with health-care delivery in the community setting, two options can be deleted from consideration. If you know one concept (either secondary or rehabilitation) that is not related to health-care delivery in the community setting, two options can be deleted from consideration.

① **Primary care is associated with health promotion, screening, education, and protection. Although tertiary care is associated with specialized diagnostic and therapeutic care generally delivered in the acute-care setting, it also includes specialized services such as rehabilitation and hospice services, which are most often delivered in community settings.**

② Although primary health-care activities generally take place in the community setting, secondary health care activities take place in the acute-care setting and generally not in the community setting.

③ Although tertiary care is associated with specialized services such as rehabilitation, rehabilitation is not a category of health-care delivery. Rehabilitation is a specialized service provided in acute-care and community settings. Activities that help people maintain or restore function after an illness are in the tertiary prevention, not primary prevention, category.

④ Rehabilitation is not considered a category of health care but rather a type of service provided in acute and community settings. Secondary health care is associated with hospital-based service (e.g., critical, emergency, and acute care).

13 **TEST-TAKING TIP** ⊙ The word "situational" modifies the word "stress" and is the clue in the stem.

① Counseling a parent experiencing empty nest syndrome is an intervention that supports a person experiencing a maturational, not a situational, stress. Maturational stresses are situations that occur during a period of growth. Maturational growth requires the mastery of tasks in a relatively predictable order and includes the assumption of new roles, according to Erikson.

② Counseling an older adult to visit the senior center is an intervention supporting a person experiencing a maturational stress, not situational stress.

③ Providing sex education to an adolescent is an intervention that supports a person experiencing a maturational, not situational stress.

④ **A situational stress is an external event that is not part of everyday living; it causes a high degree of anxiety and generally requires learning new coping mechanisms. Physical illness is always a situational stress because it is a physical and emotional assault on the "self," requires the sudden assumption of new roles, triggers behaviors that reflect an attempt to cope, and requires the learning of new coping skills to deal with the stress.**

14 **TEST-TAKING TIP** ⊙ The word "most" in the stem sets a priority.

① **Where people place themselves on the health–illness continuum is a highly individual perception based on personal expectations and values. People generally fulfill numerous roles. In the role performance model of health and wellness, people who are disabled or ill but are able to carry out their role according to personal expectations tend to view themselves as closer to the high-level wellness end of the health–illness continuum. When role performance becomes impaired, people are more likely to view themselves as disabled.**

② How people anticipate the future has a significant impact on their ability to understand their health. The nurse needs to assess what people believe and feel about their future life. The nurse must work within the context of the person's situation to best assist with the development of coping mechanisms.

③ People react in diversified ways to illness and disability. Every person is an individual, and how an individual reacts depends on many factors, such as age, gender, cultural/ethnic background, religious beliefs, economic status, previous experiences, role in the family, and support systems.

④ Assuming the sick role (passivity, social and psychologic regression, and submission to treatment regimens) is adaptive and beneficial if not taken to the extreme. Because illness is a modification in the ability to function, there is always a concurrent need to modify behavior in an attempt to rest and recover, which is adaptive. Assumption of the sick role becomes maladaptive and harmful when a person is unable to move on physically and emotionally after the crisis is resolved.

15 **TEST-TAKING TIP** ⊙ The word "most" in the stem sets a priority.

① **By 2020, the number of people over the age of 65 will increase to 50 million individuals in the United States; this is the fastest growing segment of the population.**

② Diversity is increasing, not decreasing, in the United States.

③ Although this is a true statement, it does not have the same impact on the health-care needs of the society as the individuals mentioned in another option.

④ The number of people living in poverty is increasing, not decreasing, in the United States.

16 TEST-TAKING TIP ○ The word "most" in the stem sets a priority. The words "basic needs" and "Maslow's Hierarchy of Needs" are the clues in the stem. Option 1 is unique because it includes the word "for" while the other 3 options include the word "the."

(1) **Meals on Wheels delivers meals daily to those at home who need assistance with preparing nutritious meals. Adequate nutrition (food) is essential for survival and is a first-level (physiologic) need according to Maslow's Hierarchy of Needs.**

(2) This relates to self-actualization, which is the highest level in Maslow's Hierarchy of Needs.

(3) Removing throw rugs protects a person from falls. According to Maslow's Hierarchy of Needs, safety and security needs become significant after basic physiologic needs are met.

(4) Encouraging socialization helps to support the need to belong to a group, which is a third-level need according to Maslow's Hierarchy of Needs. When people feel that they belong and are appreciated for who they are, love and belonging needs are being met.

17 TEST-TAKING TIP ○ The word "most" in the stem sets a priority. The word "coalition" in the stem is related to words such as *partnership*, *alliance*, and *unification*. The definition of the word "coalition" should lead you to the word "share" in Option 3.

(1) A "wellness program" and a "community coalition" are two different concepts. A wellness program is a type of health promotion program that focuses on the reduction of risks and the development of positive health habits.

(2) Growing diversity speaks to the increasing differences in culture and ethnicity in the population. People of different cultures maintain cultural values, traditions, and beliefs that contribute to the texture and complexity of a community. Although a group of people from one cultural or ethnic group may share a common purpose, this concept is different from community coalition.

(3) **Synonyms for the word "coalition" include *alliance*, *unification*, and *combination*. A community coalition is the unification of individuals and groups to address issues related to a shared purpose.**

(4) "Home care" and "community coalition" are two different concepts. Home care is associated with providing services for a patient in the individual's place of residence.

18 (1) Pressure ulcers should be measured at least weekly whether the patient is in the hospital or in the home. It may be done more frequently depending on the needs of the individual.

(2) The frequency of changing the dressing on a wound is individualized depending on the patient's needs. The setting is irrelevant.

(3) **Sterile technique is used when a hospitalized person needs a wound dressing change to prevent the occurrence of a hospital-acquired infection. The risk of infection for a hospitalized person is increased at several stages of the chain of infection. Medical aseptic technique alone often is used when changing a wound dressing in the home. People are usually further along in recovery and less susceptible to infection, and people have built up a resistance to the "familiar microorganisms" in the home environment.**

(4) Both bulb and piston syringes can be used in either home or acute-care settings.

19 TEST-TAKING TIP ○ The words "lowest-level need" and "Maslow" are the clues in the stem.

(1) Identifying hazards in the environment is a health promotion activity that supports the safety of employees. The needs for safety and security are second-level needs according to Maslow's Hierarchy of Needs.

(2) **Assessing the health of an employee includes identifying the physical status of the individual, which addresses first-level needs, such as air, food, water, shelter, rest, sleep, and activity, necessary for survival.**

(3) An immunization program is a specific health protection activity that helps to keep a person safe from a specific disease. The needs for safety and security are second-level needs according to Maslow's Hierarchy of Needs.

(4) Promoting social adaptation addresses people's love and belonging needs. The need to feel loved and the need to attain a place within a group are third-level (love and belonging) needs according to Maslow's Hierarchy of Needs.

20 (1) The *size* of a community is the total number of people in the community.

(2) ***Density* refers to the number of people who live within a square mile. High- and low-density areas have their own commonalities (e.g., high-density areas are usually more stressful; low-density areas may have a decreased availability of health services).**

(3) *Mobility* refers to how frequently people move in and out of the community.

(4) The *composition* of a community includes factors such as the age, gender, marital status, and occupations of people in the community.

21 ① This represents a simple count of the number of people with a disease.

② Calculating the prevalence rate over a period of time is called a *period prevalence rate*. It is calculated with the formula:

$$\text{Period Prevalence Rate} = \frac{\text{Number of Persons with a Characteristic During Period of Time}}{\text{Total Number in the Population}}$$

③ *Prevalence* refers to all people with a health condition existing in a given population at a given point in time. It is calculated with the formula:

$$\text{Prevalence Rate} = \frac{\text{Number of Persons with a Characteristic on a Particular Day}}{\text{Total Number in the Population}}$$

④ This reflects an *incidence rate*. It is calculated with the formula:

$$\text{Incidence} = \frac{\text{Number of Persons Developing a Disease}}{\text{Total Number at Risk per Unit of Time}}$$

22 TEST-TAKING TIP ◉ The word "most" in the stem sets a priority. Options 2 and 4 are equally plausible because they both relate to respiratory assessments.

① **The leading cause of death in the older adult is heart disease. Assessments of rate and rhythm of heartbeats are essential.**

② Although COPD is a major health problem in older adults, it is not the leading cause of death.

③ Chronic liver disease is a common cause of death in adults 45 to 64 years of age.

④ Same as #2.

23 TEST-TAKING TIP ◉ The word "most" in the stem sets a priority. The word "adolescent" is the clue in the stem. Options 1 and 2 are equally plausible; they both are childhood communicable diseases.

① Mumps and measles occur most often in toddlers and young school-age children. With the measles, mumps, and rubella (MMR) vaccine, the incidence of these diseases has declined considerably.

② Same as #1.

③ Although child abuse occurs in teenagers, it is most commonly identified in toddlers and young school-age children.

④ **Substance abuse (e.g., alcohol, cigarettes, illegal drugs, inhalants) is a health problem commonly associated with adolescents. Complex physical, emotional, cognitive, and social changes, along with the desire to take risks and the need to develop a self-identity, all influence behavior.**

24 TEST-TAKING TIP ◉ The word "most" in the stem sets a priority. The concept "activities of daily living" is associated with the concept of "assisted living" and is a covert clang association.

① Group homes are for specific populations, such as people who are developmentally disabled, mentally ill, or recovering from alcohol or drug abuse.

② A nursing home provides skilled nursing care, which this patient does not need.

③ This patient needs more care than can be provided in a daycare center. This person needs assistance with toileting, grooming, dressing, and eating which all occur before arrival at the daycare center.

④ **Assisted-living facilities help with ADLs, prepare meals, and dispense medications as needed.**

25 Answer: 2, 3, 1, 5, 4.

② **Examine own beliefs and values. Nurses must explore their own beliefs and values before caring for others. This activity supports the advice, "Know Thyself."**

③ **Remain open to other peoples' views. Nurses must remain open to the thoughts, beliefs, values, etc of patients; a nonjudgmental attitude is essential for patients to feel accepted.**

① **Listen attentively. Once the nurse has a self awareness and conveys an openness to others, then the nurse must actively listen to hear the content and feeling tone of messages from others.**

⑤ **Assist patients and family members to problem solve. After complete collection of data is accomplished, then identifying problems and exploring possible solutions to the problems can be attempted.**

④ **Elicit the support of community resources. Once potential solutions are identified, appropriate community resources can be explored and selected to assist with the resolution of the problem.**

Pharmacology

• • •

This section encompasses questions related to how drugs physiologically and biochemically affect the body (pharmacodynamics) and how drugs are absorbed, distributed, metabolized, and eliminated from the body (pharmacokinetics). The questions include such topics as the therapeutic and side effects of classifications of drugs, medication toxicity, peak and trough values, factors affecting drug action, common assessments before and after drug administration, use of the nursing process in drug therapy, and the role of the nurse in patient teaching and adherence to the medication regimen.

Questions

Please fill in the circle to mark your answer choice.

1   The nurse identifies that an age-related alteration in the older adult that may affect the absorption of an oral hypoglycemic agent is:
   ① A decrease in hydrochloric acid production
   ② An increase in mesenteric blood flow
   ③ An increase in subcutaneous fat
   ④ An increase in cardiac output
   TEST-TAKING TIP ○ Identify the unique option.

2   Which cathartic acts as a wetting agent to soften stool and is most effective in preventing straining during defecation?
   ① Colace
   ② Dulcolax
   ③ Mineral oil
   ④ Milk of Magnesia
   TEST-TAKING TIP ○ Identify the key word in the stem that sets a priority.

3   Which drug should the nurse identify as being most effective in the immediate treatment of anaphylaxis?
   ① Prednisone
   ② Solu-Cortef
   ③ Epinephrine
   ④ Solu-Medrol
   TEST-TAKING TIP ○ Identify the key word in the stem that sets a priority. Identify the word that is a clue in the stem. Identify the options that are equally plausible. Identify the unique option.

4   A patient receiving a cardiac glycoside is "digitalized." The nurse understands that digitalization means:
   ① Large doses of the drug were administered to quickly reach the therapeutic window.
   ② An excessive amount of the drug was given and unacceptable side effects occurred.
   ③ Blood levels of the drug have been maintained at acceptable levels over time.
   ④ The therapeutic window was exceeded and toxicity has occurred.
   TEST-TAKING TIP ○ Identify the equally plausible options.

5   The nurse anticipates which group of drugs is most likely to be ordered when a patient has difficulty sleeping?
   ① Benzodiazepines
   ② Barbiturates
   ③ Analgesics
   ④ Opioids
   TEST-TAKING TIP ○ Identify the key word in the stem that sets a priority. Identify the options that are equally plausible.

6 A patient is receiving prednisone, a glucocorticoid. The nurse should monitor the patient's electrolytes for:
① Hypokalemia and hyponatremia
② Hypokalemia and hypernatremia
③ Hyperkalemia and hyponatremia
④ Hyperkalemia and hypernatremia

TEST-TAKING TIP ◉ Identify the duplicate facts among the options. Identify the options that are opposites.

7 Which group of medications has a high risk for a drug interaction with digoxin (Lanoxin)?
① Glucocorticoids
② Sulfonamides
③ Antibiotics
④ Antacids

TEST-TAKING TIP ◉ Identify the word in the stem that sets a priority. Identify the options that are equally plausible.

8 After administering a cathartic, the nurse identifies that the drug is effective when the patient:
① Has a bowel movement
② Describes pain relief
③ Falls asleep
④ Voids urine

9 The nurse is administering heparin to a patient daily. The nurse should assess for which undesirable clinical response that indicates the need to discontinue the heparin therapy?
① International normalized ratio of 2.5
② Platelet count of 100,000/mm³
③ Hematuria
④ Gastritis

TEST-TAKING TIP ◉ Identify the word in the stem that indicates negative polarity.

10 The nurse understands that the classification of drugs that can precipitate superinfections is:
① Diuretics
② Antibiotics
③ Vasopressors
④ Thrombolytics

11 The physician orders an antibiotic intravenous piggyback every 12 hours. What time should the nurse schedule a blood sample to be drawn to determine a trough level for this patient when the drug is administered at 2:00 PM?
① 3:00 PM
② 8:00 PM
③ 1:30 AM
④ 2:30 AM

TEST-TAKING TIP ◉ Identify the options that are opposites.

12 The nurse is evaluating a patient's response to an antitussive. The patient response that indicates that the antitussive is effective is a decrease in:
① Fever
② Nasal congestion
③ Mucus viscosity
④ Frequency of coughing

13 When performing a health history a patient states, "I take 1 package of Metamucil every day no matter what." Which drug effect should the nurse most likely expect to occur?
① Tolerance
② Synergistic

③ Habituation
④ Idiosyncratic

TEST-TAKING TIP ○ Identify the key word in the stem that sets a priority.

14 The patient is receiving an antibiotic that has a 4 to 10 μg/mL (micrograms per milliliter) therapeutic range, an optimum peak value of 8 to 10 μg/mL, and a minimum trough level of 0.5 μg/mL. The value that requires the nurse to notify the physician is a:
① Peak value of 5 μg/mL
② Peak value of 9 μg/mL
③ Trough value of 0.3 μg/mL
④ Trough value of 0.7 μg/mL

TEST-TAKING TIP ○ Identify the words in the stem that indicate negative polarity. Identify the options that are opposites.

15 The nurse administers an expectorant to a patient. Which adaptation indicates to the nurse that the patient is experiencing a therapeutic response to the medication?
① Reduced fever
② Productive cough
③ Relieved nasal congestion
④ Dilation of respiratory airways

16 The blood serum level of the therapeutic range for an antibiotic is 4 to 10 μg/mL. The nurse concludes that the implication of a peak level of 12 μg/mL is that the:
① Drug dose is safe
② Drug dose is subtherapeutic
③ Patient is at risk for drug accumulation
④ Patient's next dose should be given over a longer period of time.

TEST-TAKING TIP ○ Identify the unique option.

17 The nurse identifies which physiologic change in the older adult contributes to prolonged drug half-life?
① Reduced subcutaneous tissue
② Reduced glomerular filtration rate
③ Decreased hydrochloric acid production
④ Decreased gastrointestinal absorptive surface

18 A patient is receiving a neuroleptic antipsychotic medication. Extrapyramidal reactions are significant undesirable responses associated with this classification of drugs. Therefore, the nurse should assess the patient for which adaptations?
① Respiratory depression and diarrhea
② Akathisia and respiratory depression
③ Spasm of the muscles of the face and akathisia
④ Diarrhea and spasms of the muscles of the face

TEST-TAKING TIP ○ Identify the duplicate facts among the options.

19 When caring for a patient receiving an analgesic, the nurse should assess for which therapeutic response?
① Temperature within expected range
② Less labored breathing
③ Nausea has subsided
④ Pain is tolerable

TEST-TAKING TIP ○ Identify the key word in the stem that sets a priority.

20 The patient is receiving an antibiotic that has a 4 to 10 μg/mL therapeutic range, an optimum peak value of 8 to 10 μg/mL, and a minimum trough level of 0.5 μg/mL. When monitoring the patient's response to therapy, which value should the nurse consider acceptable?
① Peak value of 8 μg/mL
② Peak value of 11 μg/mL
③ Trough value of 0.1 μg/mL
④ Trough value of 0.3 μg/mL

21 Which statement by the patient receiving digoxin (Lanoxin) 0.25 mg every day indicates that the nurse needs to provide further teaching?
① "I should not take antacids with digoxin."
② "I should call the doctor if I have nausea, vomiting, or weakness."
③ "If I forget to take my digoxin, I should take 2 pills the next day."
④ "I should not take the digoxin if my apical pulse is below 60 beats per minute."

TEST-TAKING TIP ○ Identify the words in the stem that indicate negative polarity. Identify the option that is unique.

22 The nurse understands that opioid (narcotic) analgesics limit pain by:
① Diminishing peripheral pain reception
② Modifying the patient's perception of pain
③ Competing with receptors for sensory input
④ Closing the gating mechanism for impulse transmission

23 A patient is receiving an antibiotic, an antiemetic, an antihistamine, and an antihypertensive. Considering this patient's risk for falls, which medication commonly causes postural hypotension?
① Antibiotic
② Antiemetic
③ Antihistamine
④ Antihypertensive

TEST-TAKING TIP ○ Identify the clues in the stem.

24 The nurse is collecting a health history for a patient who will be receiving intravenous heparin therapy. Which statement by the patient needs further exploration by the nurse?
① "I stopped taking my daily aspirin tablet about five days ago."
② "I always experience heavy menstrual periods."
③ "I eat a lot of green, leafy vegetables."
④ "I may be pregnant."

TEST-TAKING TIP ○ Identify the words in the stem that indicate negative polarity.

25 To best promote intestinal peristalsis, the nurse should encourage a patient to:
① Use a bulk cathartic weekly
② Take castor oil once a month
③ Eat whole-grain foods every day
④ Self-administer a stool softener daily

TEST-TAKING TIP ○ Identify the key word in the stem that sets a priority. Identify the option that is unique.

26 Which drug is palliative in its therapeutic action?
① Calcium
② Demerol
③ Penicillin
④ Synthroid

27 After the physician orders an antidepressant for a patient, the patient asks the nurse, "How long will it take before I feel better?" Before answering, the nurse recalls that an emerging therapeutic response to an antidepressant medication usually takes:
① 2 hours
② 2 days
③ 2 weeks
④ 2 months

TEST-TAKING TIP ○ Identify the word in the stem that is a clue.

28 The nurse understands that antipsychotics potentiate the effects of:
① Amphetamines
② Anticoagulants
③ Opioid analgesics
④ Oral hypoglycemic agents

29 The nurse is administering vincristine sulfate (Oncovin), an antineoplastic drug, to a patient with cancer. For which neurologic system side effects should the nurse assess this patient?
① Decreased red and white blood cells
② Alternating constipation and diarrhea
③ Electrolyte imbalances and renal failure
④ Peripheral neuropathies and paralytic ileus

   TEST-TAKING TIP ○ Identify the word in the stem that provides a clue.

30 A patient is receiving a diuretic. Which patient assessments reflect therapeutic responses to the diuretic? Check all that apply.
① _____ Decreased weight
② _____ Increased appetite
③ _____ Increased urinary output
④ _____ Increased blood pressure
⑤ _____ Decreased white blood cells

290 Pharmacology
Answers and Rationales

1 **TEST-TAKING TIP** ○ Options 2, 3, and 4 all relate to concepts that increase something and begin with the word "An." Option 1 is unique because it begins with "A" and it is the only option with the word decrease.
① Hydrochloric acid production decreases as the body ages.
② Mesenteric blood flow decreases as the body ages.
③ **As the body ages, there is a decrease in subcutaneous fat.**
④ Cardiac output decreases as the body ages.

2 **TEST-TAKING TIP** ○ The word "most" in the stem sets a priority.
① **Docusate sodium (Colace) is a detergent that lowers the surface tension of feces, allowing penetration by water and fat, which soften stool.**
② Bisacodyl (Dulcolax) is a stimulant cathartic because it irritates the intestinal mucosa, increasing intestinal motility.
③ Mineral oil lubricates the fecal mass, facilitating defecation; regular use interferes with the absorption of the fat-soluble vitamins A, D, E, and K.
④ Magnesium hydroxide (Milk of Magnesia) is a saline or osmotic agent that draws water into the fecal mass.

3 **TEST-TAKING TIP** ○ The word "most" in the stem sets a priority. The word "immediate" in the stem is a clue. Options 1, 2, and 3 are all plausible because they are all corticosteroids. Option 2 is unique because it is the only option that is not a corticosteroid.
① Prednisone is a corticosteroid. Corticosteroids, which have an anti-inflammatory action, are generally administered to prevent the recurrence of symptoms.
② Solu-Cortef is a corticosteroid.
③ **Epinephrine (Adrenalin) is administered as soon as possible after a person demonstrates adaptations of systemic anaphylaxis or as a preventive measure in a person who is highly allergic and who has been exposed to an allergen. Epinephrine quickly stimulates alpha (α)- and beta (β)-adrenergic receptors of the autonomic nervous system, causing vasoconstriction and bronchodilation.**
④ Solu-Medrol is a corticosteroid.

4 **TEST-TAKING TIP** ○ Options 2 and 4 are equally plausible because they both relate to toxicity.
① **Large loading doses are administered quickly to promote the desired clinical effects. The therapeutic blood level for digoxin is 0.5 to 2.0 ng/mL. Values that are 2.4 ng/mL or greater indicate toxicity.**
② Toxicity occurs when the therapeutic range is exceeded and is associated with unacceptable side effects. This is a non-therapeutic effect.
③ This relates to maintenance doses of the drug; a maintenance dose is sufficient to replace the amount of drug eliminated from the body between doses.
④ Same as #2.

5 **TEST-TAKING TIP** ○ The word "most" in the stem sets a priority. Options 3 and 4 are equally plausible.
① **Benzodiazepines, such as temazepam (Restoril) and zolpidem (Ambien), are a group of nonbarbiturate sedative-hypnotics. They influence the neurons in the central nervous system that suppress responsiveness to stimuli, thereby decreasing levels of arousal.**
② Barbiturates, such as sodium pentobarbital (Nembutal) and secobarbital (Seconal), have many side effects and have been replaced by benzodiazepines as the first drugs of choice to induce sleep.
③ Analgesics are primarily administered to reduce pain, not to induce sleep.
④ Opioids are primarily administered to reduce pain, not to induce sleep.

6 **TEST-TAKING TIP** ○ The question is asking about potassium and sodium imbalances as a result of glucocorticoid therapy. If you know at least one electrolyte imbalance that can occur, two options can be eliminated from consideration. Options 2 and 3 are opposites.
① Although hypokalemia may occur, hypernatremia, not hyponatremia, may occur.
② **Prednisone, a glucocorticoid, has significant water- and sodium-retaining (mineralocorticoid) activities. As sodium is retained, potassium is depleted.**
③ The opposite may occur. The patient may experience hypokalemia and hypernatremia.
④ Although hypernatremia may occur, hypokalemia, not hyperkalemia, may occur.

7 **TEST-TAKING TIP** ○ The word "high" in the stem sets a priority. Options 2 and 3 are equally plausible. Sulfa drugs are antibiotics.
① **Prednisone, a glucocorticoid with mineralocorticoid activity, can precipitate hypokalemia. Hypokalemia increases the sensitivity of the myocardium to digitalis. Hypokalemia can precipitate digitalis toxicity, even if digoxin serum levels are in the therapeutic range of 0.5 to 2.0 ng/mL.**

(2) Sulfonamides do not interact with digoxin.

(3) Antibiotics do not interact with digoxin.

(4) Antacids do not interact with digoxin.

8 (1) **Cathartics, also called laxatives, induce defecation.**

(2) Analgesics relieve pain. Also, some cathartics may cause slight abdominal discomfort due to increased intestinal peristalsis.

(3) Sedatives and hypnotics promote sleep.

(4) Diuretics increase urinary output.

9 **TEST-TAKING TIP** ◉ The word "undesirable" in the stem indicates negative polarity.

(1) An international normalized ratio (INR) value is obtained to assess the effectiveness of warfarin sodium (Coumadin) therapy, not heparin therapy. An activated partial thromboplastin time (APTT) is one test that is performed to assess the effects of heparin therapy.

(2) A low platelet count (thrombocytopenia) occurs in 5 to 10 percent of patients receiving heparin therapy. Platelets can fall to 100,000 units from the expected range of 195,000 to 400,000/mm³. This often resolves without intervention even with continued heparin therapy.

(3) **Hematuria (blood in the urine) is a serious side effect of heparin therapy that requires the temporary termination of therapy. If severe bleeding is identified, protamine sulfate is administered as an antidote.**

(4) Heparin is administered parenterally, not by mouth, and does not cause gastritis.

10 (1) Diuretics increase the formation and excretion of urine. They can cause dehydration and electrolyte imbalance, but they do not precipitate superinfection.

(2) **Prolonged or inappropriate use of antibiotics can stimulate bacterial growth as normal flora of the gastrointestinal tract and skin are destroyed. Infections that occur while a patient is receiving antimicrobial therapy are called *superinfections*.**

(3) Vasopressors constrict the blood vessels; they cause hypertension, not superinfections.

(4) Thrombolytics dissolve thrombi or emboli; they also prolong the coagulation processes, which may increase the risk of bleeding. Thrombolytics do not precipitate superinfections.

11 **TEST-TAKING TIP** ◉ Options 3 and 4 are opposites. One is 30 minutes before the drug is administered and the other is 30 minutes after the drug is administered.

(1) This is too soon for a trough level. This time is appropriate for a peak level.

(2) This is too soon for a trough level. This time is half way between two doses.

(3) **The blood level of an antibiotic is at its lowest level just before the next scheduled dose.**

(4) After the drug is administered, the blood level of the drug rises. A value taken at 30 minutes after the drug is administered does not reflect the lowest serum level, which is the purpose of identifying a trough level.

12 (1) Antipyretics reduce a fever; antitussives do not.

(2) Nasal decongestants reduce nasal congestion; antitussives do not.

(3) Mucolytics reduce mucus viscosity; antitussives do not.

(4) **Antitussives reduce the frequency and intensity of a cough. They act on the central or peripheral nervous system or on the local mucosa.**

13 **TEST-TAKING TIP** ◉ The word "most" in the stem sets a priority.

(1) Tolerance occurs when an individual requires increases in the dosage of a drug to maintain its therapeutic effect.

(2) A synergistic effect occurs when the effect of two medications given together is greater than the effect of the medications when given individually.

(3) **Drug habituation occurs when an individual develops a mild form of psychologic dependence and relies on the use of a substance.**

(4) An idiosyncratic effect occurs when a person's response to a drug is an underresponse, an overresponse, or a different response from that which is expected.

14 **TEST-TAKING TIP** ◉ "Notify the physician" are the words that reflect negative polarity. The question is asking, "Which blood level result is unacceptable?" Options 2 and 3 are opposites.

(1) Although this falls below the optimal peak value of 8 to 10 μg/mL, it is within the therapeutic window of 4 to 10 μg/mL, which is acceptable.

(2) This falls within the optimal peak value range of 8 to 10 μg/mL, which is acceptable.

(3) **The physician should be notified to increase the dose of the antibiotic. A value of 0.3 μg/mL is below 0.5 μg/mL, which is the lowest trough value of the antibiotic necessary to inhibit bacterial growth.**

(4) A value of 0.7 μg/mL is higher than 0.5 μg/mL, which is the minimum trough value necessary for a dose to be effective.

15 ① An antipyretic reduces a fever; an expectorant does not.

② **Expectorants cause a cough to be more productive by decreasing viscosity of mucus and increasing the flow of respiratory tract secretions.**

③ A nasal decongestant relieves nasal congestion; an expectorant does not.

④ A bronchodilator dilates airways of the respiratory tract; an expectorant does not.

16 TEST-TAKING TIP ◉ Option 3 is unique. It is the only option that does not include the word "dose."

① The drug dose is not safe. A peak level of 12 μg/mL indicates that the drug dose is too high and needs to be reduced by the physician. The optimum peak value should be between 8 to 10 μg/mL.

② If the value were subtherapeutic, it would be below 4 μg/mL.

③ **A value of 12 μg/mL is 2 μg/mL higher than is necessary to be effective and contributes to drug accumulation and toxicity if it continues for 3 to 5 days.**

④ The dose needs to be adjusted by the physician and not just given at a slower rate.

17 ① Reduced subcutaneous tissue is unrelated to drug accumulation.

② **A reduced glomerular filtration rate contributes to reduced excretion of a drug, thereby prolonging drug half-life.**

③ Drugs that rely on gastric acid for absorption are less effective when there is a reduction in hydrochloric acid production in older adults.

④ Diminished absorptive surface reduces the absorption of drugs.

18 TEST-TAKING TIP ◉ This question is associating four possible effects of neuroleptics: respiratory depression, diarrhea, akathisia, and spasms of the muscles of the face. If you know just one effect, unrelated or related to neuroleptics, you can delete two options from consideration.

① Respiratory depression is associated with opioid analgesics, not neuroleptics. Constipation, not diarrhea, is a common anticholinergic effect of neuroleptics.

② Although akathisia can occur with neuroleptics, respiratory depression is often seen with opioid analgesics, not neuroleptics.

③ **Spasms of the muscles of the face (tardive dyskinesia) and restlessness/agitation (akathisia) occur in response to dopamine blockage or depletion in the basal ganglia. These undesirable responses are common to most neuroleptic drugs and occur within the first few days of therapy.**

④ Although tardive dyskinesia occurs with neuroleptics, constipation, not diarrhea, is a common anticholinergic effect of neuroleptics.

19 TEST-TAKING TIP ◉ The word "main" in the stem sets a priority.

① Antipyretics are a group of drugs designed to reduce fever. Although some analgesics also may have an antipyretic effect, when given as analgesics, they reduce pain.

② Bronchodilators dilate respiratory airways, facilitating breathing.

③ Antiemetics are designed to minimize nausea and vomiting.

④ **Analgesics are given mainly to reduce pain and discomfort. There are three types of analgesics: nonnarcotic and nonsteroidal anti-inflammatory drugs (NSAIDs), narcotic analgesics or opioids, and adjuvants or coanalgesics.**

20 ① **A peak value of 8 μg is acceptable because it is within the therapeutic range of 4 to 10 μg/mL and optimum peak value of 8 to 10 μg/mL.**

② A peak level of 11 μg/mL is not acceptable because it exceeds the therapeutic range and optimum peak value of 10 μg/mL.

③ A trough level of 0.1 μg/mL is not acceptable because it is below the minimum trough level of 0.5 μg/mL.

④ A trough level of 0.3 μg/mL is not acceptable because it is below the minimum trough level.

21 TEST-TAKING TIP ◉ The words "further teaching is necessary" in the stem indicate negative polarity. Option 3 is unique because it does not begin with the words "I should."

① Antacids can interfere with the absorption of digoxin and should not be taken at the same time.

② Nausea, vomiting, and weakness are signs of toxicity. The patient needs a test to determine digoxin serum blood level.

③ **This action is unsafe and could lead to toxicity. If a dose is missed, it should be taken within 12 hours of the scheduled dose.**

④ Digoxin slows the heart rate and strengthens cardiac contractions. If the apical pulse is below a predetermined parameter set by the physician (frequently between 50 to 60 beats per minute), the dose should be held.

22 (1) Local anesthetics, not narcotics, diminish localized sensation and the perception of pain by inhibiting nerve conduction.

(2) **Opioids act on the higher centers of the brain to modify pain perception.**

(3) This is the theory related to using distracting sensory input to inhibit pain perception.

(4) Opioids do not close synaptic gates; stimulation of large nerve fibers, via methods such as transcutaneous electrical stimulation, closes synaptic gates.

23 **TEST-TAKING TIP** ○ The words "postural hypotension" and "common" in the stem are the clues.

(1) Postural hypotension is not a common side effect of antibiotics.

(2) Postural hypotension is not a common side effect of antiemetics.

(3) Postural hypotension is not a common side effect of antihistamines.

(4) **Most antihypertensives contribute to postural hypotension because of actions such as peripheral vasodilation, decreased peripheral resistance, decreased heart rate, and decreased cardiac contraction.**

24 **TEST-TAKING TIP** ○ The words "needs further exploration" in the stem indicate negative polarity.

(1) Although aspirin can prolong bleeding time when given with heparin, 5 days is sufficient time to be aspirin free for safe administration of heparin.

(2) **Heavy menstrual periods is a contraindication for the use of heparin because of an increased risk of prolonged bleeding during menstruation.**

(3) Eating a lot of green, leafy vegetables can contribute to the ineffectiveness of warfarin sodium (Coumadin), not heparin sodium.

(4) Heparin does not cross the placental barrier and has no effects on the fetus or newborn.

25 **TEST-TAKING TIP** ○ The word "best" in the stem sets a priority. Options 1, 2, and 4 all focus on taking a cathartic (laxative) to promote intestinal peristalsis. Option 3 is unique because it indicates a dietary approach to prevent constipation and promote defecation.

(1) The routine intake of cathartics (laxatives) should be avoided to prevent dependence.

(2) The routine use of castor oil should be avoided to prevent dependence.

(3) **Whole grains provide fiber and bulk, which distend the bowel lumen, promoting intestinal peristalsis.**

(4) Routine use of a stool softener should be avoided to prevent dependence.

26 (1) Mineral supplements are considered restorative, not palliative; they return the body to health.

(2) **Demerol is an opioid that relieves the symptoms of a disease (palliative action) but does not alter the disease process itself.**

(3) Penicillin is an antibiotic that kills pathogenic organisms; a drug that kills an organism is considered to have a curative, not palliative, action.

(4) Synthroid replaces the thyroxin that is deficient in hypothyroidism. When a drug replaces body fluids or substances, it is substitutive, not palliative, in its therapeutic action.

27 **TEST-TAKING TIP** ○ The word "emerging" modifies the words "therapeutic response" in the stem and is the clue.

(1) 2 hours is too short a time to achieve a therapeutic response to an antidepressant.

(2) 2 days is too short a time to experience a therapeutic response to antidepressants.

(3) **Generally patients demonstrate an initial response 1 to 3 weeks after the start of antidepressant therapy; it takes this long to establish a therapeutic plasma level.**

(4) One or 2 months may be necessary to achieve a maximal, not initial, response to antidepressant therapy.

28 (1) Antipsychotics decrease, not potentiate, the effectiveness of amphetamines.

(2) Antipsychotics decrease the effectiveness of anticoagulants.

(3) **Antipsychotics potentiate the effects of other central nervous system depressants such as opioid analgesics.**

(4) Antipsychotics decrease the effectiveness of oral hypoglycemic agents.

29 **TEST-TAKING TIP** ○ The word "neurologic" in the stem is a clue. The word "neurologic" in the stem and the word "neuropathies" in Option 4 are closely related. Consider Option 4 carefully. In this question, it is the correct answer.

(1) Red and white blood cells are part of the hematopoietic, not the neurologic, system.

(2) Constipation and diarrhea are related to the gastrointestinal, not neurologic, system.

(3) Electrolyte imbalances and renal failure are related to the renal, not neurologic, system.

(4) **A peripheral neuropathy occurs in almost every patient, particularly depression of the Achilles tendon reflex. Decreased innervation of the bowel causes a paralytic ileus, resulting in constipation or obstipation.**

30 ① __X__ A diuretic enhances the selective excretion of water and various electrolytes. One liter of fluid is equal to 2.2 pounds. A rapid decrease in weight indicates fluid loss.

② ____ A diuretic increases urinary output, not appetite.

③ __X__ A diuretic enhances the selective excretion of water and various electrolytes by affecting renal mechanisms for tubular secretion and reabsorption, thereby increasing urinary output.

④ ____ As excess fluid is excreted from the body, the blood pressure should decrease, not increase.

⑤ ____ Diuretics are not antibiotics and therefore will not destroy microorganisms resulting in a decrease in white blood cells.

Comprehensive Final Book Exam

This test is provided to give you an opportunity to practice your test-taking skills. It is designed to measure your knowledge of nursing content and motivate you to continue with your efforts to succeed in testing situations.

When self-administering this 100 question practice test, set aside 2 hours of uninterrupted time. This will allow approximately 1 minute per question with 20 minutes for review. To simulate a testing environment, you must sit at a table and select a time when you will not be disturbed. If you spend less than 1 minute on a question, you can use this time for the questions you find more difficult or add it to the time you have reserved for your review at the end of the test. Use the full 2 hours to complete this practice test. If your school allots more or less time than 1 minute per question, adjust your time accordingly. If your examinations are not timed, use all the time you need to complete the test.

To record your answer, fill in the bubble in front of the option you have selected. Answer every question. If you do not know the answer to a question, attempt to eliminate as many options as you can using test-taking skills and then make an educated guess. If you are preparing for a computer-administered test that does not permit you to return to previous questions, answer each question before moving on to the next question. Do not go back to answer or change the answer to a previous question.

After you complete this practice test, compare your answers to the answers and rationales provided at the end of the chapter. Evaluate your performance by following the directions in Chapter 10, Analyze Your Test Performance. This will help you diagnose information processing errors and identify knowledge deficits; the chapter also provides suggestions for corrective actions. Do not be tempted to avoid this important step in taking a practice test. It is through this self-analysis that you can eventually maximize your strengths and address your educational needs in preparation for your next test.

Two Comprehensive Course Exit Exams appear on the enclosed disk. Each examination consists of 75 questions and includes the correct answers and rationales for all the options. These exams provide additional opportunities for applying your test-taking skills as well as simulate taking a test on a computer.

Questions

1 A debilitated patient is admitted to the hospital with the diagnoses of heart failure and osteoporosis. What should the nurse do to help prevent injury to this patient with bone demineralization?
   ① Apply emollients to the skin every day
   ② Encourage walking in the hall once daily
   ③ Have the patient drink several liters of fluid daily
   ④ Support joints when changing the patient's position

2 The nurse educator is teaching a class about patient hygiene and grooming to nursing assistants. The nurse instructs the nursing assistants to brush patients' hair daily to prevent:

① Pediculosis
② Dandruff
③ Alopecia
④ Tangles

3 A patient has a progressive, debilitating disease. Although usually pleasant, the patient begins to complain that the doctor is incompetent, the nurses are uncaring, the room is too cold, and the food is terrible. The patient is coping by using the defense mechanism of:

① Displacement
② Projection
③ Denial
④ Anger

4 The nurse is routinely monitoring a patient's blood pressure. What should the nurse do first when an assessment reveals a change in the patient's blood pressure?

① Report the change to the charge nurse
② Document the observed change
③ Obtain the other vital signs
④ Notify the physician

5 Which action by a patient should the nurse report to the physician because the patient may need a restraint?

① Climbing off the end of the bed at night
② Wandering into other patients' rooms
③ Picking at lint on bed linens
④ Pulling out an IV line

6 A comatose patient begins to vomit while lying in bed. The nurse's initial response should be to position the patient in the:

① Supine position
② Lateral position
③ High-Fowler's position
④ Dorsal recumbent position

7 A patient whose spouse recently died begins to cry. The nurse's best response is to:

① Arrange for grief counseling
② Explain that being sad is normal
③ Look away when the patient cries
④ Sit down while touching the patient's hand

8 The nurse is assessing a patient who is having difficulty sleeping. The nurse concludes that an adequate night's sleep was attained when the patient:

① Has the ability to remember dreams
② Demonstrates renewed strength
③ Sleeps at night without waking
④ Slept seven hours

9 Differentiating among facts, inferences, and opinions is essential for critical thinking when providing nursing care. Put an X in front of the statements that are inferences.

① _____ The patient weighs 265 pounds.
② _____ The patient will lose weight when eating fewer calories.
③ _____ The patient needs to lose weight because he is too heavy.
④ _____ The patient is not following his diet because he gained 4 pounds.

10 A patient has left-sided hemiparesis because of a stroke (brain attack). When feeding this patient, the nurse should:
① Offer fluids to assist with swallowing of food
② Place the patient in a low-Fowler's position
③ Insert food on the strong side of the mouth
④ Tuck a towel under the patient's chin

11 A patient has a left-sided hemiplegia as the result of a cerebrovascular accident (brain attack). While being dressed, the patient states in a disgusted tone of voice, "I feel like a 2-year-old. I can't even get dressed by myself." The nurse's BEST response is:
① "It's hard to feel dependent on others."
② "Most people who have had a stroke feel this way."
③ "It must be terrible not being able to move your arm."
④ "You are feeling down today, but things will get better."

12 A newly admitted patient complains of not having had a good bowel movement in 10 days. To identify the possibility of a fecal impaction, the nurse should ask:
① "Have you had small amounts of liquid stool?"
② "What types of food with fiber do you eat?"
③ "Do you notice a bad odor to your breath?"
④ "Are you having any vomiting?"

13 A patient is on Droplet Precautions. The *most* effective way to reduce the transmission of microorganisms at meal times for patients who are on Droplet Precautions is by:
① Washing and rinsing the dishes with hot water
② Having patients wash their hands after eating
③ Isolating used trays in the dirty utility room
④ Using disposable dishes and utensils

14 The nurse observes that a nursing assistant is using inappropriate body mechanics when the nursing assistant is:
① Holding clean equipment close to the body when walking
② Flexing the knees when lifting an object from the floor
③ Placing the feet apart when transferring a patient
④ Bending from the waist when making a bed

15 Which intervention is an example of primary disease prevention?
① Self-examination of the testes
② Mammography screening
③ Use of a bicycle helmet
④ Testing of well water

16 The nurse is providing a bed bath for a bed-bound patient. Which should the nurse wash last?
① Legs
② Feet
③ Axilla
④ Rectum

17 An older bed-bound adult has a stage I pressure ulcer in the sacral area. To relieve pressure and promote circulation to the sacral area, the nurse should position the patient in the:
① Dorsal recumbent position
② Semi-Fowler's position
③ Lateral position
④ Supine position

18 The physician orders ear drops for a 2-year-old child with otitis media. When instilling eardrops into the ear of this 2-year-old child, the nurse should:
   ① Pull the pinna of the child's ear downward and backward while instilling the drops
   ② Maintain the lateral position with the affected ear down after instilling the drops
   ③ Apply pressure to the tragus of the ear while instilling the drops
   ④ Hyperextend the child's head before instilling the drops

19 The bed of a patient who has an indwelling urinary catheter (Foley) is found wet with urine. After determining that the catheter is patent, the nurse should:
   ① Insert a larger-size catheter
   ② Provide perineal care whenever necessary
   ③ Position a waterproof pad under the patient's buttocks
   ④ Tell the patient to use the bedpan when there is an urge to void

20 The nurse is assessing a patient in pain. The location and description of pain are important for the nurse to explore when determining its:
   ① Duration
   ② Etiology
   ③ Intensity
   ④ Threshold

21 The nurse should use a class A fire extinguisher to put out a fire in a:
   ① Toaster oven
   ② Wastepaper basket
   ③ Stove in the pantry
   ④ Maintenance closet

22 The nurse is caring for a patient in a coma because of a traumatic brain injury. What should the nurse do when providing mouth care for this patient?
   ① Explain to the patient what will be done
   ② Apply petroleum jelly to the tongue and lips
   ③ Use glycerin and lemon swabs to cleanse the mouth
   ④ Position the patient in the dorsal recumbent position

23 Across the spectrum of wellness and illness, the nurse understands that *most* older adults view themselves as:
   ① Frail
   ② Tired
   ③ Healthy
   ④ Dependent

24 A patient's therapeutic serum level for an ordered antibiotic should be between 4 and 10 µg/mL (micrograms per milliliter). When a patient's peak level is 12 µg/mL, the nurse should conclude that the:
   ① Drug dose is safe.
   ② Drug dose is subtherapeutic.
   ③ Patient is at risk for drug accumulation.
   ④ Patient's next dose should be administered over a longer period of time.

25 A patient with kidney failure is placed on a fluid restriction of 1000 mL of fluid in 24 hours. The nurse should:
   ① Eliminate liquids between meal times
   ② Indicate the order for clear liquids in the patient's plan of care
   ③ Divide the fluids equally among the hours the patient is awake
   ④ Give proportionally more fluids during the day than during the night

26 The nurse is making patient rounds at the beginning of a shift. Which patient assessment made by the nurse requires immediate intervention?
① 10 respirations per minute by a sleeping patient
② Rattling sounds in the pharynx of an unconscious patient
③ Slight shortness of breath after returning from the bathroom
④ Expectorating large amounts of thick mucus from the mouth

27 Which action by the nurse supports a patient's right to privacy?
① Leaving a crying patient alone
② Addressing a patient by the last name
③ Providing information about patient care
④ Closing the door when interviewing the patient

28 Identify the range of motion being performed in the following diagram.
① Flexion
② Inversion
③ Adduction
④ Circumduction

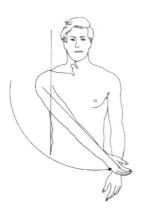

29 When washing the penis of an uncircumcised patient, the nurse should:
① Wash down the shaft toward the meatus
② Retract the foreskin completely
③ Employ a very light touch
④ Use a rubbing motion

30 The nurse is providing preoperative teaching for a patient. To prevent pulmonary complications postoperatively, the nurse should teach the patient to perform:
① Incisional splinting
② Progressive ambulation
③ Diaphragmatic breathing
④ Range-of-motion exercises

31 A patient is scheduled for an elective surgical procedure. Which is not verified when the nurse witnesses the signing of the consent by the patient? That the patient:
① Signs the consent voluntarily in the presence of the nurse
② Is the person who signed the consent in front of the nurse
③ Was explained the risks and benefits of the procedure by the nurse
④ Appears alert and competent to give a consent as determined by the nurse

32 The nurse administers an antiemetic to a patient. Adaptations that indicate to the nurse that the patient is experiencing a therapeutic response to the drug are a decrease in:
① Nausea and anxiety
② Vomiting and nausea
③ Coughing and anxiety
④ Vomiting and coughing

33 The physician orders daily weights for the purpose of evaluating a patient's fluid loss or gain. The nurse should weigh the patient:
① Twice a day
② One hour before meals
③ At the same time each day
④ Before urinating in the morning

34 The nurse identified reactive hyperemia over a bony prominence occurred in response to:
① Applying a warm soak
② Using an effleurage massage technique
③ Pulling a patient up in bed without using a pull sheet
④ Turning a patient who was in one position for several hours

35 The nurse is assessing a variety of patients with respiratory problems. The presence of which adaptation causes the most concern?
① Inspiratory stridor
② Pleural friction rub
③ Expiratory wheezing
④ Nonproductive cough

36 A nursing student graduates from an educational program that prepares people to be registered professional nurses. To pursue licensure, it is important that the graduate understand that licensure of registered nurses in the United States is:
① Governed by each state
② Controlled by federal law
③ Regulated by constitutional law
④ Authorized by the American Nurses Association

37 The primary nurse is responsible for a group of patients. Which two patients should the nurse attend to before the others? Check the two that apply.
① _____ A patient who is awaiting to be escorted to the lobby after being discharged.
② _____ A patient admitted for hypertension who wants pain medication for a headache.
③ _____ A patient who five days after surgery states, "Something feels very strange in my belly."
④ _____ A patient who got dizzy when the nursing assistant was transferring the patient from a wheelchair to the bed.
⑤ _____ A patient who is anxious to have an IV removed after being informed by the physician that it can be discontinued.

38 A female patient who has cancer that has metastasized to the bone experiences pain when moving. What should the nurse do when the patient refuses to move?
① Reassure her that she will not be hurt
② Complete nursing care as quickly as possible
③ Let her perform her own activities of daily living
④ Touch her gently when assisting with required care

39 A medication is delivered by the Z-track method when the nurse:
① Uses a special syringe designed for Z-track injections
② Pulls laterally and downward on the skin before inserting the needle
③ Administers the injection in the muscle on the anterior lateral aspect of the thigh
④ Injects the needle in a separate spot for each dose on a Z-shaped grid on the abdomen

40 The nurse is caring for a patient with a hearing deficit. What is the most significant intervention to ensure that the patient heard what the nurse said?
① Face the patient
② Speak distinctly
③ Obtain feedback
④ Raise the volume of speech

41 When preparing a soapsuds enema for an adult, how much fluid should the nurse use to effectively stimulate the bowel?
① 250 mL
② 500 mL
③ 700 mL
④ 900 mL

42 The nursing assistant informs the nurse that a patient's pulse seems irregular. The nurse should monitor this patient's pulse:
① At the carotid
② With a Doppler
③ For a full minute
④ At two different sites

43 Before administering medications, it is important for the nurse to assess the patient's ability to excrete drugs from the body. Therefore, impairment in which organ is of most concern to the nurse?
① Liver
② Lungs
③ Kidneys
④ Intestines

44 The nurse is teaching oral care to a patient with a history of gingivitis and dental plaque. To prevent dental plaque, the nurse should teach the patient to:
① Rinse the mouth with diluted hydrogen peroxide
② Have the teeth cleaned by a dental hygienist once a year
③ Brush the biting surface of the teeth using a forward and backward motion
④ Vibrate the toothbrush while holding it at a forty-five degree angle where the teeth meet the gum line

45 Home care is designed to assist individuals and families in all realms except:
① Acute care
② Respite care
③ Hospice care
④ Restorative care

46 Which action associated with restraint use can the nurse delegate to an unlicensed nursing team member?
① Assessment of a patient's safety needs
② Evaluation of a patient's response to restraint use
③ Selection of the appropriate type restraint to meet a patient's needs
④ Performance of range of motion to a patient's joints after release of a restraint

47 A patient on a bladder-retraining program is incontinent at 1:00 AM every day. What should the nurse do to promote continence?
① Toilet the patient at 1:30 AM.
② Toilet the patient at 12:30 AM.
③ Limit the patient's intake of fluid after dinner.
④ Position the patient's call bell within easy reach.

48 The nurse is implementing nasotracheal suctioning in an adult. What should the nurse do?
① Apply intermittent suction during removal of the catheter.
② Use wall suction with a pressure setting below 90 mm Hg.
③ Suction the nasotracheal area after the oropharyngeal area.
④ Employ continuous suction for 20 seconds during removal of the catheter.

49 The nurse is caring for patients from culturally diverse populations. Which is the best action by the nurse to facilitate communication?
① Honor cultural differences when communicating
② Facilitate communication by asking family members to interpret
③ Convey the meaning of nursing interventions by using a picture book
④ Learn important phrases in different languages of cultural groups in the community

50 A patient is admitted to the Post Anesthesia Care Unit (PACU) after a prostatectomy. The patient's vital signs are blood pressure 150/90, pulse 88 and bounding, respirations 24 with some crackles. The nurse makes the inference that the patient is experiencing:
① Hypervolemia
② Hyperkalemia
③ Hyponatremia
④ Hypoglycemia

51 The nurse in the hospital is assigned the responsibility of administering medications to all the patients on the unit. The nurse understands that the primary reason many oral drugs are administered with food is to:
① Prevent drug interactions
② Protect the gastric mucosa
③ Stimulate biotransformation
④ Reduce the risk of gastric reflux

52 A woman who has dependent edema is shopping for a jar of prepared pasta sauce. Which ingredient that appears on the Nutrition Facts label is of most concern for this person?
① Protein
② Sodium
③ Calories
④ Cholesterol

53 The nurse is preparing an intradermal injection that is ordered for a patient. Which factor is related to an intradermal injection?
① 3-mL syringe
② 26-gauge needle
③ 1-inch needle length
④ 30-degree angle of insertion

54 Nurses are required by law to:
① Stop at the scene of an accident
② Report all situations concerning rape
③ Notify authorities about instances of child abuse
④ Obtain parental consent if a 16-year-old seeks an abortion

55 A patient who was in an automobile collision is at risk for internal hemorrhage. For which sign should the nurse monitor this patient?
① Decreased respiratory rate
② Fall in blood pressure
③ Bradycardia
④ Warm skin

56 When transferring a patient from the bed to a chair, the nurse sits the patient on the side of the bed for several minutes primarily to:
① Allow the patient to regain energy expended while sitting
② Enable the body to adapt to a drop in blood pressure
③ Provide time for the heart rate to return to normal
④ Permit the patient to take several deep breaths

57 The physician orders sublingual nitroglycerin for a patient with the diagnosis of angina pectoris (chest pain related to transient cardiac ischemia). When teaching the patient about this medication, the nurse should instruct the patient to:
① "Take only 1 dose of nitroglycerin. If the pain continues, call 911."
② "Take 1 dose every 3 minutes as often as necessary until pain is relieved."
③ "Double the dose of nitroglycerin 5 minutes after the first dose if there is no relief from pain."
④ "You can repeat the dose of nitroglycerin every 5 minutes for 3 doses. If the pain is unrelieved, get immediate medical attention."

58 When auscultating a patient's breath sounds, the nurse should:
① Move the stethoscope systematically from the apices to the bases of the lungs
② Place the stethoscope over the ribs along the midclavicular line
③ Instruct the patient to breathe deeply through the nose
④ Position the patient in a low-Fowler's position

59 A terminally ill patient appears sad and withdrawn. The nurse should respond by being:
① Animated
② Cheerful
③ Present
④ Aloof

60 When caring for a patient with an indwelling urinary catheter (Foley), it is most important for the nurse to:
① Provide perineal care after defecation
② Reinsert a new catheter every 72 hours
③ Increase the oral intake to 1500 mL of fluid in 24 hours
④ Ensure that the balloon is inflated by tugging gently on the catheter daily

61 The nurse is assessing a patient for a systemic adaptation to an inflammatory response; therefore, the nurse should monitor the patient for:
① Pain
② Fever
③ Edema
④ Erythema

62 The nurse is evaluating a patient's use of a liquid metered-dose inhaler. Which behavior indicates an inappropriate technique?
① Shaking the drug before pressing down on the inhaler
② Pressing down on the inhaler while inhaling quickly
③ Holding the breath at the height of inhalation
④ Tilting the head back slightly

63 A patient tells the nurse, "I have such problems with constipation." When teaching this patient about appropriate foods to include in the diet to address this problem, the nurse should convey that an excellent source of fiber is:
① Apples
② Cherries
③ Apricots
④ Pineapples

64 The nurse identifies an excoriated perineal area in a patient with diarrhea. Which step of the nursing process has the nurse performed?
① Analysis
② Evaluation
③ Assessment
④ Implementation

65 When caring for patients in a culturally competent manner, it is most important for the nurse to:
1. Recognize beliefs and attitudes about one's own culture and the culture of others
2. Learn what people of common cultures believe about health and illness practices
3. Behave in an ethnocentric manner when interacting with people of other cultures
4. Focus on the cultural aspects that are more similar rather than those that are different

66 On the third day of hospitalization, a patient communicates a preference to shower at night. To best promote continuity of care, the nurse should:
1. Explain that AM care is given in the morning
2. Orally inform the other health team members
3. Indicate this preference on the patient's plan of care
4. Initially encourage a modification of personal routines while hospitalized

67 When planning care to relieve pain, the nurse can use an intervention that incorporates the gate-control theory of pain such as:
1. Promoting rest
2. Encouraging activity
3. Administering a narcotic
4. Applying a warm compress

68 The nurse is teaching a preoperative patient about leg exercises. The nurse encourages these exercises to be performed after surgery primarily to:
1. Promote venous return
2. Limit joint contractures
3. Prevent muscle atrophy
4. Increase muscle strength

69 A patient with a large pressure ulcer is being cared for in the home by a spouse. To promote wound healing, the nurse teaches the spouse about foods high in vitamin C. Which food selected by the spouse indicates that the teaching is understood?
1. Sunflower seeds
2. Green peppers
3. Black beans
4. Beef liver

70 Which is an example of a community health practice that directly remedies an unhealthy situation?
1. Providing health care to the homeless
2. Providing for fluoridation of water
3. Supporting rehabilitation services
4. Supporting vaccination programs

71 To best understand human behavior, the nurse needs to identify the impact of Erikson's theory of personality development which includes the concept that:
1. Basic level needs have to be met before higher level needs
2. Biologic needs must be met before fulfillment of one's unique potential
3. Once a developmental stage is passed it cannot be revisited and relearned
4. Cultural and interpersonal tasks have to be accomplished to grow developmentally

72 The nurse is making rounds at the beginning of a shift and assesses a patient who has an IV infusion in progress. Which data does the nurse need to know to ensure that the correct IV solution is running? Check the data that apply.
1. _____ Tubing drop factor
2. _____ Drip rate per minute
3. _____ Solution indicated on the IV bag
4. _____ Volume of solution in the IV bag
5. _____ Solution ordered by the physician

73 The nurse should remove a dirty sheet from an unoccupied bed by:
1. Pushing the sheet together
2. Rolling the sheet into itself
3. Sliding the sheet to the side of the bed
4. Fanfolding the sheet to the foot of the bed

74 When assessing a patient for an emotional response to stress, the nurse should monitor the patient for:
1. Pain
2. Irritability
3. Headaches
4. Hypertension

75 When planning a preoperative teaching class, the nurse understands that most patients do not want to take postoperative analgesics primarily because they are afraid of:
1. Losing control
2. Receiving an injection
3. Becoming dependent on them
4. Experiencing negative side effects

76 The nurse assesses that the patient understands the teaching about diaphragmatic breathing when the patient says, "I should:
1. Feel my abdomen flatten on inspiration."
2. Raise my shoulders and chest when I inhale."
3. Hold my breath for 3 seconds at the height of inspiration."
4. Use my hands to put pressure against the abdomen when I inhale."

77 The nurse must develop a teaching plan that addresses issues in the affective domain. Which is the most important patient factor that the nurse must assess before developing the teaching plan?
1. Intelligence
2. Strengths
3. Maturity
4. Values

78 The nurse is caring for a patient who is nauseated and vomiting. After the patient is done vomiting, the nurse should:
1. Always contain the vomitus in a medical waste container
2. Pour the vomitus down the sink in the dirty utility room
3. Save a specimen of the vomitus for testing
4. Discard the vomitus in the toilet

79 Which statement by a patient experiencing insomnia indicates that the nurse must provide further education?
1. "I like to take a walk after dinner."
2. "I always have a snack just before I go to bed."
3. "I set my bedroom temperature at a cool setting at night."
4. "I drink a few glasses of wine while I watch television at night."

80 The nurse is administering heparin intravenously to a patient with a deep vein thrombosis. Which is most important for the nurse to have readily available on the unit while the patient is receiving heparin intravenously?
1. Potassium chloride
2. Protamine sulfate
3. Prothrombin
4. Plasma

81 Which nursing action interferes with the chain of infection at the level of transmission?
1. Covering the nose when sneezing
2. Repositioning a patient every two hours
3. Disposing of any item that touches the floor
4. Applying a sterile dressing over a contaminated wound

82 According to Kübler-Ross's theory on death and dying, people:
1. Ultimately reach the stage of acceptance
2. Generally pass through the stages smoothly
3. Can move back and forth between the stages
4. Always move progressively forward through the stages

83 A patient tells the nurse about problems with constipation. The nurse should teach the patient to avoid eating:
1. Cheese and broccoli
2. Yogurt and cheese
3. Broccoli and peas
4. Peas and yogurt

84 The nurse evaluates that the patient understands the teaching about how to self-administer a rectal suppository when the patient:
1. Bears down during insertion of the suppository
2. Requests sterile gloves to insert the suppository
3. Allows the suppository to warm to room temperature
4. Inserts the suppository immediately after its removal from the refrigerator

85 When planning nursing interventions to prevent falls in older adults in a hospital, the nurse recognizes that the frequency of falls increases:
1. At night
2. Before meals
3. After surgery
4. During visiting hours

86 Community health practice, unlike acute health care, is:
1. Family focused
2. Individual focused
3. Population focused
4. Geographically focused

87 A patient ingests a 2000-calorie meal consisting of 60 gm of fat. What percentage of calories came from fat?
1. 12%
2. 27%
3. 35%
4. 48%

88 The nurse in the intensive care unit is caring for a group of patients with a variety of health problems. In relation to the general adaptation syndrome (GAS), the nurse understands that all patients who are exposed to a stressful event will:
1. Adapt in a unique way
2. Experience an iatrogenic stress
3. Eventually achieve homeostasis
4. Have an autonomic nervous system response

89 Which action violates a principle of surgical asepsis?
1. Recapping a syringe after withdrawing medication from a vial
2. Holding a wet sterile gauze with sterile forceps while the handle is higher than the tip

③ Failing to wipe the rubber port of a newly opened sterile multiple-dose vial with an alcohol swab
④ Pouring Betadine on gauze that is lying in its opened sterile paper wrapper while on an overbed table

90 To BEST evaluate peripheral circulation in the lower extremities, the nurse should assess the patient's:
① Pedal pulses and hair on the toes
② Hair on the toes and blood pressure
③ Capillary refill in the toenails and pedal pulses
④ Blood pressure and capillary refill in the toenails

91 A patient, who had a brain attack, has hemiparesis. What should the nurse do to **best** prevent this patient from developing contractures?
① Teach the patient to perform active ROM exercises.
② Transfer the patient to a chair twice a day.
③ Support the patient's joints with pillows.
④ Reposition the patient every two hours.

92 The nurse should teach a female patient with the diagnosis of a urinary tract infection that women have a higher incidence than men because:
① Urine flows toward the rectum via gravity when women void
② Women use bedpans, which harbor microorganisms
③ Women must sit, rather than stand, when toileting
④ The rectum is closer to the urinary meatus

93 A confused patient is incontinent of urine and stool. To BEST prevent skin breakdown in this patient, the nurse should:
① Check the perineal area frequently and wash if necessary
② Instruct the patient to always call the nurse when soiled
③ Place sheepskin on the bed and apply a diaper
④ Reposition the patient frequently

94 A patient has an order for oxycodone 1 tablet every 4 hours prn for pain after abdominal surgery. The nurse identifies that the oxycodone is effective when the patient:
① Is able to cough with a tolerable level of discomfort
② Does not ask for another tablet for pain
③ Requests another tablet in 3 hours
④ Has a decrease in the respiratory rate

95 A school-age child is to be hospitalized for several weeks. To enhance achievement of the developmental task associated with this age group, the nurse should encourage the parents to:
① Have siblings visit several times a week
② Bring a favorite stuffed animal from home
③ Plan for schoolwork to be brought to the hospital
④ Arrange for the television to be turned on in the room

96 The nurse is caring for a patient who has a history of urge incontinence. To provide for the elimination needs of this patient, the nurse should:
① Toilet the patient every four hours
② Toilet the patient immediately on request
③ Encourage the patient to stay near the bathroom
④ Ask the patient to limit fluid intake in the evening

97 The school nurse is teaching a health class about nutrition. The nurse should include that protein foods are used primarily by the body for:
① Energy
② Growth
③ Excretion
④ Catabolism

98 What should the nurse do when assisting a blind patient to walk?
   ① Walk in front of the patient while the patient uses the corridor handrail.
   ② Stand next to the patient and have the patient hold the nurse's arm.
   ③ Stand behind the patient and provide verbal directions.
   ④ Walk on the side while holding the patient's elbow.

99 The nurse is caring for a patient with a nasogastric tube. What should the nurse do to assess for correct placement of the tube?
   ① Auscultate the lungs
   ② Aspirate stomach contents
   ③ Place the end of the tube in water
   ④ Instill a small amount of normal saline

100 A patient has metastatic lung cancer and the physician discusses the diagnosis and prognosis in detail with the patient. After a severe episode of coughing and shortness of breath later in the day, the patient says to the nurse, "This is just a cold. I'll be fine once I get over it." The nurse's best response is:
   ① "Tell me more about your illness."
   ② "It's really not a cold, it's lung cancer."
   ③ "The doctor had some bad news for you today."
   ④ "Remember what the doctor told you this morning."

Answers and Rationales

1 (1) Emollients hold moisture in the skin, making it supple; they do not prevent bone injury.
(2) Weight-bearing helps limit bone demineralization, but it will not prevent bone injury.
(3) An intake of 2500 mL of fluid daily flushes the kidneys and limits calculi formation, which can occur because of the high level of calcium salts in the urine as a result of demineralization. It does not prevent bone injury.
(4) Bone demineralization (osteoporosis) causes the bones to become weak, brittle, and fragile; supporting joints when turning or moving limits the stress that could cause a fracture.

2 (1) Pediculosis is caused by direct contact with lice or their eggs (nits); brushing the hair will not prevent head lice.
(2) Shampooing the hair and rubbing the scalp help to limit dandruff.
(3) Loss of hair can be caused by nutritional, emotional, iatrogenic, and genetic factors; it is not prevented by brushing.
(4) Brushing separates tangles and evenly distributes secretions and oils down the hair shafts.

3 **(1) The patient is anxious and is reducing anxiety by transferring emotions from something stressful to substitutes that are less anxiety producing.**
(2) Projection is the attribution of unacceptable thoughts or actions to another.
(3) Denial is a defense mechanism used to avoid emotional conflicts and to refuse to cope with unpleasant realities by keeping them out of conscious awareness.
(4) Anger is a behavior that is an adaptive response; it defends the individual, but is not known as a defense mechanism.

4 (1) This may be done later; it is not the priority at this time.
(2) Same as #1.
(3) Because of the interrelationships among the circulatory system, respiratory system, and the basal metabolic rate, all the vital signs should be obtained for an accurate assessment.
(4) Same as #1.

5 (1) This behavior can be addressed by interventions other than a restraint.
(2) Wandering should be controlled by observation, not a restraint.
(3) Picking at the gown and bed linens is not unsafe behavior that requires application of a restraint.
(4) Physical or chemical restraints may be necessary to protect the patient from self-harm. Pulling out an IV can cause tissue injury and will interrupt medical therapy.

6 (1) This position is contraindicated because it promotes aspiration by allowing vomitus to flow to the posterior oral pharynx and enter the trachea.
(2) The lateral position prevents aspiration because it allows vomitus to drain out of the mouth via gravity.
(3) A high-Fowler's position provides inadequate support for an unconscious patient.
(4) Same as #1.

7 (1) Grief counseling may be done later; it is not the priority at this time.
(2) Although feeling sad is a common response to a loss, the nurse is making an assumption the patient is sad without knowing the patient-spouse relationship; the tears may indicate other feelings such as relief or joy.
(3) Avoiding eye contact may give the patient the message that it is not acceptable to cry.
(4) Sitting down and touching the patient's hand communicates acceptance and caring.

8 (1) Remembering dreams is unrelated to adequate sleep.
(2) The purpose of sleep is to rest and restore the body, which generally is evidenced by renewed strength.
(3) Although a person sleeps at night without waking, the length of the sleep or the length of REM sleep may be insufficient to restore or renew the body.
(4) Seven hours may or may not be enough sleep because each person has unique needs and a biologic clock for determining sleeping intervals.

9 (1) ____ "The patient weighs 265 pounds" is a fact. A fact is checkable and can be confirmed and verified through investigation.
(2) _X_ "If the patient eats fewer calories, the patient will lose weight" is an inference. An inference is a conclusion drawn from logic derived from deductive or inductive reasoning.
(3) ____ "The patient needs to lose weight because he is too heavy" is an opinion. An opinion reflects the beliefs of the speaker and may fit the facts but can also be a miscalculation or error.
(4) _X_ "The patient is not following his diet because he gained 4 pounds" is an inference. An inference is a conclusion drawn from logic derived from deductive or inductive reasoning.

10 ① Offering fluids to assist with swallowing will promote aspiration and is contraindicated. Fluids should be taken after a mouthful of food is swallowed.

② A low-Fowler's position could promote aspiration; the patient should be placed in a high-Fowler's position to allow gravity to facilitate swallowing.

③ **Placing food on the strong side of the mouth allows the unaffected muscles to control chewing, moves the bolus of food to the posterior oral cavity, and facilitates swallowing.**

④ This should be avoided because it has the same implication as a bib; the patient may feel childlike.

11 ① **This statement identifies the patient's feelings and provides an opportunity for further discussion.**

② This statement is a generalization that may not be true; also, it cuts off communication.

③ This statement focuses on the inability to move rather than feelings of helplessness, dependence, and regression.

④ This statement is false reassurance because the nurse does not know if things will get better.

12 ① **A fecal impaction is an obstruction in the large intestine; peristalsis behind the obstruction initially increases in an attempt to move the mass, causing liquid stool to pass around the area of the impaction.**

② This question is not significant at this time; foods with fiber promote intestinal peristalsis, which prevents constipation.

③ A bad odor to the breath is unrelated to a fecal impaction; it may be related to a small bowel obstruction.

④ People with a fecal impaction may experience rectal pressure, bloating, and nausea, but rarely do they vomit; nausea and vomiting occur more frequently with small bowel obstructions.

13 ① Washing and rinsing are ineffective.

② The hands should be washed before eating.

③ Used trays from an isolation room will contaminate the dirty utility room.

④ **Contaminated disposable articles can be bagged and discarded, which prevents the spread of microorganisms.**

14 ① Weight carried close to the center of gravity helps maintain balance.

② Using the strong muscles of the legs to carry a load helps prevent back strain.

③ The wider the base of support and the lower the center of gravity, the greater the stability of the nurse.

④ **Bending from the waist puts stress on the vertebrae and muscles of the back because it does not distribute the work among the largest and strongest muscle groups of the legs.**

15 ① This action is associated with secondary disease prevention, not primary prevention. Secondary prevention activities are associated with early detection and encouragement of treatment, when actions may contribute to control or elimination of an already present risk factor, illness, or disease.

② Same as #1.

③ **Primary prevention, such as use of a bicycle helmet, is associated with health teaching and actions that relate to specific protection and prevention of disease or injury. Primary prevention activities precede disease or dysfunction and include actions generally applied to a healthy population.**

④ Same as #1.

16 ① This area is cleaner than the perianal area, and if washed last, will become more contaminated from microorganisms and fecal material from the rectum.

② Same as #1.

③ Same as #1.

④ **The perianal area has fecal material and microorganisms that can contaminate other parts of the body; therefore, the perianal area should be washed last.**

17 ① In the dorsal recumbent or supine position, pressure will still be on the sacrum because it is a back-lying position.

② In the semi-Fowler's position, pressure will still be on the sacrum, and with the head elevated, shearing force may occur if the patient were to slide down in bed.

③ **In the lateral position, the iliac crest and greater trochanter, not the sacrum, bear the body's weight.**

④ Same as #1.

18 ① **The pinna is pulled downward and backward to straighten the ear canal in a child less than 3 years; this provides direct access to the deeper external ear structures. With children older than 3 years and adults the ear is pulled backward and upward to straighten the external ear canal.**

② A lateral position with the affected ear down will allow the ear drops to flow out of the ear by gravity. The affected ear should be on the upper side for a minimum of 3 minutes to allow complete distribution of the medication.

③ Applying pressure to the tragus of the ear prevents the drops from entering the ear canal. This may be done after instillation of the drops to disperse the medication.

④ Hyperextending the child's head is done for the instillation of nose drops, not eardrops.

19 (1) **Urine is leaking around the urinary retention catheter and a larger-size catheter is required; once ordered, it is within the role of the nurse to select the appropriate size catheter and perform the insertion.**

(2) With a urinary retention catheter in place, the patient should not be wet with urine because it is a closed system from the bladder to the collection bag.

(3) A waterproof pad should be unnecessary because with an adequate-size catheter there should be no leaking of urine.

(4) The presence of a retention catheter negates the need to void.

20 (1) The location and description of pain are not significant in determining the duration of pain.

(2) **The location of pain is often related to the underlying disease or illness; the quality or subjective description of pain often have commonalities related to specific illness, such as burning epigastric pain associated with gastric ulcers and crushing chest pain associated with myocardial infarctions.**

(3) This is totally individual and unreliable for determining relationships among location and description of pain.

(4) Same as #3.

21 (1) A Class A fire extinguisher contains water and is contraindicated in an electrical fire because water conducts electricity.

(2) **A Class A fire extinguisher contains water, which safely and effectively puts out fires composed of burning wood, paper, or cloth.**

(3) Water should not be used because it causes grease to spatter; also the stove might be an electric stove.

(4) A maintenance closet usually contains flammable materials; water is contraindicated because it dilutes flammable liquids, which spreads the fire.

22 (1) **Hearing is the last sense to deteriorate, and the patient may hear the nurse; all patients have a right to know what will be done and why.**

(2) A petrolatum-based lubricant is for external, not internal, use.

(3) Glycerin and lemon swabs, if used, should be applied after the mouth is cleansed. Many nurses no longer use lemon and glycerin swabs because they cause drying of the mucous membranes.

(4) A dorsal recumbent position will promote aspiration and is contraindicated. A side-lying position is appropriate.

23 (1) The majority of older adults are or perceive themselves as being independent, healthy, and active even if they have several chronic illnesses.

(2) Although people lead more sedentary lifestyles as they age, they are still active; most older adults do not view themselves as tired.

(3) **Most older adults perceive themselves as healthy because they measure their health in relation to how well they function rather than by the absence or presence of disease.**

(4) Most older adults view themselves as independent, not dependent.

24 (1) The drug dose is too high, as indicated by a peak serum level higher than the therapeutic serum level range.

(2) The drug dose is too high, not too low.

(3) **12 µg/mL is 2 µg/mL higher than is necessary to be effective and may contribute to drug accumulation and toxicity if this continues for 3 to 5 days.**

(4) The dose is too high and should be reduced, not just administered at a slower rate.

25 (1) Liquid intake should be dispersed over the hours when the patient is awake and not just ingested with meals.

(2) Fluid restriction is concerned with limiting the volume of fluid, not the type of fluid.

(3) Patients should have more fluids during the day and evening than at night, when they are usually asleep.

(4) **The patient and nurse should make a fluid schedule, taking into consideration factors such as periods of wakefulness, number of meals, oral medications, personal preferences, and so on. An appropriate schedule might be 500 mL between 8 AM and 4 PM, 400 mL between 4 PM and 11 PM, and the remainder of the fluid, 100 mL, during the night.**

26 (1) While a person is awake, normal respiratory rates are usually between 12 and 20 per minute; when a person is asleep, the need for oxygen declines, resulting in a decrease in the respiratory rate and an increase in the depth of respirations.

(2) **Rattling sounds in the pharynx indicate mucus is in the airway; suctioning may be necessary to maintain a patent airway because an unconscious patient cannot cough voluntarily.**

(3) Slight shortness of breath is an expected response to activity.

(4) Coughing and expectorating are actions that maintain a patent airway.

27 (1) Leaving abandons the patient; a crying patient needs support, not isolation.

(2) Calling the patient by name supports the patient's need for identity, dignity, and respect, not privacy.

(3) Providing information supports the patient's right to know what is going to be done and why, not privacy.

(4) **This provides a personal, secluded environment for a confidential discussion.**

28　①　Flexion is the decrease in the angle between the bones forming a joint.
　　②　Inversion is turning the sole of the foot medially.
　　③　**Adduction of the shoulder occurs when the arm and hand are brought across the midline in the front of the body with the elbow straight.**
　　④　Circumduction is movement of a ball and socket joint in a full circle.

29　①　Washing should move secretions and debris away from the urinary meatus, preventing infection.
　　②　**Smegma collects under the foreskin, which must be retracted to permit thorough cleaning.**
　　③　A light touch may be too stimulating; a gentle but firm touch is more effective.
　　④　A rubbing motion may injure delicate perineal tissue and be too stimulating.

30　①　This limits incisional pain and prevents dehiscence.
　　②　Although ambulation increases the respiratory rate, its primary purpose is to prevent circulatory complications such as thrombosis.
　　③　**Diaphragmatic breathing promotes alveolar expansion and facilitates oxygen–carbon dioxide exchange.**
　　④　Range-of-motion exercises prevent contractures.

31　①　Consent must be given freely and without coercion, and the consent form is signed in the presence of the nurse.
　　②　The person receiving the treatment or a legally accepted alternative, such as the parent of a child, legal guardian, or spouse, must sign the consent form in front of the nurse.
　　③　**It is the responsibility of the practitioner, not the nurse, to provide this information. Patients have a legal right to have adequate and accurate information to make knowledgeable decisions about their treatment.**
　　④　If the nurse determines that a patient is incapable of signing a consent form because of an impaired decision-making ability, such as a lowered level of consciousness, confusion, or lack of touch with reality, the physician should be notified immediately.

32　①　Although antiemetics reduce nausea, anxiolytics reduce anxiety.
　　②　**Antiemetics block the emetogenic receptors to prevent or treat nausea or vomiting.**
　　③　Antitussives reduce the frequency and intensity of coughing. Anxiolytics reduce anxiety.
　　④　Although antiemetics reduce vomiting, antitussives reduce coughing.

33　①　Weighing a patient twice a day is unnecessary. Weight varies over the course of the day depending on food and fluids ingested and the weight of clothing being worn. These factors produce information that is not comparable.
　　②　Weighing a patient one hour before meals is unnecessary. Meal times may vary from day to day, and the information collected will not be comparable.
　　③　**To obtain the most accurate comparable data, patients should be weighed at the same time every day (preferably first thing in the morning), after toileting, wearing the same clothing, and using the same scale. This controls as many variables as possible to make the daily measurements an accurate reflection of the patient's weight.**
　　④　Weighing the patient before urinating in the morning collects information influenced by the volume of urine in the urinary bladder. Weights should always be measured after, not before, voiding to obtain the most accurate, comparable measurements. One liter of fluid is equal to 2.2 pounds.

34　①　Heat causes vasodilation that increases circulation to the area and results in erythema, not reactive hyperemia.
　　②　Effleurage, light stroking of the skin, simulates the peripheral nerves and should not change skin coloration.
　　③　Pulling a patient up in bed without using a pull sheet exerts a shearing force that can injure blood vessels and tissues resulting in a friction burn.
　　④　**Compressed skin appears pale because circulation to the area is impaired. When pressure is relieved, the skin takes on a bright red flush as extra blood flows to the area to compensate for the period of impeded blood flow.**

35　①　**An inspiratory stridor is an obvious audible shrill, harsh sound caused by laryngeal obstruction. Obstruction of the larynx is life-threatening because it prevents the exchange of gases between the lungs and atmospheric air.**
　　②　Although pleural friction rub reflects a problem, it is not as life-threatening as a condition in another option. A pleural friction rub is a grating, rubbing sound that is heard by auscultating over the base of the lung. It is caused by inflamed pleura (pleurisy) rubbing together.
　　③　Although respiratory wheezing reflects a problem, it is not as life-threatening as a condition in another option. Expiratory wheezing is the presence of high-pitched musical sounds caused by high-velocity movement of air through narrowed airways. It is associated with asthma, bronchitis, and pneumonia.
　　④　Although a nonproductive cough reflects a problem, it is not as life-threatening as a condition in another option. A non-productive cough is coughing without mobilizing or expectorating sputum.

36 ① **The power to grant licenses to professional health-care providers is reserved for the states. An individual must meet minimum proficiency standards to receive a license, thus protecting the public.**
② Nurse Practice Acts, not federal law, govern the practice of nursing and licensure.
③ Nurse Practice Acts, not constitutional law, govern the practice of nursing and licensure.
④ The American Nurses Association (ANA) is the national professional organization for nursing in the United States. It fosters high standards of nursing practice; it does not grant licensure.

37 ① ____ This is not a priority.
② _X_ **The headache may indicate that the blood pressure is too high, which may precipitate a brain attack (stroke).**
③ _X_ **This may indicate evisceration (protrusion of viscera through separated wound edges), which needs immediate action to prevent extension of the wound separation and to limit invasion of microorganisms.**
④ ____ Orthostatic hypotension is a common occurrence when moving from a sitting to standing position. The patient is safe in bed at this time. This concern can be addressed later after patients who need immediate attention receive care.
⑤ ____ Although this needs to be done, it is not life-threatening and can wait.

38 ① This is false reassurance; this is something the nurse cannot promise.
② This can intensify pain; also, it can tire the patient, which may potentiate pain.
③ The patient refuses to move now and will probably avoid any self-care that requires movement.
④ **This conveys that the nurse recognizes the patient's need to move slowly, gently, and carefully; a gentle touch with slow movements contributes to the patient's comfort.**

39 ① A special syringe is not needed for administering a medication via Z-track. The barrel of the syringe must be large enough to accommodate the volume of solution to be injected (usually 1 to 3 mL) and the needle long enough to enter a muscle.
② **Pulling laterally and downward on the skin before inserting the needle creates a zigzag track through the various tissue layers that prevents backflow of medication up the needle track when simultaneously removing the needle and releasing the traction on the skin.**
③ The use of the vastus lateralis muscle for a Z-track injection may cause discomfort for the patient. Z-track injections are tolerated better when the well-developed gluteal muscles are used.
④ The needle is inserted into a muscle, not subcutaneous tissues, for a Z-track injection. The Z represents the zigzag pattern of the needle track that results when the skin traction and the needle are simultaneously removed.

40 ① This ensures that the speaker's lips and facial expression can be seen, which helps the patient to decode the message.
② Clear, accurate articulation allows the patient to decode the combination of vowels and consonants.
③ **The patient is the only person who can tell the nurse whether the message was heard and understood.**
④ Raising the voice does not make the message clearer; it may actually make it more difficult to understand. In addition, shouting can be demeaning.

41 ① 250 mL is too little fluid; this is the recommended amount for a toddler.
② 500 mL is too little fluid; this is the recommended amount for a large school-age child or small adolescent.
③ 700 mL is too little fluid for an adult. 700 mL is the recommended volume for an average-sized adolescent.
④ **The range of 750 to 1000 mL, with an average of 900 mL, is the suggested volume of solution for a soapsuds or tap water enema administered to an adult to stimulate effective evacuation of the bowel. It provides enough fluid to fill the bowel and apply pressure to the intestinal mucosa to stimulate defecation.**

42 ① The apical, not the carotid, pulse should be obtained when the pulse is irregular.
② A Doppler is unnecessary; a stethoscope is adequate.
③ **Taking the pulse for a full minute is necessary to obtain an accurate count. Taking the pulse for 15 seconds and multiplying by 4 or taking the pulse for 30 seconds and multiplying by 2 may result in inaccurate readings and is unsafe.**
④ Initially the response should be to obtain an apical rate. Ultimately, the apical and radial rates are compared to determine if there is a pulse deficit.

43 ① The liver is involved with the biotransformation, not excretion, of a drug.
② The majority of drugs are not excreted by the lungs, although some drugs, such as general anesthetic agents, are excreted via the respiratory tract.
③ **The majority of drugs and their metabolites are excreted through the kidneys. Decreased kidney function can result in drug toxicity because of accumulation of the drug within the body.**
④ The majority of drugs are not excreted through the intestines.

44

(1) Rinsing the mouth with diluted hydrogen peroxide does not provide the necessary friction needed to remove debris that contributes to the formation of plaque.

(2) A dental hygienist will use various dental instruments to remove tartar, which is hardened plaque.

(3) Although this is an integral part of dental hygiene, it removes debris from the biting surface of the teeth, not plaque where the teeth and gums meet.

(4) **Plaque, composed of bacteria and saliva, forms on the teeth primarily at the gum line. A vibrating toothbrush provides friction that helps to dislodge plaque from the teeth.**

45

(1) **Acute care is provided by institutions with the highly skilled, intensive, specialized services that are provided by hospitals.**

(2) Respite care provides services so that caregivers can get relief from the stress of their responsibilities. Respite care can be provided in the home or nursing home setting.

(3) Hospice care offers services that enable dying persons to stay at home with the support needed to die with dignity.

(4) Efforts that seek to reduce disability and restore function are related to rehabilitation. Recovering lost functions or developing new compensating skills commonly is accomplished in the home setting.

46

(1) Assessment of patient needs requires the knowledge and judgment of a registered nurse. This task has great potential for harm if the caregiver misassesses the patient's condition. In addition, it requires an assessment of numerous systems and risk factors, a complex level of interaction with the patient, problem solving, and innovation in the form of an individually designed plan of care that provides for the patient's safety.

(2) The skill of evaluation requires the knowledge and judgment of a registered nurse. This task has great potential for harm if the caregiver misassesses the patient's response. In addition, it requires an assessment of numerous systems and risk factors; a complex level of interaction with the patient, problem solving, and innovation in the form of an individually designed nursing plan of care that provides for the patient's safety.

(3) The choice of the type of restraint is based on the physician's order.

(4) **Performing range of motion exercises is not complex, requires simple problem-solving skills, and employs a simple level of interaction with the patient. It is within the scope of practice of an unlicensed nursing assistant and does not require the more advanced competencies of a registered nurse.**

47

(1) This is too late.

(2) **This provides the patient with the opportunity to void before becoming incontinent; if effective, it contributes to self-esteem and personal hygiene.**

(3) This decreases the volume of urine voided; it does not prevent incontinence.

(4) The patient may not have time to communicate the need to void or may be unaware of the need to void before being incontinent.

48

(1) **This prevents trauma to any one section of the respiratory mucosa because of prolonged suction pressure.**

(2) For wall suctioning to be effective when suctioning an adult, it should be maintained at 100 to 120 mm Hg.

(3) The opposite is the acceptable technique. The nasotracheal area is considered sterile and is suctioned before the oropharyngeal area, which is considered clean; this minimizes contamination of the sterile area.

(4) Suction is applied on removal, not insertion, of the catheter. Intermittent suctioning should not exceed 10 seconds to prevent hypoxemic complications induced by the suctioning.

49

(1) **The nurse needs to interact with individuals from different cultures in a way that observes cultural differences. For example, the nurse needs to be aware of the impact of eye contact, touch, and invasion of personal space because they have different meanings in different cultures.**

(2) The question does not indicate that the patient does not speak English. However, if the patient does not speak English, the nurse needs to use a nonpartisan interpreter. The patient may not be willing to share delicate information with the nurse in the presence of family members.

(3) The question does not indicate that the patient does not speak English. Although helpful, it is not the best answer for this question.

(4) Same as #3.

50

(1) **These are signs of fluid volume excess; fluids are administered during surgery to maintain an adequate circulating blood volume. Occasionally, intraoperative IV fluids may be excessive and is a complication that must be monitored for by the nurse in the post anesthesia care unit.**

(2) Hyperkalemia is indicated by muscle weakness, areflexia, decreased heart rate, irregular pulse, irritability, apathy, confusion, and a serum potassium level more than 5.0 mEq/L.

(3) Hyponatremia is indicated by lethargy, confusion, apprehension, muscle cramps, anorexia, nausea, vomiting and a serum sodium level less than 135 mEq/L.

(4) Hypoglycemia is indicated by fatigue, dizziness, restlessness, hunger, sweating, palpitations, tremors, nausea, and a capillary blood glucose level of less than 70 mg/dL.

51 (1) Drug interactions are not prevented by the presence of food. They occur as long as the modification of a drug occurs in the presence of another drug.

(2) **Food protects the gastrointestinal mucosa from being irritated by a drug. Gastrointestinal irritation may result in mucosal erosion and bleeding.**

(3) Biotransformation, the detoxification of a drug in the liver, occurs after a drug is absorbed through the gastrointestinal tract. Biotransformation is unrelated to the presence of food when an oral drug is ingested.

(4) The presence of food when an oral drug is administered prevents gastric irritability, not gastric reflux.

52 (1) Protein intake is not directly related to an increase in interstitial edema.

(2) **An increase in dietary sodium will increase interstitial edema in this patient. This patient should identify the number of milligrams of sodium contained in a serving of the pasta sauce and determine if this amount of sodium is acceptable on the ordered diet.**

(3) Calories are not directly related to an increase in interstitial edema.

(4) Cholesterol intake is not directly related to an increase in interstitial edema.

53 (1) An intradermal injection usually involves a small volume of fluid (e.g., 0.1 mL). A 1-mL syringe, rather than a syringe that can accommodate larger volumes, permits a more precise measurement of a small volume of fluid.

(2) **A 26-gauge needle has a narrow diameter and short bevel that is conducive to the formation of the wheal associated with an intradermal injection.**

(3) An intradermal injection is usually administered with a needle that is ½ inch in length.

(4) This angle is too extreme and results in an injection that is too deep to form a wheal.

54 (1) Stopping at the scene of an accident is an ethical responsibility, not a legal requirement.

(2) It is the responsibility of the injured person to report an incident of rape.

(3) **The law requires professionals, such as teachers, certain health-care professionals, and social workers, to report suspicions of child abuse to the authorities.**

(4) In June 1992, the Supreme Court of the United States upheld the constitutional right of a woman to control her own body to the extent that she can abort a fetus in the early stages of pregnancy. However, the decision stipulated that each state may legislate its own reasonable restrictions. It is likely that some states require parental notification if the woman seeking an abortion is a minor. Notification should not be confused with consent.

55 (1) The respiratory rate will increase, not decrease, in an effort to bring more oxygen to body cells.

(2) **The patient will become hypotensive with the loss of blood because of hypovolemia.**

(3) The heart rate will increase, not decrease, in an effort to increase cardiac output and bring more oxygen to body cells.

(4) The skin will be cool and clammy because of the sympathetic nervous system response.

56 (1) Allowing the patient to regain energy is not the primary reason for sitting on the side of the bed before transfer.

(2) **Orthostatic hypotension is a condition that contributes to impaired stability. When moving to a sitting or standing position from lying or sitting, cerebral circulation is reduced, resulting in light-headedness and dizziness; sitting on the side of the bed allows the peripheral blood vessels to constrict in response to the vertical position.**

(3) Providing time for the heart rate to return to normal is not the primary reason for sitting on the side of the bed before transfer.

(4) Although the patient might take several deep breaths, it is not the main reason for sitting on the side of the bed before transfer.

57 (1) Sublingual nitroglycerin has a rapid onset and a relatively short duration of action. One dose may not be enough.

(2) Excessive administration of nitroglycerin can cause severe hypotension and death; when a therapeutic response does not occur after following the prescribed nitroglycerin protocol, medical attention is necessary because the person may be experiencing a cardiac event.

(3) Doubling the dose may precipitate severe or even life-threatening hypotension.

(4) **Sublingual nitroglycerin has a rapid onset and a relatively short duration of action. Three doses may be necessary to achieve a desired therapeutic response. However, if pain persists beyond 15 minutes, it may indicate the presence of an acute cardiac event that requires emergency medical intervention.**

58 (1) **The systematic sequence for assessment of breath sounds facilitates a thorough assessment that allows for comparison of similar lung fields on the right and left sides of the thorax.**

(2) Bone interferes with the transmission of breath sounds. Placing the stethoscope over intercostal spaces enhances the volume and quality of breath sounds.

(3) Breathing through the nose can cause turbulence that can imitate adventitious breath sounds. Mouth breathing can augment the volume of breath sounds.

(4) A low-Fowler's position interferes with placement of the stethoscope over the lung fields on the back. An upright position, such as sitting or high-Fowler's, is preferred because it promotes chest excursion and permits placement of the stethoscope.

59 ① An animated demeanor may be overwhelming for the patient. The patient is in the fourth stage of grieving, depression; during this stage people become quiet and withdrawn.

② Cheerfulness denies the patient's feelings and cuts off communication.

③ **The patient is developing a full awareness of the impact of dying and is expressing sorrow; this stage of coping should be supported by the quiet presence of the nurse.**

④ This is a form of abandonment; the nurse must be present and accessible.

60 ① **Perineal care after defecation removes microorganisms, mucus, and fecal material containing enzymes that can injure delicate perineal tissue. The warm, moist environment of the perineal area promotes the multiplication of microorganisms that can ascend the outside of the catheter into the bladder, resulting in a urinary tract infection.**

② Reinserting a catheter every 72 hours is unnecessary. The catheter usually is changed every 4 to 6 weeks or when crusting or sediment collects inside the tubing.

③ An oral intake of 1500 mL in 24 hours is too little. A patient with a urinary catheter should have a fluid intake of at least 2000 to 2500 mL daily.

④ Tugging gently on the catheter daily can cause trauma to the bladder and urethra and should be avoided. When a urinary catheter is inserted and immediately after the balloon is inflated, slight tension, not tugging, is applied to the catheter until resistance is felt; this ensures that the balloon is inflated adequately and the catheter is anchored in the bladder.

61 ① Pain is a local adaptation to stimulation of nerve endings; it is a localized response of the central nervous system to the stimulus of pain.

② **The inflammatory response is stimulated by trauma or infection, which increases the basal metabolic rate; with infection, fever results from the effect of pyrogens on the temperature-regulating center in the hypothalamus.**

③ Edema is a local adaptation resulting from local vasodilation and increased vessel permeability.

④ Erythema is a local adaptation resulting from increased circulation and local vasodilation in the involved area.

62 ① Shaking the drug before inhalation is an acceptable practice because it mixes the medication within the solution so that the aerosol drug concentration is even.

② **When using an MDI, inhalation should be slow; this limits bronchial constriction and promotes a more even distribution of the aerosolized medication.**

③ Holding the breath at the height of inhalation is desirable because it allows tiny drops of aerosol spray to reach deeper branches of the airway.

④ Tilting the head back slightly while using a metered-dose inhaler is desirable because it maximizes airway exposure to medication from the inhaler.

63 ① **Apples are an excellent source of fiber. One medium apple supplies 3.5 grams of dietary fiber.**

② Ten cherries provide only 1.2 grams of dietary fiber.

③ Five halves of dried apricots provide only 1.2 grams of dietary fiber.

④ A ½ cup of pineapple provides only 1.1 gram of dietary fiber.

64 ① In the analysis step of the nursing process, the nurse interprets data, determines the significance of data, and formulates a nursing diagnosis.

② Evaluation involves determining patient responses to nursing interventions, identifying whether goals and outcomes are met, and revising the plan of care when necessary.

③ **Observation of human responses is part of the assessment phase of the nursing process; assessment involves collecting, verifying, clustering, and communicating objective and subjective data.**

④ Implementation involves carrying out the plan of care and documenting the care provided.

65 ① **The nurse has to clarify personal values and beliefs before understanding and accepting nonjudgmentally the cultural beliefs and practices of others.**

② Although learning about what people of common cultures believe about health and illness practices may be helpful, the nurse needs to understand that each person is an individual who may or may not embrace some or all of the values and beliefs identified with one's cultural heritage. Stereotyping (the assigning of a trait existing in some members of the group to all members of the group) must be avoided if care is to be culturally competent.

③ An ethnocentric manner interferes with the nurse's ability to be culturally competent. Ethnocentrism is the view that one's own attitudes, beliefs, customs, and culture are better than those of another.

④ Although different cultures share common elements, they may be demonstrated through different behaviors and customs. Recognizing only the similarities denies the differences that make cultures unique.

66 (1) Hygiene care is not done only in the morning.
(2) Oral instructions may not reach all members of the nursing team.
(3) Indicating the patient's preference on the patient's plan of care provides a written plan of care of what should be done for the patient; it supports communication among health team members, contributes to continuity, and individualizes care.
(4) Encouraging a modification of personal routines is not necessary; care should be individualized.

67 (1) Rest, sleep, and relaxation associated with pain relief are not based on the gate-control theory.
(2) Activity uses distraction to focus attention on stimuli other than the pain. When in pain, patients often do not have the physical or emotional energy to concentrate on activities.
(3) Narcotics act on the higher centers of the brain to modify the perception of pain.
(4) The gate-control theory assumes that pain fibers that originate in the peripheral areas of the body have synapses in the gray matter of the dorsal horns of the spinal cord. Large nerve fibers stimulated by heat, cold, and touch transmit impulses through the same synapses as those that transmit pain. When larger fibers are stimulated, they close the gate to painful stimuli, and the perception of pain is reduced.

68 **(1) Circulatory stasis occurs after surgery because postoperative patients are not as active as they were before surgery; leg exercises promote venous return and prevent the formation of thrombi and thrombophlebitis.**
(2) Although leg exercises may prevent contractures, that is not the primary reason for performing leg exercises postoperatively.
(3) Although leg exercises prevent muscle atrophy, that is not the primary reason for performing leg exercises postoperatively.
(4) Same as #3.

69 (1) Sunflower seeds contain only trace amounts of vitamin C.
(2) Green peppers are an excellent source of vitamin C (ascorbic acid). One pepper contains 95 mg of vitamin C.
(3) Black beans contain no vitamin C.
(4) Beef liver contains no vitamin C.

70 **(1) Homeless individuals have more difficulty meeting their basic physiologic needs, which increases their risk of illness; in addition, they are unlikely to enter the health-care system early in a disease process.**
(2) Nonfluoridated water is not an unhealthy situation because fluoride can be obtained from other sources.
(3) Although rehabilitation services may contribute to an increase in the quality of one's life, the lack of rehabilitation services is not an unhealthy situation.
(4) Supporting a vaccination program may contribute to prevention of disease; but it will not correct an already unhealthy situation.

71 (1) This statement reflects Maslow's Hierarchy of Needs, not Erikson's Stages of Psychosocial Development.
(2) This statement reflects Maslow's Hierarchy of Needs, not Erikson's Stages of Psychosocial Development.
(3) Erikson emphasized that a person might regress to an earlier stage to seek comfort and reduce anxiety when unable to cope with a stressful event, situation, or illness.
(4) Erikson emphasized the importance of environment as being extremely influential in achievement or nonachievement of developmental tasks. Culture and social and family relationships are factors that have tremendous impact on one's environment.

72 (1) _____ This is necessary to know to calculate the IV drip rate, not to determine if the correct IV solution is running.
(2) _____ The drip rate per minute indicates the current rate at which the IV is running, not whether the correct IV solution is running.
(3) _X_ The nurse needs to have two pieces of data to determine if the correct IV solution is running. First, what is the solution the physician ordered and then what solution is in the IV bag? These solutions must be identical to administer ordered IV solutions safely.
(4) _____ This is necessary to know to calculate the IV drip rate.
(5) _X_ The administration of IV fluids is a dependent function of the nurse. The solution ordered by the physician must be verified.

73 (1) This will not secure loose ends; debris could fall on the floor.
(2) This secures loose ends and keeps debris contained within the center of the sheet.
(3) Same as #1.
(4) Same as #1.

74 ① Pain is a physiologic response to stress.
② **Irritability is a behavioral-emotional response; the body is using physical and emotional energy to reduce stress.**
③ Headache is a physiologic response to pain.
④ Hypertension is a physiologic response to stress.

75 ① Although fear of losing control is a concern of some patients, it is not the primary concern of most patients.
② Although fear of receiving an injection is a concern for some patients, it is not the primary concern of most patients.
③ **Postsurgical patients avoid or limit the intake of pain medication for fear of becoming physically or psychologically dependent; however, the drug dosage and ordered time intervals are insufficient to cause dependence over a short period of time after surgery.**
④ Although a fear of experiencing negative side effects is a concern for some patients, it is not the primary concern of most patients.

76 ① The abdomen rises on inspiration.
② These accessory muscles should not be involved consciously with diaphragmatic breathing. The abdomen should rise and fall rather than the shoulders; the chest naturally expands and recoils.
③ **Diaphragmatic breathing involves a pattern of a slow deep inhalation followed by a slow exhalation with a tightening of the abdominal muscles to aid exhalation; the patient should hold the breath for 2 to 3 seconds at the height of inhalation, just before the exhalation.**
④ Pressure against the abdomen will interfere with the amount of air that is drawn into the lungs on inspiration.

77 ① A general assessment of intelligence is common to all learning domains. It is important to design learning content and strategies based on the learner's level of intellectual ability to avoid teaching below or above the learner's intellectual capabilities.
② An assessment of a patient's strengths is common to all learning domains. Prior knowledge needs to be determined so the nurse knows where to begin teaching new content. Learning is most effective when built upon prior learning.
③ A general assessment of a learner's level of maturity is common to all learning domains. Teaching and learning is fundamentally different during various phases of the life span. The level and amount of information should be geared to the learner's developmental stage and cognitive level.
④ **In the affective domain, learning is concerned with values, feelings, emotions, beliefs, and attitudes.**

78 ① Vomitus should be flushed down a toilet, not contained in a medical waste container.
② It is unnecessary to remove vomitus from the room; vomitus should be poured down a toilet rather than a sink.
③ Saving vomitus for a specimen is generally unnecessary. Although a physician may request that vomitus be assessed, it is rarely sent for laboratory analysis.
④ **Discarding vomitus in the toilet represents the most practical action when disposing of vomitus; it dilutes and contains it and removes the vomitus from the environment.**

79 ① Activity during the day or early evening stimulates physical functioning and increases mental activity. Activity performed 2 hours before bedtime is appropriate.
② A snack is appropriate because it prevents hunger and promotes sleep if it contains the amino acid L-tryptophan.
③ Although excessively cold environmental temperatures will cause frequent awakenings, a cool environmental temperature usually is comfortable for sleeping.
④ **Alcohol shortens sleep onset but its rapid metabolism causes rebound arousal, resulting in shortened REM sleep. It also causes early morning awakenings secondary to a full bladder because alcohol acts as a mild diuretic.**

80 ① Potassium chloride is used for the treatment or prevention of potassium deficiency and is unrelated to heparin therapy.
② **Protamine sulfate can chemically combine with heparin, neutralizing its anticoagulant action; it should be kept readily available for the treatment of heparin overdose.**
③ Prothrombin is a plasma protein coagulation factor synthesized by the liver, not a drug that should be used as an antidote to heparin.
④ Plasma may be ordered after the antidote is given. Packed red blood cells will more likely be ordered than plasma.

81 ① Covering the nose when sneezing interferes with the chain of infection at the portal of exit stage, not at the transmission stage.
② Turning and positioning contribute to maintaining skin integrity. An intact skin interrupts the chain of infection at the portal of entry stage, not the transmission stage, of the chain of infection.

(3) Disposing of any item that touches the floor is an action that interferes with the transmission of microorganisms in the chain of infection. Items that touch the floor are contaminated and must be disposed of in a manner that contains the spread of microorganisms.

(4) Applying a sterile dressing over a contaminated wound interferes with the chain of infection at the reservoir or source of the infection. It interrupts the chain of infection at the portal of exit stage.

82 (1) Some people never progress past denial, the first step in Kübler-Ross's theory of grieving.

(2) Although passing through the stages may be smooth for some people, it is not smooth for most individuals; the intensity and speed of progression depend on many factors such as extent of loss, level of growth and development, cultural and spiritual beliefs, gender roles, and relationships with significant others.

(3) The stages are not concrete, and the patient's behavior changes as different levels of awareness and/or coping occur. Kübler-Ross's theory of grieving is behaviorally oriented.

(4) Progression is not always forward. Patients tend to move back and forth among stages or may remain in one stage.

83 (1) Although cheese can contribute to constipation, broccoli facilitates defecation.

(2) Dairy products are low in roughage and lack bulk; they produce too little waste to stimulate the defecation reflex. Low-residue foods move more slowly through the intestinal tract, permitting increased fluid uptake from stool, resulting in hard-formed stools and constipation.

(3) Both broccoli and peas provide bulk that increases peristalsis, which facilitates defecation.

(4) Although yogurt contributes to constipation, peas provide bulk (undigested residue), which facilitates fecal elimination.

84 (1) Bearing down is contraindicated. When people hold their breath, they tend to perform the Valsalva maneuver. The Valsalva maneuver increases intra-abdominal pressure, which makes it more difficult to insert and retain a suppository; the increased pressure can expel the suppository.

(2) Inserting a rectal suppository is not a sterile procedure.

(3) Warming the suppository will cause it to melt, which interferes with insertion.

(4) Cold suppositories maintain their shape for ease of insertion; it is safe and easy to insert a suppository that has been refrigerated.

85 (1) Because of a dark, unfamiliar environment at night, older adults may become confused and disoriented, which contributes to the occurrence of falls.

(2) The time before meals generally is unrelated to falls. The incidence of falls may increase after meals because the gastrocolic reflex increases peristalsis causing a need to defecate. Walking to the bathroom may result in a fall.

(3) All patients, including postoperative patients, should be assisted when ambulating until they are able to ambulate safely on their own; therefore, these patients should not fall.

(4) Visiting hours generally are unrelated to falls.

86 (1) The family is included in both acute care and community health care.

(2) Individuals are included in both acute care and community health care; in addition, community health care focuses on the needs of groups and society.

(3) A characteristic of community health is that it focuses on the health status of people in an aggregate (people who, as a group, form a distinct population).

(4) Neither acute care nor community health care is focused solely by geographic area. People who are served may come from different geographic areas, and groups can be identified by a variety of factors such as common interests (e.g., citizens concerned about air pollution) or similar problems (e.g., homelessness, single-parent families).

87 (1) This is an incorrect calculation.

(2) Each gram of fat equals 9 calories. 60 grams of fat × 9 = 540 calories. 540 ÷ 2000 = 0.27 or 27%.

(3) Same as #1.

(4) Same as #1.

88 (1) The GAS is a common physiologic response to stress that follows a uniform, not unique, pattern in everyone.

(2) An iatrogenic stress is a stimulus caused by a treatment or diagnostic procedure. It is a stress that can stimulate the GAS.

(3) Not everyone achieves homeostasis. Some individuals reach the stage of exhaustion.

(4) Stressors precipitate the GAS, which is a neuroendocrine response and part of the autonomic nervous system.

89 (1) Recapping a sterile syringe that has not had contact with a patient or a nonsterile surface does not violate surgical asepsis; the needle of a syringe and the area inside the needle cap are both sterile and pose no microbiologic risk of contamination.

(2) This is correct technique. Fluids flow in the direction of gravity. When the tip is held lower than the handle, fluid remains at the level of the gauze and the tip of the forceps; this area is considered sterile. If the nurse

raises the tip of the forceps higher than the handle, fluid flows up the handle onto the hand and becomes contaminated. When the tip of the forceps is then lowered, the contaminated fluid flows back down the length of the forceps, contaminating the forceps and the gauze.

(3) When the metal protective ring and cap are removed from around the top of a multiple-dose vial, the rubber port surface is sterile until it is touched by something nonsterile. The rubber stopper does not have to be wiped with alcohol the first time the vial is accessed with a sterile syringe.

(4) **Although the inside of a sterile gauze wrapper is sterile, when the paper wrapper becomes wet, capillary action transfers microorganisms from the nonsterile surface of the table to the inside of the wrapper; the gauze then becomes contaminated, which violates sterile technique.**

90 (1) Pedal pulses are assessed to determine circulation to the feet. A lack of, not presence of, hair on the feet and lower legs may be caused by prolonged hypoxia. In addition, other factors such as genetic endowment may cause a lack of hair in the lower extremities.

(2) Lack of hair on the feet and lower legs may indicate prolonged hypoxia. A blood pressure does not evaluate peripheral circulation in the lower extremities as does inspection and palpation.

(3) **Applying pressure causes blanching, and when the pressure is released, the normal color should return quickly (within 1 to 2 seconds), indicating adequate arterial perfusion. Assessing pedal pulses measures the adequacy of circulation to the feet.**

(4) Although capillary refill assesses adequacy of peripheral circulation, blood pressure does not evaluate peripheral circulation in the lower extremities as does inspection and palpation.

91 (1) **Range-of-motion exercises maximally stretch all muscle groups; this prevents shortening of muscles, which can result in contractures.**

(2) Although movement of joints experienced during activity will contribute to preventing contractures, it will not move all joints through their full range; also, prolonged sitting can cause flexion contractures of the hips and knees.

(3) Although supporting joints contributes to maintaining functional alignment, which can help prevent contractures, it is not the best intervention.

(4) Turning and repositioning a patient every 2 hours will reduce pressure, not prevent contractures.

92 (1) Urine that flows toward the rectum rarely causes infection; however, bacteria from the rectal area can cause urinary tract infections.

(2) If properly cleaned after use, bedpans are not a source of infection.

(3) The act of sitting when toileting should not increase the prevalence of infection.

(4) **Stool wiped toward the urinary meatus can cause urinary tract infections; *Escherichia coli*, a common bacteria in stool, causes urinary tract infections.**

93 (1) **When patients are incontinent, they should be cleaned immediately; feces contain digestive enzymes and urine contains ammonia and other irritating substances that cause skin breakdown.**

(2) This is an unrealistic instruction for this patient; a cognitively impaired patient will have difficulty with this task.

(3) Sheepskin and an incontinence pad (the word "diaper" should be avoided because it is demeaning) hold moisture next to the skin, and their use should be avoided.

(4) Although this should be done, it is more significant to remove urine and feces from the skin.

94 (1) **The main purpose of pain relief medication is to enable the patient to comfortably engage in necessary activity.**

(2) Some people are stoic and/or do not request medication for pain. Patients' pain should be assessed and pain medication offered if necessary.

(3) The patient is experiencing pain before the next scheduled dose; this indicates that the patient is in pain and the intervention was ineffective.

(4) This is a side effect, not a therapeutic effect; opiates decrease respiration by depressing the respiratory center in the brainstem.

95 (1) Although visits by siblings is appropriate, it does not address the task of initiative versus guilt.

(2) A stuffed animal is appropriate for an infant or a toddler.

(3) **This is an appropriate activity for a school-age child. School-age children are interested in doing and producing.**

(4) Watching television does not support the developmental tasks of a school-age child.

96 (1) A patient with urge incontinence generally will be unable to wait 4 hours between voidings.

      (2) Toileting the patient immediately upon request supports continence because the person with urge incontinence must immediately void or lose control.

      (3) Encouraging the patient to stay near the bathroom promotes isolation and should be avoided.

      (4) Limiting fluid intake during the early evening and night may be part of a toileting program to provide uninterrupted sleep; however, it does not address the patient's need to urinate immediately when feeling the urge to void.

97 (1) Carbohydrates, not protein, are the main fuel source for energy. Athletes competing in endurance events often adhere to a diet that increases carbohydrates to 70% of the diet for the last three days before a race (carbohydrate loading) to maximize muscle glycogen storage.

      (2) Anabolism, the process by which the body's cells synthesize protoplasm for growth and repair, requires amino acids, which are the essential components of protein.

      (3) Although adequate amounts of food from all the food groups are necessary for maintaining healthy functioning systems within the body, it is really effective kidney functioning and an adequate fluid balance that are necessary for excretion. The increased load of nitrogenous wastes associated with an excessive protein intake burden, rather than facilitate, excretion.

      (4) Protein is ingested to prevent, not promote, catabolism. Catabolism occurs when complex substances break down into simpler substances, releasing energy.

98 (1) Corridor rails are not continuous, and standing in front does not position the nurse in a way that will protect the patient; this method does not inspire confidence.

      (2) Instructing the blind patient to hold onto the nurse's arm allows the nurse to guide and the patient to follow; it supports the patient's comfort and promotes confidence.

      (3) The patient cannot see and should not lead.

      (4) Walking on the side while holding the patient's elbow is one method used to assist a patient who has a mobility, not visual, deficit.

99 (1) The tube is in the stomach, not the lungs.

      (2) The tube is in the stomach, and application of negative pressure to the tube will cause gastric contents to be pulled up the tube and into the syringe.

      (3) This is unsafe; if the tube is in the respiratory system rather than the stomach, a deep inhalation may cause an aspiration of fluid.

      (4) This is unsafe; if the tube is in the wrong place (e.g., esophagus, trachea), it may result in aspiration of the fluid.

100 **(1) This provides an opportunity to discuss the illness; eventually, a developing awareness occurs, and the patient probably will move on to other coping mechanisms.**

      (2) This response may take away the patient's coping mechanism, is demeaning, and cuts off communication; the patient is using denial to cope with the diagnosis.

      (3) Same as #2.

      (4) Same as #2.

Bibliography

Adams, AK: The Home Book of Humorous Quotations. New York, Dodd, Mead & Company, 1969.

Alfaro-LeFevre, R: Critical Thinking in Nursing: A Practical Approach, ed 3. Philadelphia, W. B. Saunders Company, 2004.

American Association of Colleges of Nursing, AACN White Paper: Distance Technology in Nursing Education. Available at *http://www.aacn.nchc.edu/Publications/positions/whitepaper.htm*

American Philosophical Association: Critical Thinking: A Statement of Expert Consensus for Purposes of Educational Assessment and Instruction. The Delphi Report: Research Findings and Recommendations Prepared for the Committee on Pre-College Philosophy. (ERIC Document Reproduction Service No. ED 315–423), 1990.

Bowers, B, and McCarthy, D: Developing analytic thinking skills in early undergraduate education. Journal of Nursing Education 32:107–113, 1993.

Brookfield, DD: Developing Critical Thinkers. San Francisco, Jossey-Bass, 1991.

Case, B: Walking around the elephant: A critical-thinking strategy for decision making. The Journal of Continuing Education in Nursing 25:101–109, 1994.

Chaffee, J: Thinking Critically, ed 8. Boston, Houghton Mifflin, 2006.

Daly, W: Critical thinking as an outcome of nursing education. What is it? Why is it important to nursing practice? Journal of Advanced Nursing 28:323–331, 1998.

Erikson, EH: Childhood and Society. New York, Norton, 1993.

Gordon, M: Nursing Diagnosis: Process and Applications, ed 3. St. Louis, Mosby, 1994.

Holmes, TH, and Rahe, RH: The social readjustment rating scale. Journal of Psychosomatic Research 11:213–218, 1967.

Kataoka-Yahiro, M, and Saylor, C: A critical thinking model for nursing judgment. Journal of Nursing Education 33:351–356, 1994.

Kübler-Ross, E: On Death and Dying. New York, Macmillan, 1969.

Loving, GL: Competence validation and cognitive flexibility: A theoretical model grounded in nursing education. Journal of Nursing Education 32:415–421, 1993.

Maslow, AH: Motivation and Personality, ed 2. New York, Harper & Row, 1970.

Nugent, P, and Vitale, B: Fundamentals Success: A Course Review Applying Critical Thinking to Test Taking, ed. 2. Philaadelphia, F. A. Davis, 2008.

Paul, RW, and Heaslip, PH: Critical thinking and intuitive nursing practice. Journal of Advanced Nursing 22:40–47, 1995.

Pless, BS: Clarifying the concept of critical thinking in nursing. Journal of Nursing Education 32:425–428, 1993.

Pond, EE, and Bradshaw, MJ: Teaching strategies for critical thinking. Nurse Educator 15:18–22, 1991.

Safire, W, and Safir, L: Good Advice. New York, Times Books, 1982.

Selye, H: The Stress of Life, rev ed. New York, McGraw Hill, 1976.

Simpson, E, and Courtney, M: Critical thinking in nursing education: Literature review. International Journal of Nursing Practice 8:89–98, 2001.

Snyder, M: Critical thinking: A foundation for consumer-focused care. The Journal of Continuing Education in Nursing 24:206–210, 1993.

Stevenson, B: The Home Book of Questions Classical and Modern, ed 10. New York, Dodd, Mead & Company, 1967.

Taggart, W, and Torrance, PE: Administrator's Manual for the Human Information Processing and Survey. Bensenville, IL, Scholastic Testing Service, 1984.

Venes, D (ed): Taber's Cyclopedic Medical Dictionary, ed 20. Philadelphia, F. A. Davis, 2005.

Vitale, B: NCLEX-RN: Core Review and Exam Prep. F. A. Davis, Philadelphia, 2007.

Index